P9-DHR-987

Taste of Home
Guilt Free
cooking

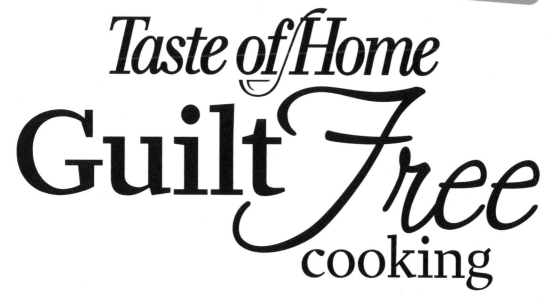

Taste of Home
B O O K S

REIMAN MEDIA GROUP, INC. • GREENDALE, WISCONSIN

Taste of Home — Reader's Digest

A TASTE OF HOME/READER'S DIGEST BOOK

©2008 Reiman Media Group, Inc.
5400 S. 60th St., Greendale WI 53129
All rights reserved.

Taste of Home and Reader's Digest are registered trademarks
of The Reader's Digest Association, Inc.

Editor:	Janet Briggs
Art Director:	Edwin Robles, Jr.
Layout Designers:	Catherine Fletcher
	Emma Acevedo
Proofreader:	Linne Bruskewitz
Editorial Assistant:	Barb Czysz
Recipe Asset Management System:	Coleen Martin, manager;
	Sue A. Jurack, specialist
Food Director:	Diane Werner RD
Recipe Testing and Editing:	Taste of Home Test Kitchen
Food Photography:	Reiman Photo Studio
Cover Art Direction:	Rudy Krochalk
Cover Photo Photographer:	Rob Hagen
Cover Photo Food Stylist:	Julie Herzfeldt
Cover Photo Set Stylist:	Jennifer Bradley Vent
Senior Editor/Books:	Mark Hagen
Creative Director:	Ardyth Cope
Chief Marketing Officer:	Lisa Karpinski
Vice President, Executive Editor/Books:	Heidi Reuter Lloyd
Senior Vice President, Editor in Chief:	Catherine Cassidy
President, Consumer Marketing:	Dawn Zier
President, Food & Entertaining:	Suzanne M. Grimes
President and Chief Executive Officer:	Mary G. Berner

Pictured on front cover: Very Berry Pie (page 220).
Pictured on back cover: Canadian Bacon Potato Skins (page 30),
Turkey Noodle Soup (page 40), Spiced Beef Roast (page 114).
Pictured on spine: Strawberry Slush (page 33).

International Standard Book Number (10): 0-89821-613-3
International Standard Book Number (13): 978-0-89821-613-4
Library of Congress Control Number: 2008926168

For other Taste of Home books and products,
visit www.tasteofhome.com.
For more Reader's Digest products and information,
visit www.rd.com (in the United States)
www.rd.ca (in Canada)

Printed in China
1 3 5 7 9 10 8 6 4 2

Table of *Contents*

Introduction   4

Chapter 1 Breakfast & Brunch   9

Chapter 2 Snacks & Beverages   25

Chapter 3 Soups & Stews   39

Chapter 4 Breads & Rolls   55

Chapter 5 Side Dishes   71

Chapter 6 Beef Favorites   91

Chapter 7 Poultry Classics   115

Chapter 8 Pork Pleasers   141

Chapter 9 Fish & Seafood   163

Chapter 10 Meatless Main Dishes   187

Chapter 11 Cookies & Bars   205

Chapter 12 Just Desserts   219

Index   249

Guilt Free Made Easy

Welcome back to Flavor!
With the **all-time favorites** in this cookbook, you'll reach your **health goals**...*deliciously.*

Cheesy lasagna piping hot from the oven, thick cream soups bursting with flavor and rich chocolate cake piled high with frosting...now you can indulge in these longtime favorites while keeping your healthy eating goals intact. All you need are the right recipes, and thanks to *Taste of Home Guilt Free Cooking*, you're holding those recipes now!

That's right! Say "good-bye" to guilt and "hello" to the mouthwatering classics you enjoy most. Whether you're following a weight-loss plan, on a restricted diet or you simply want to eat healthy, the 356 dishes found here satisfy cravings with fewer calories, fat or sodium. Best of all, the incredible items in this collection don't cut back on flavor, so you can dig into all of those comforting staples you just can't seem to do without.

In addition to offering hundreds of luscious foods, *Guilt Free Cooking* includes Nutrition Facts and Diabetic Exchanges with every recipe. Not only do these numbers help you create balanced meals, but they offer the information needed for anyone involved in a point-based weight-loss system. (See *A Guide to Guilt Free Cooking* on page 7 for an explanation behind the Nutrition Facts.)

You'll also notice two icons that highlight recipes that are particularly lower in fat ⌊⌊⌊⌊ and sodium ⌊⌊⌊⌊. You'll find these tools to be great time-savers if you're following a special diet. And because many of today's cooks need to get out of the kitchen quickly, all of the dishes that are table-ready in 30 minutes or less are highlighted with an icon (🕐) too.

Practicing Portion Control

One of the keys to enjoying your favorite foods guilt free is controlling the serving sizes. That's why all of the recipes in this book specifically note the total yield of the dish as well as the individual serving size on which the Nutrition Facts are based.

It's important to control portion sizes for several reasons. For one thing, it's easy to forget that the amount of food you eat is just as important as the type of food, particularly with the super-sized portions we've grown accustomed to today.

The serving sizes in *Guilt Free Cooking* are generous and will leave you satisfied. However, it's all right to occasionally eat more than one serving of any food as long as it is accounted for and fits into an overall daily plan. Simply balance a slight indulgence by skimming back on serving sizes later in the day. For example, if you'd like to enjoy an extra slice of pizza at lunch, you may want to consider skipping your afternoon snack that day or turning down dessert after dinner.

It's important to remember that getting enough vitamins and minerals is essential to your well-being. However, eating too much of anything without burning excess calories will likely result in weight gain.

Losing extra pounds is especially important for diabetics because doing so can help lower blood glucose. Similarly, those at risk for developing diabetes can decrease that possibility by controlling serving sizes and, therefore, maintaining a healthy weight.

Managing Weight

Losing weight all comes down to the number of calories consumed versus the number of calories burned. For instance, for every 3,500 calories you expend beyond your intake, you'll lose a pound of fat. If you consume 1,500 calories a day, and burn 2,000 calories each day, you can count on losing roughly one pound per week. Increase the calories you burn by becoming more active, and weight loss is likely to follow.

Keep the following eight tips in mind if you are trying to lose a few pounds:

Plan to Prepare. One of the biggest obstacles health-conscious cooks face is finding time to prepare nutritious dinners. Beat the clock with a meal plan. Select several recipes you'd like to try this week, then jot them down to create a meal plan that fits your schedule. (See *Guilt Free Menus* on page 8 to get you started.)

Mix Up Standbys. Eating the same things time and again can tempt anyone toward full-fat dishes. To prevent this, mix up your menus by using the recipes in this book. Not only will the different flavors satisfy you, but you're sure to find new favorites.

Brown Bag It. Curb the urge to grab a quick lunch by packing a meal that you look forward to. See the General Recipe Index that begins on page 251 and consider the sandwiches, soups and snacks *Guilt Free Cooking* offers.

Pack on Produce. Numerous studies prove that a diet rich in fruits and vegetables results in a healthier body, wards off disease and delays the effects of aging. Remember to include produce at breakfast, lunch and dinner. Enjoy some fresh, sliced vegetables as a snack and enjoy a piece of fruit sometime after supper.

Got Fiber? Most people don't get nearly the amount of fiber they need. That's unfortunate, since a high-fiber diet can lower blood pressure and cholesterol. It also reduces the risk of heart disease and diabetes, and it leaves folks feeling full and satisfied. Strive to work beans, grains and high-fiber breads and cereals into your daily menu.

Keep a Diary. Keep a daily journal of what and when you eat. It's easier to stick to goals when you are recording every nibble...and you are also less likely to scratch the whole day after one overindulgence. Review your entries from time to time to identify eating trends, and include affirming notes about goals, exercise accomplishments, etc.

Walk on By. Beat temptation by skipping the sugary sweets and salty treats at the supermarket. Keeping these foods out of the pantry may also help you find healthier snacking options. If you buy treats for the kids, purchase items that they enjoy but that don't interest you. Better yet, buy the kids healthier snacks. Avoid buying unhealthy snacks in bulk.

Snack Smartly. On the weekend, fix health-minded goodies such as Seasoned Snack Mix (p. 31) or Chocolate Cappuccino Cookies (p. 206). Munch on these low-fat treats at home and work. If you're looking for something you can grab in a hurry, consider the list of low-calorie snacking options titled 100 Calories or Less! on page 8.

> *"It's important to remember that getting enough vitamins and minerals is essential to your well-being."*

A large part of following a well-rounded diet is avoiding saturated and trans fats. The FDA estimates that the average American consumes about 6 grams of trans fat a day, with the majority of that amount coming from purchased baked goods. Other culprits are margarine, fried potatoes and snacks such as chips.

Most of these foods contain partially hydrogenated vegetable oils. The dishes in *Guilt Free Cooking* primarily use liquid oils such as olive and canola oil that are free of trans fat. You'll also find that the recipes for baked goods in this book typically call for small amounts of butter or reduced-fat margarine, which contain only a minimal amount of trans fat.

Daily Nutrition Guide

	Women 30-50	Women over 50	Men 50-65
Calories	2,000	1,800	2,400
Fat	65 g or less	60 g or less	80 g or less
Saturated Fat	22 g or less	20 g or less	27 g or less
Cholesterol	300 mg or less	300 mg or less	300 mg or less
Sodium	2,300 mg or less	2,300 mg or less	2,300 mg or less
Carbohydrates	300 g	270 g	360 g
Fiber	28 g	25 g	34 g
Protein	50 g	45 g	60 g

This chart is only a guide. Calorie requirements vary, depending on age, weight, height and amount of activity. Children's dietary needs vary as they grow.

Skim Back on Salt and Sugar

The reason *Guilt Free Cooking* highlights lower-sodium recipes with an icon is that many cooks are concerned about the amount of salt and sodium in the foods they serve their families.

Much has been written about the health benefits of low-sodium diets. In the past, there were debates as to whether or not salt affects blood pressure. However, several studies now indicate that as many as 30-50 percent of the population is salt-sensitive, meaning that salt intake can cause blood pressure to rise in some individuals. Older people, African-Americans and those who already have high blood pressure, diabetes or chronic kidney conditions tend to be more salt-sensitive than others; however, it is wise for everyone to monitor their sodium intake.

In addition to the amount of salt that comes from the salt shaker, processed foods contain an incredible amount of sodium. Cheese, pasta sauce, lunchmeat, frozen dinners, canned vegetables, etc. contain hundreds of milligrams (or more) of sodium per serving. The best way to cut sodium is to eat unprocessed foods, which means preparing hearty meals at home.

Similarly, baking at home also allows family cooks to keep an eye on the amount of sugar they use. Monitoring sugar intake is nothing new. Whether as children we limited sugar to protect our teeth or as adults we reduce it to lose weight, folks from coast to coast have battled sugar's sweet temptations for decades.

Doctors once solely blamed sugar for rapidly increasing blood glucose. Studies later revealed that sugar has the same effect on blood glucose as other carbohydrates, so experts now recommend monitoring the total amount of carbs in a meal plan as opposed to focusing on sugar alone.

This means that most diabetics can enjoy a sensible amount of sugar in their diets. Some eat small portions of baked goods while others cut back on sugar by using a sugar substitute when baking.

Today's sugar substitutes are up to 600 times sweeter than the real deal, so less sugar is needed in a recipe. This is a great benefit because using less sugar frees up more carbs in meal plans.

Make It a Double

Folks usually remain calorie-conscious when deciding what to eat for dinner, but we don't always give much thought to what we are pouring into our glasses. And that's unfortunate, because beverages can be filled with good-for-you nutrients...or merely empty calories that ultimately pack on pounds.

Most everyone is aware that the more water they consume, the better. If you're looking for another nutritious beverage, however, low-fat milk is a no-brainer. After all, milk is a powerhouse of essential nutrients.

Milk's most notable benefit, however, is the amount of calcium it offers—and it is usually fortified with vitamin D, which helps the body absorb that calcium. In fact, most adults can reach their daily calcium quota by drinking three to four 8-ounce glasses of the white stuff.

Furthermore, the National Dairy Council says that consuming three servings of milk every day can help control high blood pressure, prevent certain cancers and reduce the risk of osteoporosis.

Best of all, low-fat or fat-free milk is a health-conscious ingredient that can lighten up all of those standbys you've come to rely on. It's a snap to whip up a heart-smart chocolate shake, a smoothie or even a creamy white sauce for pasta if you use low-fat milk as opposed to the full-fat variety.

If you're looking for something a little zestier to wet your whistle, juice squeezed directly from fruits or vegetables is a great source of vitamins, minerals and the healing agents known as phytochemicals.

Chilled fresh juices found in the refrigerated section of the supermarket are extracted

A Guide to
Guilt Free Cooking

LOW FAT Lower in Fat.
Contains 5 g or less of total fat.

LOW SALT Lower in Sodium.
Contains 300 mg or less of sodium.

Quick Fix.
Table-ready in 30 minutes or less.

Nutrition Facts: When recipes offer a choice of ingredients, the first item listed is the one calculated in the Nutrition Facts. When a range is offered for an ingredient, the first amount is the one that is used in the calculation. Only the marinade that is absorbed in a food is calculated. Garnishes are usually not included in calculations.

Diabetic Exchanges are assigned to recipes in accordance with the guidelines from the American Diabetic and American Dietetic Associations.

juices that are packaged for distribution. Frozen juice concentrates are made from pasteurized juice from which the water has been extracted before the concentrated portion is frozen.

Recipe Selection

On a per-serving basis, the target nutritional content for the items in *Guilt Free Cooking* is:

400 calories or less
12 g of fat or less
1,000 mg sodium or less
100 mg cholesterol or less

So where does that leave the bevy of bottled, boxed or canned juice drinks that line grocery shelves? Many of these beverages contain artificial colors and flavors and only a small amount of real juice. Read the label carefully and look for the words "100 percent pasteurized fruit juice." Be cautious of anything labeled as a "fruit drink."

Some fruit drinks do offer calcium and vitamin C, but they are generally void of any other nutrients. Diabetics in particular need to pay attention to the sugar added to fruit drinks, as some packaged juices contain sugar equal to the amount found in soda.

Like any other food, soda isn't harmful when consumed in moderation. The problem is that too many of us sip the sugary stuff all day long.

Not only are most sodas loaded with caffeine, but the sugar and acidity can cause tooth decay. A 12-ounce can of soda can contain as many as 10 teaspoons of sugar and 150 calories, all of which are void of nutritional value. So the next time you're tempted to hit a soda fountain, you may want to consider heading toward the water fountain instead.

Whether you're watching your fat intake, cutting back on salt or keeping sugar to a minimum, enjoy the new kitchen tool you have in *Guilt Free Cooking*. Simply turn the page and get ready to dig in! You'll surely discover how easy it is to stick to your nutrition goals without sacrificing the hearty, down-home favorites that make mealtimes special. Best of all, you can enjoy each and every bite without an ounce of guilt!

Guilt Free Menus

Chicken in Creamy Gravy (p. 132)
Green Bean Corn Casserole (p. 89)
No-Bake Chocolate Cheesecake (p. 240)

Flavorful Meat Loaf (p. 107)
Mashed Potato Bake (p. 78)
Cheesy Zucchini Medley (p. 86)

Smoked Sausage with Pasta (p. 117)
Garlic Cheese Breadsticks (p. 59)
Light Tiramisu (p. 225)

Shredded Beef Barbecue (p. 104)
Home-Style Coleslaw (p. 78)
Blueberry Crumb Pie (p. 222)

Turkey Dumpling Stew (p. 45)
Molded Cranberry Fruit Salad (p. 88)
Apple Cobbler (p. 231)

100 Calories or Less!

Looking for a no-fuss nibble? Consider these easy solutions. You don't need a recipe for these ideas and each weighs in at 100 calories or less.

- 1 small banana
- 1 medium plum
- 1 small grapefruit with 2 teaspoons sugar
- 1 cup reduced-sodium V8 juice
- 3/4 cup blueberries
- 3/4 cup red grapes
- 1/2 medium pear and 1/2 ounce reduced-fat cheddar cheese
- 1/2 small baked potato with 3 tablespoons salsa
- 1/4 cup unsweetened pineapple tidbits with 1/3 cup 1% cottage cheese
- 1/4 cup dried apricots
- 1 roasted chicken drumstick, skin removed
- 1 piece string cheese
- 1 frozen fudge pop
- 1 hard-cooked egg
- 3/4 cup minestrone soup
- 1/3 cup roasted pumpkin seeds
- 3 tablespoons soy nuts
- 3 cups air-popped popcorn
- 3 graham crackers (2-1/2-inch squares)
- 3 vanilla wafers with 1/2 cup fat-free milk
- 1 crisp rice cereal bar (22 g package)
- 1 slice cinnamon-raisin toast topped with 1 teaspoon honey
- 2/3 cup Cheerios with 1/4 cup fat-free milk
- 1/3 cup miniature fish-shaped crackers
- 4 chocolate kisses

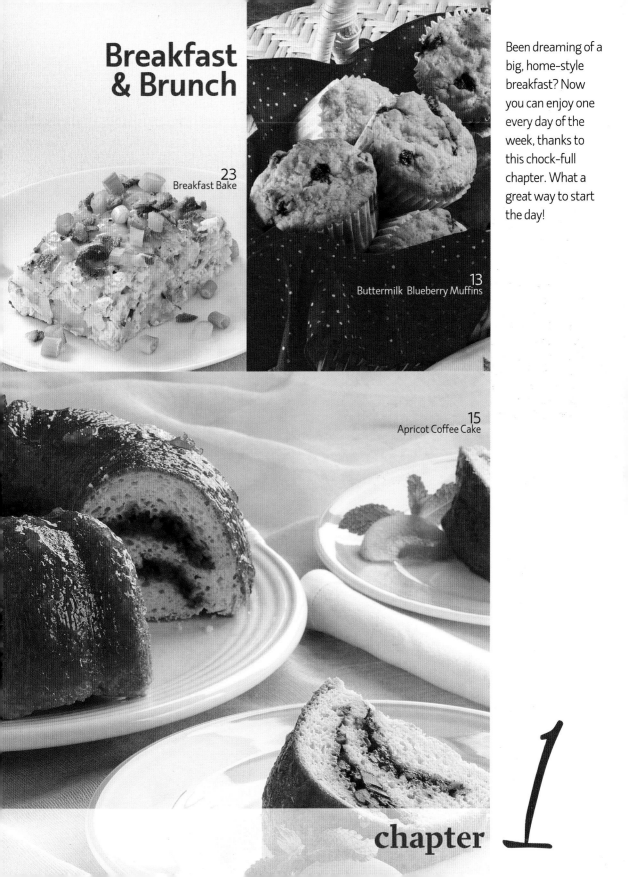

Breakfast & Brunch

23
Breakfast Bake

13
Buttermilk Blueberry Muffins

15
Apricot Coffee Cake

Been dreaming of a big, home-style breakfast? Now you can enjoy one every day of the week, thanks to this chock-full chapter. What a great way to start the day!

chapter *1*

Fruit Crepes

These fruit-topped crepes are a great way to start the day. They taste so yummy, it's hard to believe they're healthier for you.

Jean Murtagh, Solon, Ohio

PREP/TOTAL TIME
Prep: 25 min.
Bake: 15 min.
YIELD 4 servings

NUTRITION FACTS
One serving
(2 crepes) equals:
173 calories
3 g fat
0 g saturated fat
1 mg cholesterol
231 mg sodium
32 g carbohydrate
2 g fiber
7 g protein

DIABETIC EXCHANGES
1-1/2 starch
1/2 fat-free milk
1/2 fat

- 2 egg whites
- 2/3 cup fat-free milk
- 2 teaspoons vegetable oil
- 1/2 cup all-purpose flour
- 1/4 teaspoon salt
- 1/4 cup reduced-sugar orange marmalade
- 1 cup unsweetened raspberries, blackberries or blueberries

Sugar substitute equivalent to 8 teaspoons sugar

- 1/2 cup fat-free sour cream
- 1/8 teaspoon ground cinnamon

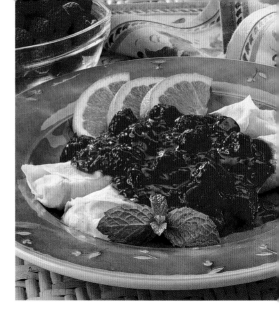

1. In a bowl, combine egg whites, milk and oil. Combine flour and salt; add to milk mixture and mix well. In a saucepan, heat marmalade until melted; remove from the heat. Fold in berries and sugar substitute; set aside. In a small bowl, combine sour cream and cinnamon; set aside.

2. Heat an 8-in. nonstick skillet coated with cooking spray; add 2 tablespoons batter. Lift and tilt pan to evenly coat bottom. Cook until top appears dry and bottom is light brown. Remove to a wire rack. Repeat with remaining batter.

3. Spread each crepe with 1 tablespoon sour cream mixture; roll up and place in an ungreased 11-in. x 7-in. x 2-in. baking dish. Spoon fruit mixture over top. Bake, uncovered, at 375° for 15 minutes.

Editor's Note: This recipe was tested with Splenda No Calorie Sweetener.

Crispy French Toast

I lighten up my morning French toast with egg substitute and fat-free milk, then flavor it with orange juice, vanilla and a dash of nutmeg. The out-of-the-ordinary cornflake coating adds a fun crunch.

Flo Burtnett, Gage, Oklahoma

PREP/TOTAL TIME
30 min.
YIELD 12 slices

NUTRITION FACTS
One serving equals
(1 slice):
147 calories
1 g fat
Trace saturated fat
Trace cholesterol
359 mg sodium
28 g carbohydrate
1 g fiber
5 g protein

DIABETIC EXCHANGE
2 starch

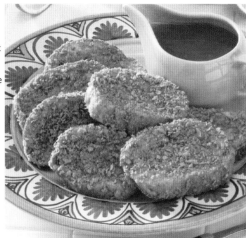

- 1/2 cup egg substitute
- 1/2 cup fat-free milk
- 1/4 cup orange juice
- 1 teaspoon vanilla extract

Dash ground nutmeg

- 12 slices day-old French bread (3/4 inch thick)
- 1-1/2 cups crushed cornflakes

1. In a shallow dish, combine the egg substitute, milk, orange juice, vanilla and nutmeg. Add bread; soak for 5 minutes, turning once. Coat both sides of each slice with cornflake crumbs.

2. Place in a 15-in. x 10-in. x 1-in. baking pan coated with cooking spray. Bake at 425° for 10 minutes; turn. Bake 5-8 minutes longer or until golden brown.

Ham and Apple Skillet

Here are all the breakfast favorites–hash browns, eggs, ham and cheese–baked together in one pan. Reduced-fat cheese, fat-free milk and lean meat help trim the fat, while chopped apple adds a touch of sweetness.

Patty Kile, Greentown, Pennsylvania

- 3 cups frozen O'Brien hash brown potatoes, thawed
- 1 large apple, peeled, cored and chopped (about 1 cup)
- 1/4 cup chopped onion
- 1/2 to 1 teaspoon rubbed sage
- 2 tablespoons water
- 1 cup diced fully cooked lean ham
- 1/2 cup shredded reduced-fat cheddar cheese, *divided*
- 4 eggs
- 1-1/2 cups fat-free milk
- 1/4 teaspoon salt

1. Press potatoes between paper towels to remove moisture; set aside. In a nonstick ovenproof skillet, cook the apple, onion and sage in water over medium heat until apple and onion are tender. Stir in potatoes and ham; heat through. Sprinkle with half of the cheese. Remove from the heat.

2. In a bowl, beat the eggs, milk and salt; pour over potato mixture (do not stir). Sprinkle with remaining cheese. Bake, uncovered, at 350° for 35-40 minutes or until center is set and a knife inserted near the center comes out clean.

FAT-FREE SAUTEING

To omit the fat when sauteing veggies or meat, use a nonstick skillet coated with cooking spray. Or, instead of cooking spray, use a couple tablespoons of water, low-sodium broth or a little fruit juice.

PREP/TOTAL TIME
Prep: 15 min.
Bake: 35 min.
YIELD 6 servings

NUTRITION FACTS
One serving (1 cup) equals:
242 calories
7 g fat
3 g saturated fat
15 mg cholesterol
541 mg sodium
29 g carbohydrate
3 g fiber
16 g protein

DIABETIC EXCHANGES
2 lean meat
1-1/2 starch
1/2 fruit

Lemon Ginger Muffins

These quick muffins are tender and have an irresistible aroma while baking. If you like lemon, you're sure to enjoy their fresh flavor.

Joyce Baker-Mabry, Hamilton, Montana

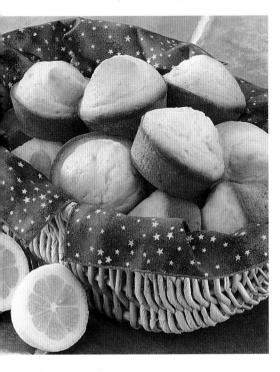

- 1/3 cup butter, softened
- 1/2 cup sugar

Sugar substitute equivalent to 1/2 cup sugar

- 4 egg whites
- 2 tablespoons minced fresh gingerroot
- 2 tablespoons grated lemon peel
- 2 cups all-purpose flour
- 1 teaspoon baking soda
- 1 cup (8 ounces) fat-free plain yogurt

1. In a large mixing bowl, beat the butter, sugar and sugar substitute until crumbly. Add the egg whites; beat well. Stir in the ginger and lemon peel. Combine the flour and baking soda; add to butter mixture alternately with yogurt.

2. Coat muffin cups with cooking spray; fill three-fourths full with the batter. Bake at 375° for 18-20 minutes or until a toothpick comes out clean. Cool for 5 minutes before removing from the pan to a wire rack. Serve warm.

Editor's Note: This recipe was tested with Splenda No Calorie Sweetener.

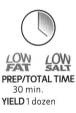

LOW FAT   LOW SALT
PREP/TOTAL TIME
30 min.
YIELD 1 dozen

NUTRITION FACTS
One serving (1 muffin) equals:
171 calories
5 g fat
3 g saturated fat
14 mg cholesterol
186 mg sodium
27 g carbohydrate
1 g fiber
4 g protein

DIABETIC EXCHANGES
2 starch
1/2 fat

Garden Frittata

PREP/TOTAL TIME
Prep: 25 min.
Bake: 45 min.+
standing
YIELD 8 servings

NUTRITION FACTS
One serving equals:
126 calories
7 g fat
4 g saturated fat
121 mg cholesterol
316 mg sodium
6 g carbohydrate
1 g fiber
11 g protein

DIABETIC EXCHANGES
1 lean meat
1 vegetable
1 fat

I created this dish one day to use up some fresh yellow squash, zucchini and tomato. It's so easy to make because you don't have to fuss with a crust. Give it a different twist by using whatever veggies you have on hand.

Catherine Michel, O'Fallon, Missouri

1 small yellow summer squash, thinly sliced
1 small zucchini, thinly sliced
1 small onion, chopped
1 cup (4 ounces) shredded part-skim mozzarella cheese
1 medium tomato, sliced
1/4 cup crumbled feta cheese
4 eggs
1 cup fat-free milk
2 tablespoons minced fresh basil
1 garlic clove, minced
1/2 teaspoon salt
1/4 teaspoon pepper
1/4 cup shredded Parmesan cheese

1. In a microwave-safe bowl, combine the squash, zucchini and onion. Cover and microwave on high for 7-9 minutes or until the vegetables are tender; drain well. Transfer to a 9-in. pie plate coated with cooking spray. Top with the mozzarella, tomato and feta cheese.

2. In a large bowl, whisk the eggs, milk, basil, garlic, salt and pepper; pour over the mozzarella and tomato layer. Sprinkle with Parmesan cheese. Bake, uncovered, at 375° for 45-50 minutes or until a knife inserted near the center comes out clean. Let stand for 10 minutes before serving.

Orange-Cinnamon French Toast

Everyone eats at the same time when you fix this citrusy, oven-baked French toast. And no one will guess that you're eating healthier!

Bernice Smith, Sturgeon Lake, Minnesota

- 2 to 4 tablespoons butter, melted
- 2 tablespoons honey
- 1/2 teaspoon ground cinnamon
- 3 eggs
- 1/2 cup orange juice
- 1/8 teaspoon salt, optional
- 6 slices bread

Additional honey, optional

1. In a bowl, combine butter, honey and cinnamon. Pour into a greased 13-in. x 9-in. x 2-in. baking pan; spread to coat the bottom of pan. In a shallow bowl, beat the eggs, orange juice and salt if desired. Dip bread into egg mixture and place in the prepared pan.

2. Bake at 400° for 15-20 minutes or until golden brown. Invert onto a serving platter; serve with honey if desired.

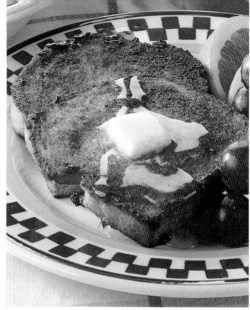

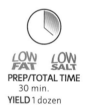

LOW FAT LOW SALT

PREP/TOTAL TIME
30 min.
YIELD 6 servings

NUTRITION FACTS
One serving (1 slice) equals:

- 158 calories
- 5 g fat
- 0 g saturated fat
- 1 mg cholesterol
- 231 mg sodium
- 23 g carbohydrate
- 0 g fiber
- 6 g protein

DIABETIC EXCHANGES
1-1/2 starch
1 fat

Buttermilk Blueberry Muffins

These golden muffins are moist, flavorful and have very little fat. You'll never make blueberry muffins from a mix again!

Jean Howard, Hopkinton, Massachusetts

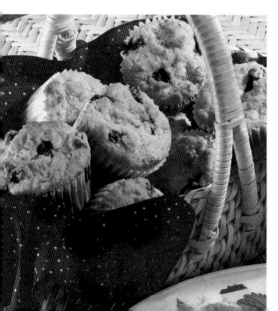

- 2 cups all-purpose flour
- 1/2 cup packed brown sugar
- 1 tablespoon baking powder
- 1 teaspoon baking soda
- 1/2 teaspoon grated lemon peel
- 1/2 teaspoon ground nutmeg
- 1 cup blueberries
- 1 cup fat-free vanilla yogurt
- 1 cup buttermilk

1. In a large bowl, combine the first six ingredients. Gently fold in blueberries. Combine yogurt and buttermilk; stir into dry ingredients just until moistened.

2. Coat muffin cups with cooking spray or use paper liners; fill two-thirds full with batter. Bake at 400° for 18-20 minutes or until a toothpick comes out clean. Cool for 5 minutes before removing from pan to a wire rack.

LOW FAT LOW SALT

PREP/TOTAL TIME
30 min.
YIELD 1 dozen

NUTRITION FACTS
One serving
(1 muffin) equals:

- 145 calories
- 1 g fat
- 0 g saturated fat
- 1 mg cholesterol
- 267 mg sodium
- 31 g carbohydrate
- 0 g fiber
- 4 g protein

DIABETIC EXCHANGE
2 starch

Sausage Breakfast Wraps

PREP/TOTAL TIME
Prep: 25 min.
Bake: 30 min.
YIELD 10 servings

NUTRITION FACTS
One serving (1 wrap)
equals:

277 calories
7 g fat
1 g saturated fat
27 mg cholesterol
893 mg sodium
30 g carbohydrate
2 g fiber
21 g protein

DIABETIC EXCHANGES
2 starch
2 lean meat
1/2 fat

I love breakfast burritos, but they're typically high in fat and cholesterol. So I created my own healthier version. Since my wraps freeze well, they make an anytime meal. Let the sausage mixture cool for about an hour before assembling and freezing the wraps.

Ed Rysdyk Jr., Wyoming, Michigan

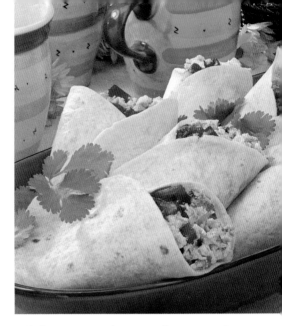

1 pound turkey Italian sausage links, casings removed

1 medium sweet red pepper, diced

1 small onion, diced

4 cartons (8 ounces *each*) frozen egg substitute, thawed

1 can (4 ounces) chopped green chilies

1 teaspoon chili powder

10 flour tortillas (8 inches), warmed

1-1/4 cups salsa

1. In a nonstick skillet, cook sausage over medium heat until no longer pink; drain. Transfer to a 13-in. x 9-in. x 2-in. baking dish coated with cooking spray. Sprinkle with red pepper and onion. Combine the egg substitute, green chilies and chili powder; pour over sausage mixture.

2. Bake, uncovered, at 350° for 30-35 minutes or until set. Break up sausage mixture with a spoon. Place 2/3 cup down the center of each tortilla; top with salsa. Fold one end of tortilla over sausage mixture, then fold two sides over.

Pecan Waffles

PREP/TOTAL TIME
30 min.
YIELD 6 waffles
(6-1/2-inch diameter)

NUTRITION FACTS
One serving
(1 waffle) equals:

233 calories
11 g fat
1 g saturated fat
37 mg cholesterol
344 mg sodium
28 g carbohydrate
2 g fiber
8 g protein

DIABETIC EXCHANGES
2 starch
2 fat

Your bunch will say a big "yes" to breakfast when these wonderful waffles are on the menu. Plus, they're quick to whip up.

Susan Bell, Spruce Pine, North Carolina

1-1/4 cups all-purpose flour

1/4 cup wheat bran

1 tablespoon sugar

2-1/2 teaspoons baking powder

1/2 teaspoon salt

1 egg

1 egg white

1-1/2 cups fat-free milk

2 tablespoons canola oil

1/3 cup chopped pecans

1. In a bowl, combine the flour, bran, sugar, baking powder and salt. In another bowl, combine the egg, egg white, milk and oil; add to the dry ingredients. Fold in pecans.

2. Bake batter in a preheated waffle iron according to the manufacturer's directions until golden brown.

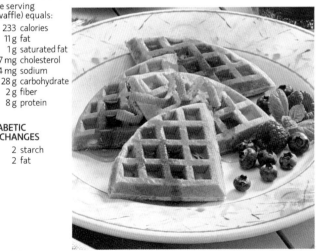

Apricot Coffee Cake

Having friends over for coffee? Serve them this scrumptious, calorie-smart coffee cake and they'll be delighted.

Taste of Home Test Kitchen

- 1 jar (10 ounces) apricot spreadable fruit, *divided*
- 3/4 cup chopped pecans

Sugar substitute equivalent to 1/3 cup sugar

- 4 teaspoons ground cinnamon

CAKE:

- 3-1/4 cups reduced-fat biscuit/baking mix

Sugar substitute equivalent to 3/4 cup sugar

- 1/8 teaspoon ground cardamom
- 2 eggs
- 1 cup fat-free milk
- 2/3 cup reduced-fat sour cream
- 1 tablespoon butter, melted

1. Place 3 tablespoons spreadable fruit in a small microwave-safe bowl; cover and refrigerate. In another bowl, combine the pecans, sugar substitute, cinnamon and remaining spreadable fruit; set aside.

2. For cake, in a large bowl, combine the biscuit mix, sugar substitute and cardamom. Combine the eggs, milk, sour cream and butter; stir into dry ingredients just until moistened. Spread a third of the batter into a 10-in. fluted tube pan coated with cooking spray. Spread with half of pecan mixture. Repeat layers. Top with remaining batter.

3. Bake at 350° for 40-45 minutes or until a toothpick inserted near the center comes out clean. Cool for 15 minutes before removing from pan to a wire rack. In a microwave, warm reserved spreadable fruit; brush over warm cake. Cool completely.

Editor's Note: This recipe was tested with Splenda No Calorie Sweetener.

PREP/TOTAL TIME
Prep: 15 min.
Bake: 40 min. + cooling
YIELD 16 servings

NUTRITION FACTS
One serving (1 slice) equals:
- 213 calories
- 8 g fat
- 2 g saturated fat
- 32 mg cholesterol
- 313 mg sodium
- 32 g carbohydrate
- 1 g fiber
- 4 g protein

DIABETIC EXCHANGES
- 1-1/2 starch
- 1 fruit
- 1 fat

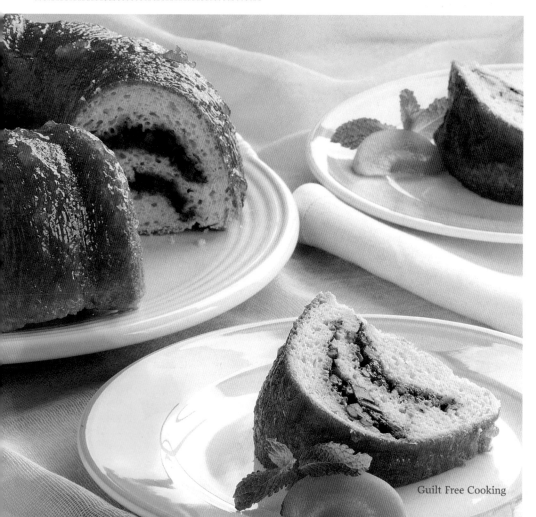

Raspberry Coffee Cake

Who says you can't eat coffee cake if you're watching your weight? This treat features bits of raspberry in every bite and a drizzle of vanilla frosting on top. Yum!

Merle Shapter, Delta, British Columbia

PREP/TOTAL TIME
Prep: 20 min.
Bake: 35 min. +
cooling
YIELD 8 servings

NUTRITION FACTS
One serving (1 piece)
equals:
178 calories
4 g fat
2 g saturated fat
35 mg cholesterol
178 mg sodium
32 g carbohydrate
2 g fiber
4 g protein

DIABETIC EXCHANGES
1 starch
1 fruit
1 fat

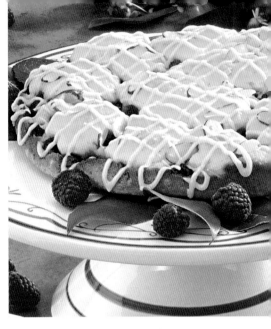

1 cup all-purpose flour
1/3 cup sugar
1/2 teaspoon baking powder
1/4 teaspoon baking soda
1/4 teaspoon salt
1 egg
1/2 cup reduced-fat plain yogurt
2 tablespoons butter, softened
1 teaspoon vanilla extract
3 tablespoons brown sugar
1 cup unsweetened fresh *or* frozen raspberries
1 tablespoon sliced almonds

GLAZE:
1/4 cup confectioners' sugar
1 teaspoon fat-free milk
1/4 teaspoon vanilla extract

1. In a bowl, combine flour, sugar, baking powder, baking soda and salt. Combine the egg, yogurt, butter and vanilla; add to dry ingredients just until moistened.

2. Spoon two-thirds of batter into an 8-in. round baking pan coated with cooking spray. Combine the brown sugar and raspberries; sprinkle over batter. Spoon remaining batter over the top. Sprinkle with almonds.

3. Bake at 350° for 35-40 minutes or until cake springs back when lightly touched and is golden brown. Cool for 10 minutes before removing from pan to a wire rack.

4. In a bowl, combine glaze ingredients. Drizzle over coffee cake. Serve warm or at room temperature.

Editor's Note: If using frozen raspberries, do not thaw before adding to batter.

Seasoned Scrambled Eggs

I frequently whip up this fluffy egg dish for two. The addition of ranch dressing, brown mustard and mozzarella cheese makes these fast-to-fix scrambled eggs something special.

Charlotte Wiley, New York City, New York

PREP/TOTAL TIME
15 min.
YIELD 2 servings

NUTRITION FACTS
One serving equals:
251 calories
16 g fat
4 g saturated fat
331 mg cholesterol
496 mg sodium
4 g carbohydrate
Trace fiber
21 g protein

DIABETIC EXCHANGES
3 lean meat
1-1/2 fat

4 egg whites
3 eggs
2 tablespoons reduced-fat ranch salad dressing
2 teaspoons spicy brown mustard
1 teaspoon minced fresh parsley
1/2 teaspoon garlic powder
1 teaspoon canola oil
1/4 cup shredded part-skim mozzarella cheese

1. In a bowl, whisk together the egg whites and eggs. Stir in the salad dressing, mustard, parsley and garlic powder. In a non-stick skillet, cook egg mixture in oil over medium heat for 2 minutes or until eggs are almost set. Stir in cheese. Cook for 1 minute longer or until eggs are set and cheese is melted. Serve immediately.

CUTTING CHOLESTEROL IN EGG DISHES

The yolk of a large egg has about 213 milligrams of cholesterol. In general, a healthy person with no dietary cholesterol restrictions may have about 300 mg per day. Seasoned Scrambled Eggs uses both egg whites and whole eggs. By substituting the whites for some of whole eggs, the serving portion can be a bit larger while still limiting the dietary cholesterol in the recipe.

Home-Style Country Sausage

My family loves sausage, but we needed to cut down on fat and calories. This version, which uses ground turkey, is spiced with garlic, sage, allspice, thyme and cayenne.

Linda Murray, Allenstown, New Hampshire

- 1 medium tart apple, peeled and shredded
- 1/2 cup cooked brown rice
- 2 tablespoons grated onion
- 2 garlic cloves, minced
- 1-1/2 teaspoons rubbed sage
- 1 teaspoon salt
- 1/2 teaspoon pepper
- 1/2 teaspoon dried thyme
- 1/8 teaspoon cayenne pepper
- 1/8 teaspoon ground allspice
- 1 pound lean ground turkey

1. In a large bowl, combine the first 10 ingredients. Crumble the ground turkey over the mixture and mix well. Shape into eight 1/2-in.-thick patties.

2. In a large nonstick skillet coated with cooking spray, cook the sausage patties for 4-6 minutes on each side or until the juices run clear.

LET'S TALK TURKEY

Did you know not all ground turkey is equal? Read the label when purchasing. Ground turkey has about 68 grams of fat in one pound, lean ground turkey about 32 grams and extra lean ground turkey about 4 grams.

LOW FAT

PREP/TOTAL TIME
20 min.

YIELD 8 patties

NUTRITION FACTS
One serving (1 patty) equals:
- 111 calories
- 5 g fat
- 1 g saturated fat
- 45 mg cholesterol
- 348 mg sodium
- 6 g carbohydrate
- 1 g fiber
- 10 g protein

DIABETIC EXCHANGE
- 2 lean meat

Crustless Spinach Quiche

My daughter is a vegetarian, so I eliminated the ham called for in the original recipe for this dish. Wedges of the lighter quiche make a flavorful brunch, lunch or supper.

Vicki Schrupp, Little Falls, Minnesota

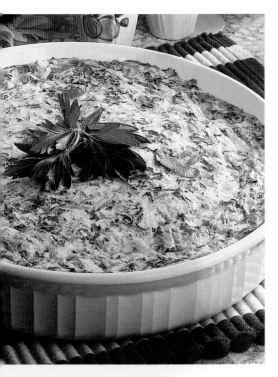

- 3 ounces reduced-fat cream cheese, softened
- 1 cup fat-free milk
- 1 cup egg substitute
- 1/4 teaspoon pepper
- 3 cups (12 ounces) shredded reduced-fat cheddar cheese
- 1 package (10 ounces) frozen chopped spinach, thawed and squeezed dry
- 1 cup frozen chopped broccoli, thawed and well drained
- 1 small onion, finely chopped
- 5 fresh mushrooms, sliced

1. In a small mixing bowl, beat cream cheese. Add milk, egg substitute and pepper; beat until smooth. Stir in remaining ingredients. Transfer to a 10-in. quiche pan coated with cooking spray. Bake at 350° for 45-50 minutes or until a knife inserted near the center comes out clean.

LOW FAT

PREP/TOTAL TIME
Prep: 15 min.
Bake: 45 min.

YIELD 8 servings

NUTRITION FACTS
One serving equals:
- 151 calories
- 5 g fat
- 0 g saturated fat
- 14 mg cholesterol
- 404 mg sodium
- 8 g carbohydrate
- 2 g fiber
- 18 g protein

DIABETIC EXCHANGES
- 1 starch
- 1 meat

PREP/TOTAL TIME
30 min.
YIELD 4 servings

NUTRITION FACTS
One serving
(3 pancakes,
calculated without
berries) equals:

   328 calories
    11 g fat
     2 g saturated fat
  58 mg cholesterol
509 mg sodium
   45 g carbohydrate
    4 g fiber
   12 g protein

**DIABETIC
EXCHANGES**
2-1/2 starch
1-1/2 fat
  1/2 reduced-fat
     milk

Hearty Oatmeal Pancakes

My husband and I are trying to fit more oatmeal into our diet, but we get tired of the usual bowlful. These moist, fluffy pancakes give us the grains that we're looking for...and they still taste like a terrific breakfast treat.

Kathy Thompson, Glendale, Kentucky

1	cup quick-cooking oats
1/2	cup all-purpose flour
1/2	cup whole wheat flour
1	tablespoon sugar
1	teaspoon baking powder
1/2	teaspoon baking soda
1/4	teaspoon salt
1	egg, lightly beaten
2	cups buttermilk
2	tablespoons canola oil
1	teaspoon vanilla extract

Assorted berries, optional

1. In a bowl, combine the first seven ingredients. In another bowl, combine the egg, buttermilk, oil and vanilla; mix well. Stir into the dry ingredients just until moistened.

2. Pour batter by 1/4 cupfuls onto a hot griddle coated with cooking spray. Turn when bubbles form on top; cook until the second side is golden brown. Serve with berries if desired.

Eggs Florentine

I wanted to impress my family with a holiday brunch but keep it on the healthier side. When I lightened up the hollandaise sauce in a classic egg recipe, everyone loved it!

Bobbi Trautman, Burns, Oregon

- 2 tablespoons reduced-fat stick margarine
- 1 tablespoon all-purpose flour
- 1/2 teaspoon salt, *divided*
- 1-1/4 cups fat-free milk
- 1 egg yolk
- 2 teaspoons lemon juice
- 1/2 teaspoon grated lemon peel
- 1/2 pound fresh spinach
- 1/8 teaspoon pepper
- 4 eggs
- 2 English muffins, split and toasted

Dash paprika

1. In a saucepan, melt margarine. Stir in flour and 1/4 teaspoon salt until smooth. Gradually add milk. Bring to a boil; cook and stir for 1-2 minutes or until thickened. Remove from the heat. Stir a small amount of sauce into egg yolk; return all to the pan, stirring constantly. Bring to a gentle boil; cook and stir for 2 minutes. Remove from the heat; stir in juice and peel. Set aside and keep warm.

2. Place spinach in a steamer basket. Sprinkle with pepper and remaining salt. Place in a saucepan over 1 in. of water.

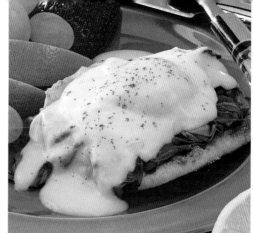

Bring to a boil; cover and steam for 3-4 minutes or until wilted and tender.

3. Meanwhile, in a skillet or omelet pan with high sides, bring 2 to 3 in. water to a boil. Reduce heat; simmer gently. Break cold eggs, one at a time, into a custard cup or saucer. Holding the dish close to the surface of the simmering water, slip the eggs, one at a time, into the water. Cook, uncovered, for 3-5 minutes or until whites are completely set and yolks begin to thicken.

4. Lift eggs out of water with slotted spoon. Place spinach on each muffin half; top with an egg. Spoon 3 tablespoons sauce on each. Sprinkle with paprika. Serve immediately.

Editor's Note: This recipe was tested with Parkay Light stick margarine.

PREP/TOTAL TIME
30 min.
YIELD 4 servings

NUTRITION FACTS
One serving equals:
229 calories
10 g fat
3 g saturated fat
267 mg cholesterol
635 mg sodium
21 g carbohydrate
2 g fiber
14 g protein

DIABETIC EXCHANGES
1 starch
1 lean meat
1 fat
1/2 fat-free milk

Cream Cheese Ham Omelet

This omelet, sized for two people, is filled with cream cheese, diced ham and onion. My husband and I are on a low-cholesterol diet, so I use an egg substitute instead of whole eggs.

Michelle Revelle, Guyton, Georgia

- 1/2 cup chopped sweet onion
- 2 teaspoons olive oil
- 1 cup egg substitute
- 1/2 cup diced fully cooked lean ham
- 1/4 teaspoon seasoned salt
- 1/8 teaspoon pepper
- 1/8 teaspoon paprika
- 3 tablespoons reduced-fat cream cheese, cubed

1. In a 10-in. nonstick skillet, saute onion in oil until tender. Reduce heat to medium; add egg substitute. As eggs set, lift edges, letting uncooked portion flow underneath.

2. When the eggs are set, sprinkle ham, seasoned salt, pepper and paprika over one side. Top with cream cheese cubes. Fold omelet over filling. Cover and let stand for 1-2 minutes or until cream cheese is melted.

PREP/TOTAL TIME
15 min.
YIELD 2 servings

NUTRITION FACTS
One serving equals:
215 calories
10 g fat
4 g saturated fat
23 mg cholesterol
905 mg sodium
7 g carbohydrate
1 g fiber
22 g protein

DIABETIC EXCHANGES
2 lean meat
1 fat
1/2 fat-free milk

PREP/TOTAL TIME
30 min.
YIELD 4 servings

NUTRITION FACTS
One serving (one omelet) equals:
239 calories
7 g fat
0 g saturated fat
9 mg cholesterol
457 mg sodium
23 g carbohydrate
0 g fiber
21 g protein

DIABETIC EXCHANGES
2-1/2 lean meat
1-1/2 starch

Hash Brown Cheese Omelet

I make a family-pleasing meal out of this fluffy omelet full of hash brown potatoes, onion and green pepper. I've found that it's also good with sliced tomatoes.

Jennifer Reisinger, Sheboygan, Wisconsin

1 medium onion, chopped
1/2 cup chopped green pepper
1-3/4 cups frozen cubed hash brown potatoes, thawed
2 cups egg substitute
1/4 cup water
1/8 teaspoon pepper
3 slices reduced-fat process American cheese product

1. In a large skillet coated with cooking spray, saute onion and green pepper. Add potatoes; cook and stir over medium heat for 5 minutes or until heated through.

2. In a bowl, beat egg substitute, water and

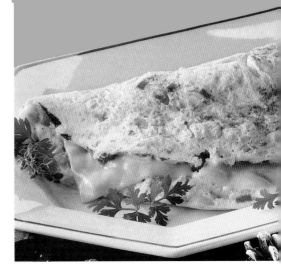

pepper; pour over vegetables. As eggs set, lift edges, letting uncooked portion flow underneath. Just before eggs are completely set, place cheese slices over half of the omelet. Fold the omelet in half and transfer to a warm serving platter.

PREP/TOTAL TIME
20 min.
YIELD 4 servings

NUTRITION FACTS
One serving (1 waffle) equals:
235 calories
5 g fat
2 g saturated fat
61 mg cholesterol
301 mg sodium
40 g carbohydrate
1 g fiber
8 g protein

DIABETIC EXCHANGES
1-1/2 starch
1 lean meat
1 fruit

Blueberry Waffles

Homemade waffles are my husband's top choice for Sunday brunch. We like them with a variety of sliced fruit on the side.

Lori Daniels, Beverly, West Virginia

1 cup all-purpose flour
2 tablespoons sugar
1 teaspoon baking powder
1/4 teaspoon salt
1 egg yolk
1/4 cup fat-free milk
1/4 cup orange juice
1 tablespoon butter, melted
1 teaspoon grated orange peel
1/8 teaspoon orange extract
4 egg whites
1 cup fresh blueberries
1 tablespoon confectioners' sugar

1. In a large bowl, combine the flour, sugar, baking powder and salt. In another bowl, whisk the egg yolk, milk, orange juice, butter, orange peel and extract; stir into dry ingredients just until combined. In a small mixing bowl, beat egg whites until stiff peaks form; fold into batter. Fold in blueberries.

2. Bake in a preheated waffle iron according to manufacturer's directions until golden brown. Sprinkle with confectioners' sugar.

SODIUM SENSE

Interested in ways to cut down the sodium in your diet? Rather than using standard baking powder, try the no-sodium variety. Look for it at health food stores.

Fruit Kabobs

Everyone enjoys fresh fruit, and it's great served with this dip. Creating kabobs is an easy way to make breakfast fun.

Cheryl Ollis, Matthews, North Carolina

- 1 medium tart apple, cut into 1-inch chunks
- 1 medium pear, cut into 1-inch chunks
- 1 tablespoon lemon juice
- 1 can (8 ounces) unsweetened pineapple chunks, drained
- 24 grapes (about 1/4 pound)
- 24 fresh strawberries

COCONUT DIP:

- 1-1/2 cups fat-free vanilla yogurt
- 4-1/2 teaspoons flaked coconut
- 4-1/2 teaspoons reduced-sugar orange marmalade

1. Toss apple and pear with lemon juice. Divide fruit into 12 portions and thread onto wooden skewers. Combine dip ingredients in a small bowl; serve with the kabobs.

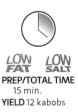

LOW FAT　**LOW SALT**

PREP/TOTAL TIME
15 min.
YIELD 12 kabobs

NUTRITION FACTS
One serving
(1 kabob) equals:
　52 calories
Trace fat
　0 g saturated fat
Trace cholesterol
10 mg sodium
　12 g carbohydrate
　0 g fiber
　1 g protein

DIABETIC EXCHANGE
　1 fruit

PREP/TOTAL TIME
Prep: 30 min. +
rising
Bake: 25 min.
YIELD 1 dozen

NUTRITION FACTS
One serving
(1 bun) equals:
193 calories
4 g fat
Trace saturated fat
Trace cholesterol
218 mg sodium
36 g carbohydrate
1 g fiber
4 g protein

DIABETIC EXCHANGES
2-1/2 starch
1/2 fat

Cinnamon Buns

With vanilla glaze, these rolls are a real taste treat.

Susan Corpman, Newhall, Iowa

1 package (1/4 ounce) active dry yeast
1 cup warm fat-free milk (110° to 115°), *divided*
3 tablespoons canola oil
1 tablespoon sugar
1 teaspoon salt
2-1/2 to 2-3/4 cups all-purpose flour
3 tablespoons dark corn syrup
3 tablespoons packed brown sugar
2 teaspoons ground cinnamon
1/8 teaspoon ground nutmeg
1/4 cup raisins

GLAZE:

1/2 cup confectioners' sugar
1/4 teaspoon vanilla extract
1 to 2 teaspoons fat-free milk

1. In a large mixing bowl, dissolve yeast in 1/4 cup warm milk. Add the oil, sugar, salt, 1-1/2 cups flour and remaining milk. Beat on medium speed for 3 minutes.

Stir in enough remaining flour to form a soft dough.

2. Turn onto a lightly floured surface; knead until smooth and elastic, about 6-8 minutes. Place in a bowl coated with cooking spray, turning once to coat top. Cover and let rise in a warm place until doubled, about 1 hour.

3. Punch dough down. Turn onto a lightly floured surface; roll into a 12-in. x 10-in. rectangle. Carefully spread corn syrup over dough to within 1/2 in. of edges. In a bowl, combine the brown sugar, cinnamon and nutmeg; sprinkle over corn syrup. Sprinkle with raisins.

4. Roll up jelly-roll style, starting with a long side; pinch seam to seal. Cut into 12 slices. Place cut side down in a 9-in. round baking pan coated with cooking spray. Cover and let rise in a warm place until doubled, about 40 minutes.

5. Bake at 350° for 25-30 minutes or until golden brown. Cool on a wire rack. For glaze, in a bowl, combine confectioners' sugar, vanilla and enough milk to achieve drizzling consistency. Drizzle over buns.

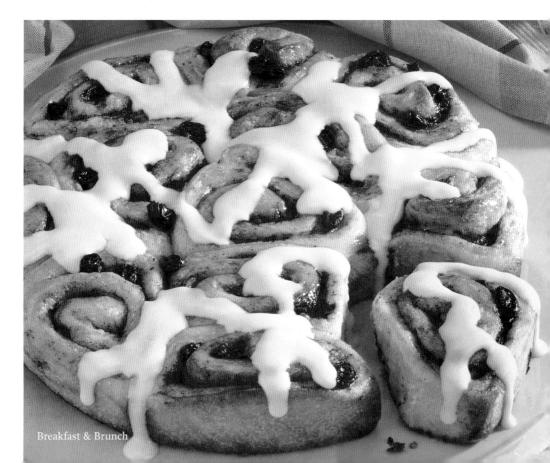

Breakfast Bake

I wanted to have hash browns and scrambled eggs one morning, and this is the dish I created. My wife thought it was great, so you can guess who's making breakfast more often!

Howard Rogers, El Paso, Texas

- 1-1/2 cups egg substitute
- 1/2 cup fat-free milk
- 3-1/2 cups frozen O'Brien hash brown potatoes, thawed
- 1-1/3 cups shredded reduced-fat cheddar cheese, *divided*
- 1/2 cup chopped sweet onion
- 4 tablespoons crumbled cooked bacon, *divided*
- 1/2 teaspoon salt
- 1/2 teaspoon salt-free seasoning blend
- 1/4 teaspoon chili powder
- 4 green onions, chopped

1. In a large bowl, whisk the egg substitute and milk. Stir in the hash browns, 1 cup cheese, onion, 2 tablespoons bacon, salt, seasoning blend and chili powder. Pour into an 8-in. square baking dish coated with cooking spray.

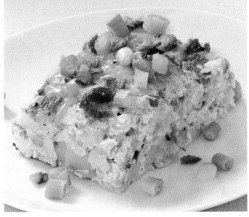

2. Bake at 350° for 45-50 minutes or until a knife inserted near the center comes out clean. Sprinkle with the remaining cheese and bacon. Bake 3-5 minutes longer or until cheese is melted. Sprinkle with green onions. Let stand for 5 minutes before cutting.

PREP/TOTAL TIME
Prep: 15 min.
Bake: 50 min.
YIELD 6 servings

NUTRITION FACTS
One serving
(1 piece) equals:
219 calories
6 g fat
4 g saturated fat
22 mg cholesterol
682 mg sodium
25 g carbohydrate
3 g fiber
17 g protein

DIABETIC
EXCHANGES
2 lean meat
1-1/2 starch

Hearty Brunch Potatoes

Our family of five enjoys this hearty dish with eggs and toast for breakfast. Leftovers are just as tasty with a salad or green beans and crusty bread for lunch or supper.

Madonna McCollough, Harrison, Arkansas

- 7 medium potatoes, peeled and cut into 1/2-inch cubes
- 1/2 cup chopped green pepper
- 1/2 cup chopped sweet red pepper
- 1/2 cup fresh *or* frozen corn
- 1 small onion, chopped
- 1 to 2 garlic cloves, minced
- 1/2 pound smoked turkey sausage links
- 2 tablespoons olive oil
- 1/4 teaspoon pepper

1. Place potatoes in a saucepan and cover with water. Bring to a boil; reduce heat. Cook, uncovered, just until tender, about 10 minutes.

2. Meanwhile, in a skillet coated with cooking spray, saute peppers, corn, onion and garlic until tender. Cut sausage into small chunks; add to vegetable mixture. Cook, uncovered, for 6-8 minutes or until heated through.

3. Drain the potatoes; add to vegetable mixture. Add oil and pepper; mix well. Transfer to an ungreased 13-in. x 9-in. x 2-in. baking dish. Bake, uncovered, at 350° for 35 minutes or until heated through.

PREP/TOTAL TIME
Prep: 25 min.
Bake: 35 min.
YIELD 12 servings

NUTRITION FACTS
One serving equals:
114 calories
3 g fat
1 g saturated fat
7 mg cholesterol
164 mg sodium
18 g carbohydrate
2 g fiber
4 g protein

DIABETIC
EXCHANGES
1 starch
1/2 vegetable
1/2 fat

Cinnamon Pecan Ring

Yogurt tenderizes the golden yeast dough in this recipe. The drizzled ring looks so scrumptious, no one will guess it's on the lighter side.

Taste of Home Test Kitchen

2-3/4 to 3-1/2 cups all-purpose flour
1/2 cup sugar, *divided*
1 package (1/4 ounce) active yeast
1 teaspoon salt
1/8 teaspoon baking soda
1/2 cup fat-free plain yogurt
1/2 cup fat-free milk
1/4 cup water
3 tablespoons butter, *divided*
3/4 cup chopped pecans, toasted
1/4 cup packed brown sugar
1 tablespoon ground cinnamon
1 egg white, lightly beaten
ICING:
1/2 cup confectioners' sugar
2 teaspoons fat-free milk
1/4 teaspoon vanilla extract

1. In a mixing bowl, combine 1 cup flour, 1/4 cup sugar, yeast, salt and baking soda. In a saucepan, heat the yogurt, milk, water and 2 tablespoons butter to 120°-130°.

Add to dry ingredients; beat on medium speed for 2 minutes. Stir in enough remaining flour to form a soft dough.

2. Turn onto a floured surface; knead until smooth and elastic, about 6-8 minutes. Transfer to a bowl coated with cooking spray; turn once to grease top. Cover and let rise in a warm place until doubled, about 1 hour.

3. Punch dough down. Roll into a 14-in. x 10-in. rectangle. Melt remaining butter; brush over dough. Combine pecans, brown sugar, cinnamon and remaining sugar; sprinkle evenly over dough to within 1/2 in. of edges. Roll up jelly-roll style, starting with a long side; pinch seam.

4. Line a baking sheet with foil; coat well with cooking spray. Place dough seam side down on prepared pan; pinch ends together to form a ring. With scissors, cut from the outside edge two-thirds of the way toward center of ring at 1-in. intervals. Separate strips slightly and twist. Cover; let rise until doubled, about 45 minutes.

5. Brush with egg white. Bake at 350° for 20-25 minutes or until golden brown. Immediately remove from pan to wire rack. Combine icing ingredients; drizzle over warm ring.

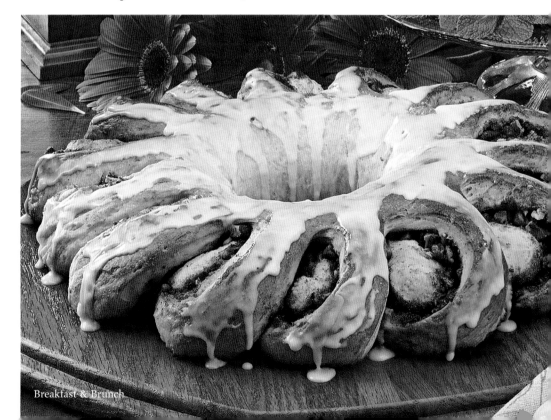

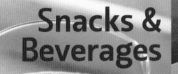

Snacks & Beverages

26
Saucy Turkey Meatballs

Think that satisfying snacks and special beverages are off-limits if you're eating healthier? You'll change your mind when you page through this appetizing chapter.

38
Chocolate Banana Smoothies

30
Canadian Bacon Potato Skins

chapter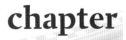

Saucy Turkey Meatballs

PREP/TOTAL TIME
Prep: 20 min.
Bake: 30 min.
YIELD 15 servings

NUTRITION FACTS
One serving
(3 meatballs) equals:
217 calories
4 g fat
1 g saturated fat
36 mg cholesterol
695 mg sodium
36 g carbohydrate
1 g fiber
10 g protein

**DIABETIC
EXCHANGES**
2 starch
1 lean meat

It's a breeze to turn lean ground turkey into these moist and tender meatballs. They're covered with a tangy-sweet sauce that everyone finds tasty.

Janell Fugitt, Cimarron, Kansas

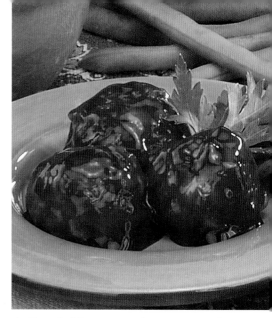

1 cup old-fashioned oats
3/4 cup fat-free evaporated milk
1 medium onion, chopped
1 teaspoon salt
1 teaspoon chili powder
1/4 teaspoon garlic salt
1/4 teaspoon pepper
1-1/2 pounds lean ground turkey
SAUCE:
2 cups ketchup
1-1/2 cups packed brown sugar
1/4 cup chopped onion
2 tablespoons Liquid Smoke, optional
1/2 teaspoon garlic salt

1. In a large bowl, combine the first seven ingredients. Crumble turkey over mixture and mix well. Shape into 1-in. balls. Place on a rack coated with cooking spray in a shallow baking pan. Bake, uncovered, at 350° for 10-15 minutes.

2. Meanwhile, combine sauce ingredients; pour over meatballs. Bake 30-35 minutes longer or until a meat thermometer reads 160° and meat is no longer pink.

Pineapple Iced Tea

PREP/TOTAL TIME
Prep: 10 min. +
chilling
YIELD 5 servings

NUTRITION FACTS
One serving
(1 cup) equals:
51 calories
0 g fat
0 g saturated fat
0 g cholesterol
1 mg sodium
13 g carbohydrate
0 g fiber
0 g protein

**DIABETIC
EXCHANGE**
1 fruit

With five teenagers, our family goes through a lot of beverages. This thirst-quenching tea is easy to mix up with five ingredients and has a sparkling citrus flavor we all enjoy.

Kathy Kittell, Lenexa, Kansas

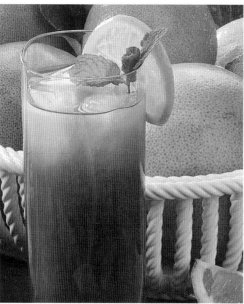

1 quart water
7 individual tea bags
1 cup unsweetened pineapple juice
1/3 cup lemon juice
2 tablespoons sugar

1. In a saucepan, bring water to a boil. Remove from the heat.

2. Add tea bags; cover and steep for 3-5 minutes. Discard tea bags. Stir in the pineapple juice, lemon juice and sugar until sugar is dissolved. Refrigerate overnight for the flavors to blend. Serve over ice.

Ranch Tortilla Roll-Ups

These zesty roll-ups are wonderful as picnic nibbles, dinner appetizers and football party munchies. When my husband's co-workers came over and tried these, they admitted that "low-fat" can be delicious.

Karen Thomas, Berlin, Pennsylvania

2 packages (8 ounces *each*) fat-free cream cheese

1 envelope ranch salad dressing mix

2 to 3 jalapeno peppers, finely chopped

1 jar (2 ounces) diced pimientos, drained

8 flour tortillas (8 inches)

1. In a small mixing bowl, combine the cream cheese, salad dressing mix, jalapenos and pimientos; mix well. Spread over tortillas.

2. Roll up tightly; wrap each in plastic wrap. Refrigerate for at least 1 hour. Unwrap and cut each tortilla into eight pieces.

Editor's Note: When cutting hot peppers, disposable gloves are recommended. Avoid touching your face.

LOW FAT

PREP/TOTAL TIME
10 min. + chilling
YIELD 16 servings

NUTRITION FACTS
One serving
(4 pieces) equals:

106 calories
2 g fat
1 g saturated fat
10 mg cholesterol
419 mg sodium
15 g carbohydrate
Trace fiber
6 g protein

DIABETIC EXCHANGES
1 fruit
1 fat

Iced Coffee

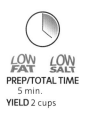

LOW FAT   LOW SALT

PREP/TOTAL TIME
5 min.
YIELD 2 cups

When my sister introduced me to iced coffee, I didn't think I'd like it. Not only did I like it, I actually wanted to try to make my own! This fast-to-fix version is really refreshing.

Jenny Reece, Lowry, Minnesota

NUTRITION FACTS
One serving (1 cup) equals:
79 calories
1 g fat
0 g saturated fat
2 mg cholesterol
76 mg sodium
15 g carbohydrate
0 g fiber
5 g protein

DIABETIC EXCHANGES
1/2 starch
1/2 fat-free milk

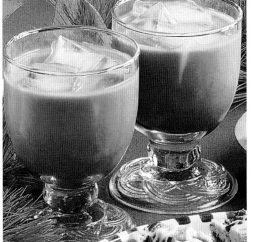

4	teaspoons instant coffee granules
1	cup boiling water
4	teaspoons sugar substitute equivalent to 4 teaspoons sugar, optional
1	cup fat-free milk
4	teaspoons chocolate syrup
1/8	teaspoon vanilla extract

Ice cubes

1. In a large bowl, dissolve coffee in the water. Add sweetener if desired. Stir in the milk, syrup and vanilla; mix well. Serve over ice.

Editor's Note: This recipe was tested with Splenda No Calorie Sweetener.

Stuffed Mushrooms

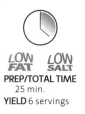

LOW FAT   LOW SALT

PREP/TOTAL TIME
25 min.
YIELD 6 servings

I first sampled these fun bites at a support group meeting for diabetics. I was amazed at how yummy the little stuffed mushrooms were. Since then, I've shared the recipe with many of my friends and co-workers.

Beth Ann Howard, Verona, Pennsylvania

NUTRITION FACTS
One serving (3 stuffed mushrooms) equals:
66 calories
3 g fat
1 g saturated fat
4 mg cholesterol
173 mg sodium
8 g carbohydrate
1 g fiber
4 g protein

DIABETIC EXCHANGES
1/2 starch
1/2 fat

1	pound large fresh mushrooms
3	tablespoons seasoned bread crumbs
3	tablespoons fat-free sour cream
2	tablespoons grated Parmesan cheese
2	tablespoons minced chives
2	tablespoons reduced-fat mayonnaise
2	teaspoons balsamic vinegar
2	to 3 drops hot pepper sauce, optional

1. Remove stems from mushrooms; set caps aside. Chop stems, reserving 1/3 cup (discard remaining stems or save for another use). In a bowl, combine the bread crumbs, sour cream, Parmesan cheese, chives, mayonnaise, vinegar, hot pepper sauce if desired and reserved mushroom stems; mix well.

2. Place mushroom caps on a baking sheet coated with cooking spray; stuff with the bread crumb mixture. Broil 4-6 in. from the heat for 5-7 minutes or until lightly browned.

MAKING CAPS

Removing the stems from mushroom caps is a snap. Hold the mushroom cap in one hand. With your other hand, grab the stem and twist to snap off.

Shrimp with Creole Sauce

Dip into this zippy Creole-style sauce, and you'll never crave seafood sauce again. Chunky and not too spicy, the tantalizing tomato blend enhances cold shrimp or cooked seafood.

Taste of Home Test Kitchen

- 1 large onion, chopped
- 1/2 cup finely chopped green pepper
- 1 celery rib with leaves, finely chopped
- 1 tablespoon canola oil
- 3 garlic cloves, minced
- 1 can (28 ounces) whole tomatoes
- 1/4 cup minced fresh parsley
- 1/4 cup water
- 1/4 cup tomato paste
- 2 tablespoons lime juice
- 1 teaspoon dried thyme
- 3/4 teaspoon salt
- 1/2 teaspoon dried oregano
- 1/4 to 1/2 teaspoon hot pepper sauce
- 1/4 teaspoon ground allspice
- 36 cooked large shrimp, peeled and deveined

1. In a large nonstick skillet, saute the onion, green pepper and celery in oil for 3-4 minutes. Add garlic; cook 1 minute longer. Drain tomatoes, reserving juice; add juice to skillet. Mash tomatoes and add to skillet.

2. Stir in the parsley, water, tomato paste, lime juice and seasonings. Bring to a boil. Reduce heat; simmer, uncovered, for 15 minutes or until thickened. Serve warm with shrimp.

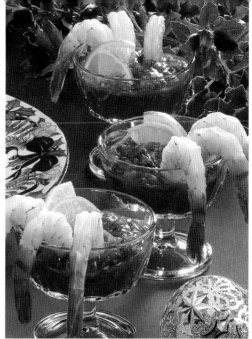

LOW FAT LOW SALT

PREP/TOTAL TIME
Prep: 10 min.
Cook: 25 min.
YIELD 12 servings

NUTRITION FACTS
One serving
(3 shrimp with 1/3 cup sauce) equals:
56 calories
1 g fat
Trace saturated fat
32 mg cholesterol
292 mg sodium
7 g carbohydrate
1 g fiber
5 g protein

DIABETIC EXCHANGES
1 very lean meat
1 vegetable

Raspberry Cream Smoothies

Frozen raspberries and banana chunks give these tasty beverages plenty of fruit flavor. They make a frosty, breakfast treat or an afternoon pick-me-up.

Nicki Woods, Springfield, Missouri

- 2 cups orange juice
- 2 cups fat-free reduced-sugar raspberry yogurt
- 2 cups frozen vanilla yogurt
- 2 small ripe bananas, cut into chunks and frozen (1 cup)
- 3 cups frozen raspberries
- 2 teaspoons vanilla extract

1. In a blender or food processor, cover and process the ingredients in batches until blended. Stir if necessary. Pour into chilled glasses; serve immediately.

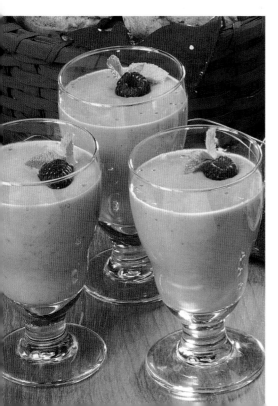

LOW FAT LOW SALT

PREP/TOTAL TIME
10 min.
YIELD 6 servings

NUTRITION FACTS
One serving (1 cup) equals:
198 calories
1 g fat
1 g saturated fat
5 mg cholesterol
98 mg sodium
40 g carbohydrate
2 g fiber
7 g protein

DIABETIC EXCHANGES
2 fruit
1 fat-free milk

NUTRITION FACTS

One serving
(3 potato skins)
equals:

211 calories
7 g fat
4 g saturated fat
21 mg cholesterol
309 mg sodium
29 g carbohydrate
5 g fiber
11 g protein

DIABETIC EXCHANGES

2 starch
1 lean meat
1/2 fat

Canadian Bacon Potato Skins

Whether you're searching for a fun appetizer or a tasty side dish, these potato skins are sure to fill the bill. I top the potato shells with Canadian bacon, tomato and cheese. Hot pepper sauce gives them a kick.

Mary Plummer, DeSoto, Kansas

6 large baking potatoes
(12 ounces *each*)

2 teaspoons canola oil

1/8 teaspoon hot pepper sauce

1 teaspoon chili powder

1 medium tomato, seeded and finely chopped

2/3 cup chopped Canadian bacon

2 tablespoons finely chopped green onion

1 cup (4 ounces) shredded reduced-fat cheddar cheese

1/2 cup reduced-fat sour cream

1. Place potatoes on a microwave-safe plate; prick with a fork. Microwave, uncovered, on high for 14-17 minutes or until tender but firm, turning once. Let stand for 5 minutes. Cut each potato in half lengthwise. Scoop out pulp, leaving a 1/4-in. shell (discard pulp or save for another use).

2. Combine oil and hot pepper sauce; brush over potato shells. Sprinkle with chili powder. Cut each potato shell in half lengthwise. Place on baking sheets coated with cooking spray. Sprinkle with the tomato, bacon, onion and cheese. Bake at 450° for 12-14 minutes or until heated through and cheese is melted. Serve with sour cream.

Editor's Note: This recipe was tested in a 1,100-watt microwave.

Cappuccino Shake

I came up with this quick and easy shake for my mother, who has been diabetic for many years. She was tickled pink!

Paula Pelis, Rocky Point, New York

> 1 cup fat-free milk
>
> 1-1/2 teaspoons instant coffee granules
>
> Sugar substitute equivalent to 4 teaspoons sugar
>
> 2 drops brandy extract *or* rum extract
>
> Dash ground cinnamon

1. In a blender, combine the milk, coffee granules, sweetener and extract. Blend until coffee is dissolved. Serve with a dash of cinnamon.

2. For a hot drink, pour into a mug and heat in a microwave.

Editor's Note: This recipe was tested with Splenda No Calorie Sweetener.

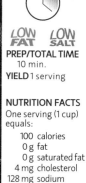

LOW FAT   **LOW SALT**

PREP/TOTAL TIME
10 min.
YIELD 1 serving

NUTRITION FACTS
One serving (1 cup) equals:
100 calories
0 g fat
0 g saturated fat
4 mg cholesterol
128 mg sodium
15 g carbohydrate
0 g fiber
9 g protein

DIABETIC EXCHANGE
1 fat-free milk

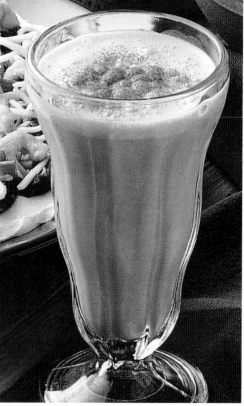

Seasoned Snack Mix

You'll never miss the oil or nuts in this crispy, well-seasoned party mix. I keep some on hand for whenever "the munchies" strike.

Flo Burtnett, Gage, Oklahoma

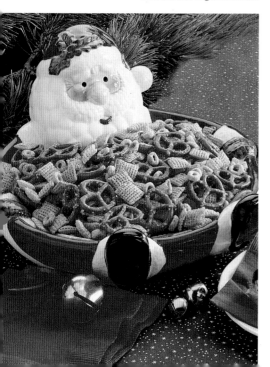

> 3 cups Rice Chex
>
> 3 cups Corn Chex
>
> 3 cups Cheerios
>
> 3 cups pretzels
>
> 2 teaspoons Worcestershire sauce
>
> 2 teaspoons butter-flavored sprinkles
>
> 1/2 teaspoon garlic powder
>
> 1/2 teaspoon seasoned salt
>
> 1/2 teaspoon onion powder

1. In a 15-in. x 10-in. x 1-in. baking pan, combine cereals and pretzels. Lightly coat with cooking spray; drizzle with the Worcestershire sauce. Combine the remaining ingredients; sprinkle over the cereal mixture.

2. Bake at 200° for 1-1/2 hours, stirring every 30 minutes. Cool completely. Store in an airtight container.

LOW FAT

PREP/TOTAL TIME
Prep: 5 min.
Bake: 1-1/2 hours
YIELD 3 quarts

NUTRITION FACTS
One serving (1 cup) equals:
115 calories
1 g fat
1 g saturated fat
0 g cholesterol
400 mg sodium
25 g carbohydrate
1 g fiber
3 g protein

DIABETIC EXCHANGE
1-1/2 starch

NUTRITION FACTS

One serving (1/4 cup dip) equals:

172 calories
11 g fat
3 g saturated fat
18 mg cholesterol
542 mg sodium
13 g carbohydrate
Trace fiber
7 g protein

DIABETIC EXCHANGES

2 fat
1 starch

Bacon Ranch Dip

I used reduced-fat ingredients to lighten up this Parmesan and bacon dip. Not only is it a snap to mix up the night before a party, but the proportions can easily be adjusted for smaller or larger groups.

Pam Garwood, Lakeville, Minnesota

1/2 cup reduced-fat mayonnaise

1/2 cup reduced-fat ranch salad dressing

1/2 cup fat-free sour cream

1/2 cup shredded Parmesan cheese

1/4 cup crumbled cooked bacon

Assorted fresh vegetables

1. In a bowl, combine the mayonnaise, salad dressing, sour cream, Parmesan cheese and bacon; mix well. Cover and refrigerate for at least 1 hour before serving. Serve with assorted fresh vegetables.

Strawberry Slush

This make-ahead slush is really refreshing on hot summer days. Pour lemon-lime soda over scoops of the strawberry blend, and you'll have a fast and fruity treat that's so thick you'll need to eat it with a spoon.

Patricia Schroedl, Jefferson, Wisconsin

- 1 quart fresh strawberries
- 2 cups fat-free vanilla ice cream, softened
- 1 package (.3 ounces) sugar-free strawberry gelatin
- 1/2 cup boiling water
- 2 teaspoons lemon juice
- 2 liters diet lemon-lime soda, chilled

Additional fresh strawberries, optional

1. In a large bowl, mash the strawberries; add the ice cream. In a small bowl, dissolve the gelatin in water; stir in the lemon juice. Add to the strawberry mixture; mix well. Pour into a 1-1/2-qt. freezer container; cover and freeze overnight.

2. Remove from the freezer 15 minutes before serving. Spoon into glasses; add soda. Garnish with strawberries if desired.

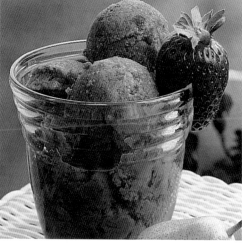

LOW FAT   LOW SALT

PREP/TOTAL TIME
15 min. + freezing
YIELD 10 servings

NUTRITION FACTS
One serving (1/2 cup serving calculated without garnish) equals:

- 63 calories
- 1 g fat
- 0 g saturated fat
- 0 g cholesterol
- 40 mg sodium
- 12 g carbohydrate
- 2 g fiber
- 2 g protein

DIABETIC EXCHANGES
1/2 starch
1/2 fruit

Smoked Salmon Spread

I'm always asked to bring this tasty spread to family gatherings, and I'm happy to oblige. Any leftovers are terrific the next day on sourdough bread with olives and tomatoes.

Susan Pettett, Vancouver, Washington

- 1 package (8 ounces) reduced-fat cream cheese
- 1 cup fat-free mayonnaise
- 2 packages (3 ounces *each*) smoked salmon, flaked
- 1/4 cup finely chopped onion
- 1 teaspoon Worcestershire sauce
- 1/2 teaspoon garlic powder
- 1/4 teaspoon lemon juice

Assorted crackers and party breads

1. In a large mixing bowl, beat cream cheese and mayonnaise until smooth. Stir in the salmon, onion, Worcestershire sauce, garlic powder and lemon juice.

2. Cover and refrigerate for at least 2 hours. Serve with crackers and breads.

FAT SAVINGS

Get in the habit of using reduced-fat, low-fat or fat-free products. By just switching from regular cream cheese to reduced-fat cream cheese, you can save about 30 calories and 4 grams of fat per ounce!

LOW FAT

PREP/TOTAL TIME
15 min. + chilling
YIELD 2-1/2 cups

NUTRITION FACTS
One serving (2 tablespoons) equals:

- 46 calories
- 3 g fat
- 1 g saturated fat
- 10 mg cholesterol
- 303 mg sodium
- 3 g carbohydrate
- 1 g fiber
- 3 g protein

DIABETIC EXCHANGES
1/2 lean meat
1/2 fat

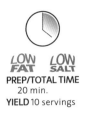

No-Yolk Deviled Eggs

Mashed potatoes are the secret ingredient in this lighter recipe, which still provides the familiar taste and look of deviled eggs.

Dottie Burton, Cincinnati, Ohio

LOW FAT **LOW SALT**

PREP/TOTAL TIME
20 min.
YIELD 10 servings

NUTRITION FACTS
One serving
(2 halves) equals:
  35 calories
  1 g fat
  0 g saturated fat
  1 mg cholesterol
  118 mg sodium
  3 g carbohydrate
  0 g fiber
  4 g protein

DIABETIC EXCHANGES
  1/2 very lean meat
  1/2 vegetable

10 hard-cooked eggs

3/4 cup mashed potatoes (prepared with fat-free milk and margarine)

1 tablespoon fat-free mayonnaise

1 teaspoon prepared mustard

2 to 3 drops yellow food coloring, optional

Paprika

1. Slice the eggs in half lengthwise; remove the yolks and refrigerate for another use. Set the whites aside.

2. In a small bowl, combine mashed potatoes, mayonnaise, mustard and food coloring if desired; mix well. Stuff or pipe into egg whites. Sprinkle with paprika. Refrigerate until serving.

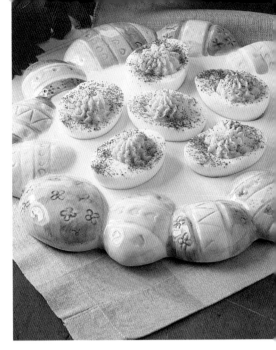

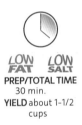

Onion Cheese Ball

My husband and our friends from church love to dig into this creamy, savory cheese ball topped with minced ham. It's a great addition to any snack buffet.

Shelby Finger, Hickory, North Carolina

LOW FAT **LOW SALT**

PREP/TOTAL TIME
30 min.
YIELD about 1-1/2 cups

NUTRITION FACTS
One serving
(2 tablespoons
calculated without
crackers or
vegetables) equals:
  24 calories
  Trace fat
  0 g saturated fat
  2 mg cholesterol
  198 mg sodium
  2 g carbohydrate
  0 g fiber
  4 g protein

DIABETIC EXCHANGE
  1/2 lean meat

1 package (8 ounces) fat-free cream cheese, softened

8 slices (3/4 ounce *each*) fat-free sharp cheddar cheese, cut into thin strips

1 small onion, diced

1 tablespoon Worcestershire sauce

1 teaspoon garlic powder

Dash hot pepper sauce

1/2 cup minced fully cooked lean ham

Fresh vegetables *or* reduced-fat crackers

1. In a mixing bowl, beat the cheeses. Add onion, Worcestershire sauce, garlic powder and hot pepper sauce; mix well. Shape into a ball and roll in ham. Cover and refrigerate for at least 1 hour. Serve with vegetables or crackers.

HAVING A BALL

The recipe for Onion Cheese Ball calls for rolling the shaped ball in minced lean ham. If you like, try rolling the ball in sesame seeds or parsley instead. You could also use chopped nuts, such as walnuts, or coarsely cracked black pepper.

Creamy Guacamole

Only four items are needed for this fabulous dip. Not only is it ideal to serve with tortilla chips, but I also spoon it over cooked chicken breasts for dinner.

Ethel Anderson, Hemlock, New York

- 1 medium ripe avocado, peeled and pitted
- 7 tablespoons fat-free sour cream
- 2 tablespoons chopped green chilies
- 1/8 teaspoon lemon-pepper seasoning

1. Cut the avocado into chunks and place in a blender; add the remaining ingredients. Cover and process until smooth. Refrigerate leftovers.

AVOCADO EASE

To peel and pit a ripe avocado, cut it in half lengthwise, then twist the halves in opposite directions to separate them. Slip a tablespoon under the seed to loosen it from the fruit. To remove the peel, scoop out the flesh from each half with a metal spoon.

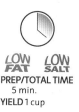

LOW FAT **LOW SALT**

PREP/TOTAL TIME
5 min.
YIELD 1 cup

NUTRITION FACTS
One serving
(2 tablespoons)
equals:
   54 calories
   4 g fat
   1 g saturated fat
   2 mg cholesterol
29 mg sodium
   4 g carbohydrate
   1 g fiber
   1 g protein

DIABETIC EXCHANGE
   1 fat

Spiced Tomato Drink

I was looking for a different beverage to serve when I remembered a tomato drink I sampled in New Guinea. I experimented until I came up with this spicy concoction, which is delicious whether it's served hot or cold.

Dorothy Anne Schultz, Dallas, Oregon

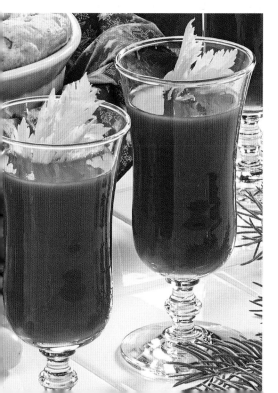

- 1 can (46 ounces) tomato juice
- 1/4 cup packed brown sugar
- 1 teaspoon ground cinnamon
- 1/2 teaspoon ground allspice
- 1/4 teaspoon salt
- 1/4 teaspoon pepper
- 1 tablespoon lemon juice

1. In a large saucepan, combine tomato juice, sugar, cinnamon, allspice, salt and pepper. Bring to a boil. Reduce heat; simmer, uncovered, for 20 minutes. Remove from the heat; stir in lemon juice. Serve warm or cold.

LOW FAT

PREP/TOTAL TIME
25 min.
YIELD 8 servings

NUTRITION FACTS
One serving
(3/4 cup) equals:
   62 calories
   Trace fat
   Trace saturated fat
   0 g cholesterol
653 mg sodium
  13 g carbohydrate
   1 g fiber
   1 g protein

DIABETIC EXCHANGES
   1 vegetable
   1/2 starch

Fudgy Fruit Dip

PREP/TOTAL TIME
5 min. + chilling
YIELD about 1/2 cup

This thick, rich, chocolaty dip is especially nice at Christmastime gatherings. I also love it with fresh-picked strawberries during summer.

Wilma Knobloch, Steen, Minnesota

NUTRITION FACTS
One serving
(2 tablespoons)
equals:
   67 calories
   1 g fat
   1 g saturated fat
   1 mg cholesterol
 32 mg sodium
 15 g carbohydrate
   1 g fiber
   1 g protein

DIABETIC EXCHANGES
  1/2 starch
  1/2 fruit

1/3   cup fat-free sugar-free hot fudge topping

1/3   cup fat-free vanilla yogurt

1-1/2   teaspoons orange juice concentrate

Fresh strawberries

1. In a bowl, combine fudge topping, yogurt and orange juice concentrate. Cover and refrigerate for at least 30 minutes. Serve with strawberries.

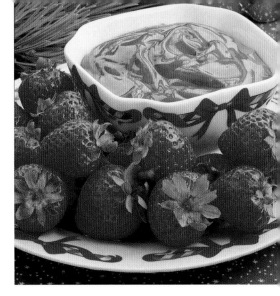

Caramel Apple Dip

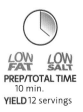

PREP/TOTAL TIME
10 min.
YIELD 12 servings

Caramel apples aren't forbidden fruit when you make them this way. People never know they're eating lighter when they dip apple slices into this warm, yummy treat.

Tami Escher, Dumont, Minnesota

NUTRITION FACTS
One serving
(2 tablespoons dip
calculated without
fruit) equals:
 102 calories
   4 g fat
   3 g saturated fat
 14 mg cholesterol
109 mg sodium
 13 g carbohydrate
   0 g fiber
   3 g protein

DIABETIC EXCHANGES
  1 starch
  1 fat

1   package (8 ounces) reduced-fat cream cheese, cubed

1/2   cup caramel ice cream topping

1/2   cup marshmallow creme

Apple slices

1. In a microwave-safe mixing bowl, combine cream cheese and ice cream topping until blended. Add marshmallow creme; mix until blended.

2. Microwave, uncovered, on 50% power for 1 minute; stir. Microwave 30-60 seconds longer, stirring every 15 seconds or until warm. Transfer to a serving dish. Serve immediately with apple slices.

Editor's Note: This recipe was tested in a 1,100-watt microwave.

FRUIT DIPPERS
Caramel Apple Dip would be great with other types of fruit dippers. For a change of pace, try banana chunks, pear slices, pineapple chunks or wedges or whole strawberries.

Shrimp Tartlets

Here in the Southwest, anything with green chilies is sure to please...and these cheesy shrimp appetizers are no exception!

Terry Thompson, Albuquerque, New Mexico

18 slices white bread

Refrigerated butter-flavored spray

FILLING:

1 cup (4 ounces) shredded part-skim mozzarella cheese

1/4 cup canned chopped green chilies

1/4 cup diced cooked shrimp

1 green onion, thinly sliced

18 whole small cooked shrimp

Paprika

1. With a rolling pin, flatten bread to 1/8-in. thickness. Using a 2-1/2-in. biscuit cutter, cut out a circle from each slice. Spritz both sides of circles with butter-flavored spray. Press into ungreased miniature muffin cups. Bake at 400° for 8-10 minutes or until lightly browned.

2. In a large bowl, combine mozzarella cheese, chilies, diced shrimp and onion; spoon into muffin cups. Top with whole shrimp and paprika. Broil 5-6 in. from the heat for 2-4 minutes or until golden brown. Serve immediately.

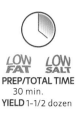

LOW FAT LOW SALT

PREP/TOTAL TIME
30 min.

YIELD 1-1/2 dozen

NUTRITION FACTS
One serving
(1 tartlet) equals:

60 calories
2 g fat
1 g saturated fat
17 mg cholesterol
168 mg sodium
7 g carbohydrate
1 g fiber
4 g protein

DIABETIC EXCHANGES
1/2 starch
1/2 meat

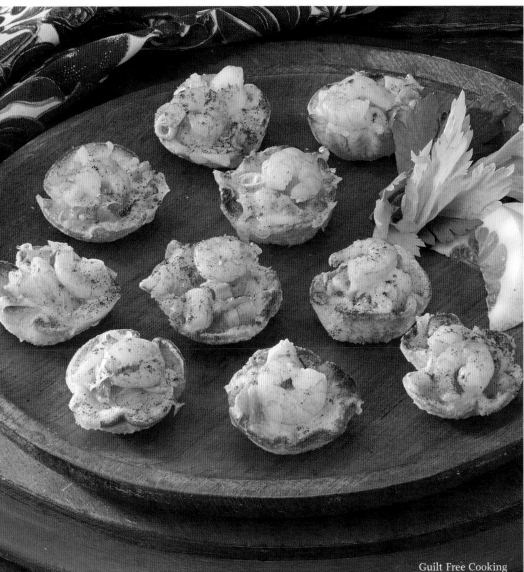

LOW FAT

PREP/TOTAL TIME
5 min. + chilling
YIELD 4 servings

NUTRITION FACTS
One serving
(1 cup) equals:

166 calories
3 g fat
2 g saturated fat
10 mg cholesterol
360 mg sodium
31 g carbohydrate
2 g fiber
6 g protein

DIABETIC EXCHANGES
1 starch
1 fat-free milk

Chocolate Banana Smoothies

When I was trying to lose weight, I wanted to find a light but satisfying beverage. I came up with this five-ingredient smoothie that's chocolaty, frosty and oh-so-good.

Katherine Lipka, Galesburg, Michigan

2 cups cold 2% milk

1 package (1.4 ounces) sugar-free instant chocolate pudding mix

2 tablespoons vanilla extract

2 large ripe frozen bananas, sliced

2 cups coarsely crushed ice cubes

1. In a blender, combine the milk, pudding mix and vanilla; cover and process until blended. Add the bananas and ice; cover and process until smooth. Pour into chilled glasses; serve immediately.

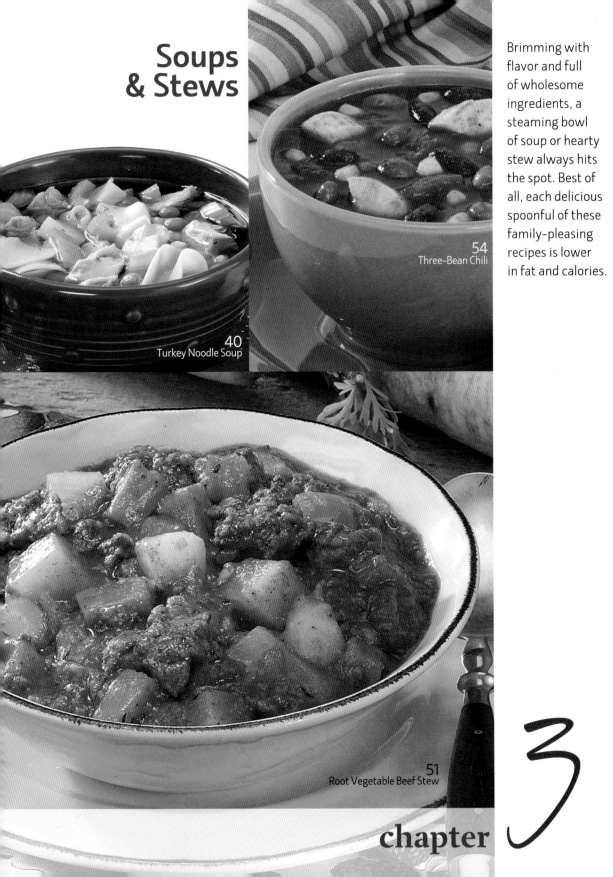

Soups & Stews

Brimming with flavor and full of wholesome ingredients, a steaming bowl of soup or hearty stew always hits the spot. Best of all, each delicious spoonful of these family-pleasing recipes is lower in fat and calories.

40
Turkey Noodle Soup

54
Three-Bean Chili

51
Root Vegetable Beef Stew

chapter 3

Beef Minestrone

This recipe proves that cutting back on fat doesn't have to mean avoiding ground beef.

Ann Lape, Richmondville, New York

PREP/TOTAL TIME
Prep: 20 min.
Cook: 1 hour
YIELD 10 servings

NUTRITION FACTS
One serving
(1 cup) equals:
141 calories
7 g fat
0 g saturated fat
31 mg cholesterol
58 mg sodium
10 g carbohydrate
0 g fiber
11 g protein

DIABETIC EXCHANGES
1 meat
1 vegetable
1/2 starch

1 pound lean ground beef
1 cup chopped onion
6 cups water
1 cup cubed peeled potatoes
1 cup chopped tomatoes
1 cup shredded cabbage
1 cup chopped carrots
1/2 cup chopped celery
1/4 cup uncooked long grain rice
1/2 teaspoon dried thyme
1 bay leaf
1/4 teaspoon pepper
5 teaspoons grated Parmesan cheese

1. In a Dutch oven, cook beef and onion over medium heat until meat is no longer pink and onion is tender; drain. Add the water, potatoes, tomatoes, cabbage, carrots, celery, rice, thyme, bay leaf and pepper; bring to a boil. Reduce the heat; cover and simmer for 1 hour.

2. Discard bay leaf. Sprinkle each serving with 1/2 teaspoon of Parmesan.

Turkey Noodle Soup

My husband is on a very low-fat diet, so I'm always experimenting to find things that will please his palate. This delicious, easy recipe makes two generous servings.

Doris Nehoda, Coos Bay, Oregon

PREP/TOTAL TIME
Prep: 15 min.
Cook: 35 min.
YIELD 2 servings

NUTRITION FACTS
One serving
(1-1/2 cups) equals:
156 calories
1 g fat
Trace saturated fat
45 mg cholesterol
659 mg sodium
18 g carbohydrate
3 g fiber
19 g protein

DIABETIC EXCHANGES
2 very lean meat
1 starch

2 cups water
3/4 cup cubed cooked turkey breast
1 celery rib with leaves, sliced
1/4 cup chopped onion
2 garlic cloves, minced
1/2 teaspoon salt
1/8 teaspoon dried marjoram
1/8 teaspoon pepper
1 bay leaf
1/2 cup cubed peeled potatoes
1/4 cup frozen peas
1/4 cup uncooked yolk-free wide noodles

Dash browning sauce, optional

1. In a large saucepan, combine the water, turkey, celery, onion, garlic, salt, marjoram, pepper and bay leaf; bring to a boil. Reduce heat; cover and simmer for 10 minutes or until celery is tender.

2. Add the potatoes, peas and noodles; cover and simmer 15 minutes longer or until potatoes are tender. Discard bay leaf. Stir in browning sauce if desired.

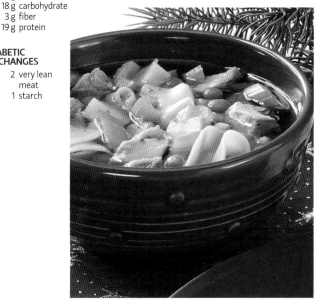

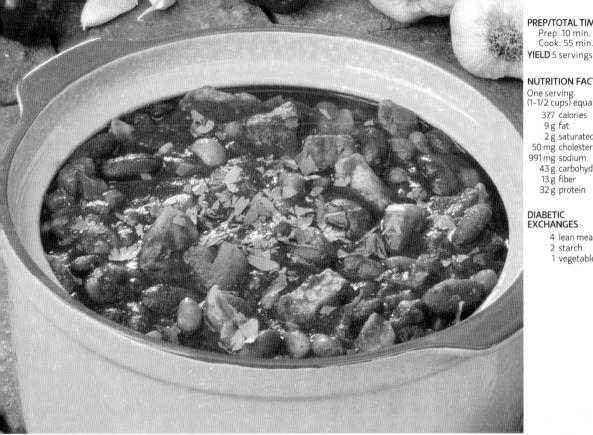

PREP/TOTAL TIME
Prep: 10 min.
Cook: 55 min.
YIELD 5 servings

NUTRITION FACTS
One serving
(1-1/2 cups) equals:
377 calories
9 g fat
2 g saturated fat
50 mg cholesterol
991 mg sodium
43 g carbohydrate
13 g fiber
32 g protein

DIABETIC EXCHANGES
4 lean meat
2 starch
1 vegetable

Mexican Pork Stew

I heat up cold evenings by serving this thick and zesty stew with corn bread. The next day, I spoon leftovers into corn tortillas with a little salsa and sour cream for a satisfying snack.

Mickey Terry, Del Valle, Texas

1   pound boneless pork loin roast, cut into 3/4-inch cubes

3   teaspoons olive oil

1   large onion, chopped

2   celery ribs, chopped

1   jalapeno pepper, seeded and chopped

1   garlic clove, minced

1-1/2   cups water

1   tablespoon chili powder

2   teaspoons brown sugar

1   teaspoon ground cumin

1/2   teaspoon salt

1/4   teaspoon pepper

1   can (6 ounces) tomato paste

1   can (16 ounces) kidney beans, rinsed and drained

1   can (15 ounces) pinto beans, rinsed and drained

1   can (14-1/2 ounces) diced tomatoes, undrained

2   teaspoons minced fresh cilantro

1. In a Dutch oven or large soup kettle over medium-high heat, brown meat on all sides in 1 teaspoon oil; drain. Remove meat and keep warm.

2. In the same pan, saute the onion, celery, jalapeno and garlic in remaining oil until tender. Stir in the water, chili powder, brown sugar, cumin, salt and pepper. Return meat to pan. Bring to a boil. Reduce heat; cover and simmer for 30 minutes.

3. Stir in the tomato paste, beans and tomatoes. Return to a boil. Reduce heat; cover and simmer 20 minutes longer or until meat is tender and beans are heated through. Sprinkle with cilantro.

Editor's Note: When cutting hot peppers, disposable gloves are recommended. Avoid touching your face.

NUTRITION FACTS

One serving
(1-1/2 cups) equals:

241 calories
7 g fat
3 g saturated fat
28 mg cholesterol
493 mg sodium
26 g carbohydrate
4 g fiber
18 g protein

DIABETIC EXCHANGES

2 lean meat
2 vegetable
1 starch

Harvest Soup

Loaded with ground beef, squash, tomatoes and two kinds of potatoes, this hearty soup makes a great family meal on a hectic night. Feel free to replace any of the vegetables with those that better suit your taste.

Janice Mitchell, Aurora, Colorado

1 pound lean ground beef

3/4 cup chopped onion

2 garlic cloves, minced

3-1/2 cups water

2-1/4 cups chopped peeled sweet potatoes

1 cup chopped red potatoes

1 cup chopped peeled acorn squash

2 teaspoons beef bouillon granules

2 bay leaves

1/2 teaspoon chili powder

1/2 teaspoon pepper

1/8 teaspoon ground allspice

1/8 teaspoon ground cloves

1 can (14-1/2 ounces) diced tomatoes, undrained

1. In a large saucepan, cook the beef, onion and garlic over medium heat until meat is no longer pink; drain well. Add the water, potatoes, squash, bouillon, bay leaves, chili powder, pepper, allspice and cloves.

2. Bring to a boil. Reduce heat; cover and simmer for 15-20 minutes or until vegetables are tender. Add the tomatoes. Cook and stir until heated through. Discard bay leaves.

Irish Stew

This classic stew is packed with potatoes, turnips, carrots and lamb. Served with Irish soda bread, it not only makes a robust supper on St. Patrick's Day but is great at any time of the year.

Lois Glezer, Cape Elizabeth, Maine

- 1-1/2 pounds lamb stew meat
- 2 teaspoons olive oil
- 4 cups water
- 2 cups sliced peeled potatoes
- 1 medium onion, sliced
- 1/2 cup sliced carrot
- 1/2 cup cubed turnip
- 1 teaspoon salt
- 1/2 teaspoon *each* dried marjoram, thyme and rosemary, crushed
- 1/8 teaspoon pepper
- 2 tablespoons all-purpose flour
- 2 tablespoons fat-free milk
- 1/2 teaspoon browning sauce, optional
- 3 tablespoons minced fresh parsley

1. In a Dutch oven, brown the lamb in oil over medium-high heat. Add the water; bring to a boil. Reduce the heat; cover and simmer for 1 hour.

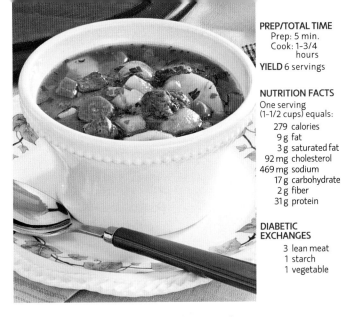

2. Add the potatoes, onion, carrot, turnip and seasonings. Bring to a boil. Reduce heat; cover and simmer for 30 minutes or until the vegetables are tender.

3. In a small bowl, combine the flour, milk and sauce if desired until smooth; stir into stew. Add parsley. Bring to a boil; cook and stir for 2 minutes or until thickened.

PREP/TOTAL TIME
Prep: 5 min.
Cook: 1-3/4 hours
YIELD 6 servings

NUTRITION FACTS
One serving (1-1/2 cups) equals:
279 calories
9 g fat
3 g saturated fat
92 mg cholesterol
469 mg sodium
17 g carbohydrate
2 g fiber
31 g protein

DIABETIC EXCHANGES
3 lean meat
1 starch
1 vegetable

Creamy Chicken Rice Soup

I combined three recipes to create this take on the classic, creamy chicken rice soup. Even with less butter and no cream, this lower-fat version is so delicious that no one ever suspects it's light.

Marge Wagner, Roselle, Illinois

- 1/2 cup chopped carrot
- 1/3 cup finely chopped onion
- 1/3 cup chopped celery
- 2 tablespoons butter
- 1/4 cup all-purpose flour
- 2 cans (14-1/2 ounces *each*) reduced-sodium chicken broth
- 2 cups cooked long grain rice
- 1 cup cubed cooked chicken
- 1/2 teaspoon salt
- 1/4 teaspoon pepper
- 1/8 teaspoon garlic powder
- 1 cup 2% milk
- 2 tablespoons lemon juice
- 1 tablespoon white wine, optional

1. In a large saucepan, saute the carrot, onion and celery in butter until tender. Stir in flour until blended. Gradually stir in broth. Add the rice, chicken, salt, pepper and garlic powder; bring to a boil. Reduce heat; cover and simmer for 10-15 minutes or until vegetables are tender.

2. Reduce heat to low. Stir in the milk, lemon juice and wine if desired. Cook and stir for 5 minutes or until heated through.

EXTRA RICE CAN SAVE SOME TIME

When cooking rice, make extra to have on hand. Cooked rice can be refrigerated for up to 7 days and frozen for up to 6 months. For convenience, package a cup or two of rice in refrigerator/freezer bags. Flatten rice out in the bags before freezing. This way it will defrost more quickly.

PREP/TOTAL TIME
30 min.
YIELD 6 servings

NUTRITION FACTS
One serving (1 cup) equals:
203 calories
6 g fat
3 g saturated fat
33 mg cholesterol
648 mg sodium
24 g carbohydrate
1 g fiber
13 g protein

DIABETIC EXCHANGES
1-1/2 starch
1 lean meat
1/2 fat

Black Bean Soup

Salsa and cumin add just the right zip to this thick chicken soup. I like to round out the meal with wedges of warm corn bread.

Mary Buhl, Duluth, Georgia

PREP/TOTAL TIME
20 min.
YIELD 10 servings
(2-1/2 quarts)

NUTRITION FACTS
One serving (1 cup)
equals:
154 calories
2 g fat
Trace saturated fat
11 mg cholesterol
878 mg sodium
21 g carbohydrate
5 g fiber
10 g protein

DIABETIC EXCHANGES
1-1/2 meat
1 starch

3/4 cup chopped celery
1 medium onion, chopped
3 garlic cloves, minced
1 tablespoon canola oil
3 cans (14-1/2 ounces *each*) chicken broth
2 cans (15 ounces *each*) black beans, rinsed and drained
1 jar (16 ounces) salsa
1 cup cubed cooked chicken breast
1 cup cooked long grain rice
1 tablespoon lime juice
1 teaspoon ground cumin

1. In a large saucepan, saute celery, onion and garlic in oil until tender. Stir in the remaining ingredients; heat through.

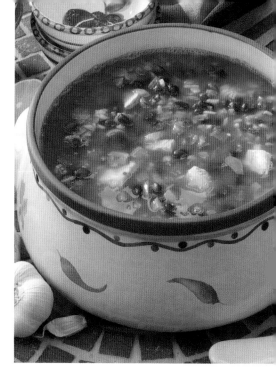

Mushroom Barley Soup

This is one of our favorites to eat while watching football games. It's delicious!

Patricia Maly, Mokena, Illinois

PREP/TOTAL TIME
Prep: 15 min.
Cook: 55 min.
YIELD 11 servings
(about
2-3/4 quarts)

NUTRITION FACTS
One serving
(1 cup) equals:
136 calories
Trace fat
Trace saturated fat
0 mg cholesterol
359 mg sodium
29 g carbohydrate
6 g fiber
6 g protein

DIABETIC EXCHANGES
1-1/2 starch
1 vegetable

1 can (49 ounces) reduced-sodium chicken broth
2 medium carrots, thinly sliced
1 medium onion, chopped
2 garlic cloves, minced
1/2 teaspoon dried basil
1/2 teaspoon dried oregano
1/2 teaspoon pepper
1-1/2 cups medium pearl barley
2 cups reduced-sodium tomato juice
1 can (14-1/2 ounces) no-salt-added diced tomatoes, undrained
1/2 pound fresh mushrooms, thinly sliced

1. In a Dutch oven or soup kettle, combine broth, carrots, onion, garlic, basil, oregano and pepper; bring to a boil. Add barley. Reduce heat; cover and simmer for 45-55 minutes or until barley is tender.

2. Add the tomato juice, tomatoes and mushrooms; cook for 10-15 minutes or until mushrooms are tender.

Turkey Dumpling Stew

My mom made this stew when I was young, and it was always a hit. I fix it on weekends for our children, who love the dumplings.

Becky Mohr, Appleton, Wisconsin

- 4 bacon strips, diced
- 1-1/2 pounds turkey breast tenderloins, cut into 1-inch pieces
- 4 medium carrots, cut into 1-inch pieces
- 2 cups water, *divided*
- 1 can (14-1/2 ounces) reduced-sodium chicken broth
- 2 small onions, quartered
- 2 celery ribs, cut into 1/2-inch pieces
- 1/4 teaspoon dried rosemary, crushed
- 1 bay leaf
- 3 tablespoons all-purpose flour
- 1/2 teaspoon salt
- 1/8 to 1/4 teaspoon pepper
- 1 cup reduced-fat biscuit/baking mix
- 1/3 cup plus 1 tablespoon fat-free milk

1. In a Dutch oven or large saucepan, cook the bacon over medium heat until crisp. Remove to paper towels; drain, reserving 2 teaspoons drippings.

2. Cook turkey in the drippings until no longer pink. Add the carrots, 1-3/4 cups water, broth, onions, celery, rosemary and bay leaf. Bring to a boil. Reduce heat; cover and simmer for 20-30 minutes or until vegetables are tender.

3. Combine flour and remaining water until smooth; stir into turkey mixture. Bring to a boil; cook and stir for 2 minutes or until thickened. Discard bay leaf. Stir in the salt, pepper and reserved bacon.

4. In a large bowl, combine the biscuit mix and milk. Drop batter in six mounds onto simmering stew. Cover and simmer for 15 minutes or until a toothpick inserted in a dumpling comes out clean (do not lift the cover while simmering).

PREP/TOTAL TIME
Prep: 10 min.
Cook: 50 min.
YIELD 6 servings

NUTRITION FACTS
One serving
(1 cup) equals:
299 calories
6 g fat
2 g saturated fat
76 mg cholesterol
787 mg sodium
26 g carbohydrate
2 g fiber
34 g protein

DIABETIC EXCHANGES
4 very lean meat
2 vegetable
1 starch
1 fat

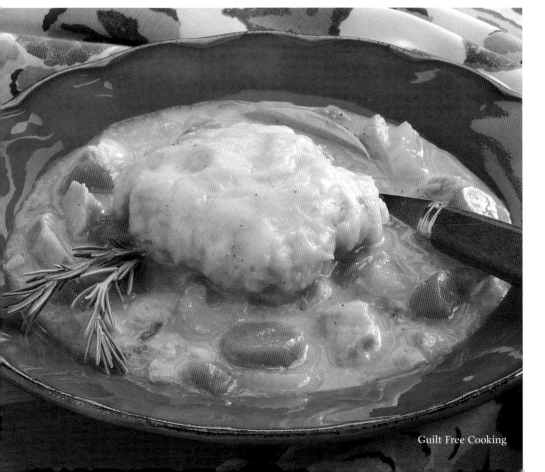

Zippy White Chili

PREP/TOTAL TIME
Prep: 15 min.
Cook: 40 min.
YIELD 4 servings

NUTRITION FACTS
One serving (1 cup
calculated without
chips) equals:
235 calories
4 g fat
0 g saturated fat
64 mg cholesterol
428 mg sodium
19 g carbohydrate
6 g fiber
29 g protein

**DIABETIC
EXCHANGES**
3-1/2 very lean
meat
1 starch
1 vegetable

*This chunky chicken chili doesn't require
any fancy preparation or exotic ingredients.
It's terrific served over crunchy tortilla chips.*

Kenny Schmidtbauer, Sioux Falls, South Dakota

1 pound boneless skinless chicken breasts, cut into cubes

1 small onion, chopped

1-3/4 cups reduced-sodium chicken broth

1 can (4 ounces) chopped green chilies

1/2 teaspoon garlic powder

1/2 teaspoon dried oregano

1/2 teaspoon minced fresh cilantro

1/8 to 1/4 teaspoon cayenne pepper

1 can (15 ounces) white kidney or cannellini beans, rinsed and drained

Baked tortilla chips, optional

1. In a saucepan coated with cooking spray, saute chicken and onion until juices run clear; drain if desired. Stir in broth, chilies, garlic powder, oregano, cilantro and cayenne. Bring to a boil. Reduce heat; simmer, uncovered, for 30 minutes.

2. Stir in beans; cook 10 minutes longer. Serve over tortilla chips if desired.

Mediterranean Seafood Chowder

PREP/TOTAL TIME
30 min.
YIELD 10 servings

NUTRITION FACTS
One serving (1 cup)
equals:
187 calories
4 g fat
1 g saturated fat
44 mg cholesterol
433 mg sodium
25 g carbohydrate
3 g fiber
12 g protein

**DIABETIC
EXCHANGES**
2 lean meat
1 starch

*My family isn't overly fond of seafood, but
everyone enjoys this rich-tasting chowder.*

Erin Nicole Morris, St. Peters, Missouri

1-1/2 cups chopped sweet yellow or red pepper

1 large onion, quartered and thinly sliced

3 garlic cloves, minced

2 tablespoons olive oil

1 can (28 ounces) crushed tomatoes

2-1/4 cups water

1 can (14-1/2 ounces) chicken broth

1 cup uncooked long grain rice

1/2 cup white wine or additional chicken broth

1/2 to 1 teaspoon dried thyme

1/2 to 1 teaspoon dried basil

1/2 teaspoon salt

1/8 teaspoon crushed red pepper flakes

8 ounces uncooked medium shrimp, peeled and deveined

8 ounces cod fillets, cut into pieces

1. In a large saucepan or Dutch oven, saute the peppers, onion and garlic in oil until tender. Add the tomatoes, water, broth, rice, wine or additional broth and seasonings. Bring to a boil. Reduce heat; cover and simmer for 15-20 minutes or until rice is tender.

2. Stir in the shrimp and cod; cover and simmer for 2-4 minutes or until shrimp turn pink and fish flakes easily with a fork.

ADD A ZIP TO THE DISH

The mighty crushed red pepper adds a kick and spicy heat to foods. If you're out of this fiery spice, substitute a few dashes of hot pepper sauce or ground red pepper.

Taco Soup

Delicious and satisfying, this thick chili-like soup has a mild taco flavor and appealing color. It also comes together quickly.

Marylou von Scheele, University Place, Washington

- 1 pound lean ground beef
- 1 medium onion, chopped
- 1 medium green pepper, chopped
- 1 envelope reduced-sodium taco seasoning
- 2/3 cup water
- 4 cups reduced-sodium V8 juice
- 1 cup chunky salsa

TOPPINGS:

- 3/4 cup shredded lettuce
- 6 tablespoons chopped fresh tomatoes
- 6 tablespoons shredded reduced-fat cheddar cheese
- 1/4 cup chopped green onions
- 1/4 cup fat-free sour cream

Tortilla chips, optional

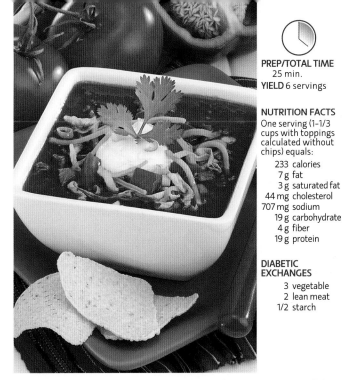

1. In a large saucepan coated with cooking spray, cook the beef, onion and pepper over medium heat until meat is no longer pink and vegetables are tender; drain. Stir in taco seasoning and water; cook and stir for 5 minutes or until liquid is reduced.

2. Add V8 juice and salsa; bring to a boil. Reduce heat; simmer, uncovered, for 5 minutes or until heated through. Top each serving with 2 tablespoons of lettuce, 1 tablespoon of tomato and cheese, and 2 teaspoons of green onions and sour cream. Serve with tortilla chips if desired.

PREP/TOTAL TIME
25 min.
YIELD 6 servings

NUTRITION FACTS
One serving (1-1/3 cups with toppings calculated without chips) equals:

- 233 calories
- 7 g fat
- 3 g saturated fat
- 44 mg cholesterol
- 707 mg sodium
- 19 g carbohydrate
- 4 g fiber
- 19 g protein

DIABETIC EXCHANGES

- 3 vegetable
- 2 lean meat
- 1/2 starch

Spiced Tomato Soup

I'm watching my sodium and frequently experiment with spices to replace the salt. The flavors of tart tomatoes and cloves really shine in this lightened-up, easy soup.

Carol Foiles, Clark, South Dakota

- 1 can (14-1/2 ounces) diced tomatoes, undrained
- 1 teaspoon reduced-sodium beef bouillon granules
- 1 cup hot water
- 1 tablespoon finely chopped onion
- 1 tablespoon sugar
- 1/8 teaspoon ground cloves
- 1/8 teaspoon dried marjoram
- 1/8 teaspoon dried thyme
- 1 bay leaf

1. In a blender or food processor, cover and process the tomatoes until pureed.

2. In a saucepan, dissolve bouillon in hot water. Add tomatoes, onion, sugar, cloves, marjoram, thyme and bay leaf. Bring to a boil, stirring occasionally. Reduce heat; cover and simmer for 20-25 minutes. Discard bay leaf before serving.

PREP/TOTAL TIME
30 min.
YIELD 2 servings

NUTRITION FACTS
One serving (1 cup) equals:

- 74 calories
- 1 g fat
- 1 g saturated fat
- 0 mg cholesterol
- 354 mg sodium
- 16 g carbohydrate
- 2 g fiber
- 2 g protein

DIABETIC EXCHANGE

- 3 vegetable

LOW FAT

PREP/TOTAL TIME
25 min.
YIELD 9 servings
(about 2 quarts)

NUTRITION FACTS
One serving
(1 cup) equals:
143 calories
2 g fat
1 g saturated fat
9 mg cholesterol
856 mg sodium
22 g carbohydrate
4 g fiber
8 g protein

DIABETIC EXCHANGES
1-1/2 starch
1 vegetable

Southwestern Broccoli Cheese Soup

A friend gave me the recipe for this chunky vegetable soup, which I've been making for years. Recently, I changed the ingredients a bit to give it some Southwestern flair.

Peggy Hendrix, Richardson, Texas

4 cups water

4 reduced-sodium chicken bouillon cubes *or* vegetable bouillon cubes

4 cups fresh broccoli florets

3 cups frozen Southern-style hash brown potatoes

1 cup chopped carrots

1 cup chopped celery

1/2 teaspoon *each* salt and pepper

3 tablespoons all-purpose flour

2 cups fat-free milk

6 ounces reduced-fat process cheese (Velveeta), cubed

1 cup chunky salsa

1. In a large saucepan, combine the water, bouillon cubes, vegetables, salt and pepper. Bring to a boil. Reduce heat; cover and simmer for 8-10 minutes or until the vegetables are tender.

2. Combine flour and milk until smooth; gradually stir into the soup. Bring to a boil; cook and stir for 2 minutes or until thickened. Reduce heat to low. Add cheese; cook and stir until cheese is melted. Add salsa; cook and stir until heated through.

Chicken Stew

Rely on this slow cooker stew on busy weekends when you'd rather not be in the kitchen. Chicken, vegetables and seasonings give every spoonful great, comforting flavor.

Linda Emery, Tuckerman, Arkansas

- 2 pounds boneless skinless chicken breasts, cut into 1-inch cubes
- 2 cans (14-1/2 ounces *each*) fat-free chicken broth
- 1 can (6 ounces) no-salt-added tomato paste
- 3 cups cubed peeled potatoes
- 1 cup chopped onion
- 1 cup sliced celery
- 1 cup thinly sliced carrots
- 1 teaspoon paprika
- 1/2 teaspoon pepper
- 1/2 teaspoon rubbed sage
- 1/2 teaspoon dried thyme
- 1/4 cup cold water
- 3 tablespoons cornstarch

1. In a 5-qt. slow cooker, combine the chicken, broth, tomato paste, potatoes, onion, celery, carrots, paprika, pepper, sage and thyme; cover and cook on high for 4 hours.

2. Mix the cold water and cornstarch until smooth; stir into the stew. Cook, covered, 30 minutes longer or until the vegetables are tender.

LOW FAT   LOW SALT

PREP/TOTAL TIME
Prep: 10 min.
Cook: 4-1/2 hours
YIELD 10 servings

NUTRITION FACTS
One serving
(1 cup) equals:
- 193 calories
- 3 g fat
- 0 g saturated fat
- 59 mg cholesterol
- 236 mg sodium
- 16 g carbohydrate
- 0 g fiber
- 24 g protein

DIABETIC EXCHANGES
- 3 very lean meat
- 2 vegetable
- 1/2 starch

Lentil Sausage Soup

This recipe makes a very large pot of hearty soup, but it freezes and reheats well. With lentils, rice and tortellini in a tomato broth, it's a tasty alternative to vegetable soup.

Melanee Van Ee-Mortensen, Fort Collins, Colorado

- 1 package (19-1/2 ounces) turkey Italian sausage links, casings removed
- 13 cups water
- 1 cup chopped carrots
- 1/2 cup chopped celery
- 2 teaspoons onion powder
- 3/4 teaspoon dried oregano
- 1/2 teaspoon garlic powder
- 1/2 teaspoon dried basil
- 1/2 teaspoon seasoning salt
- 1/4 teaspoon pepper
- 2 cups dried lentils, rinsed
- 1/2 cup uncooked long grain rice
- 2 cans (one 15 ounces, one 8 ounces) tomato sauce
- 2-1/2 cups frozen cheese tortellini

1. Crumble sausage into a nonstick skillet. Cook over medium heat until no longer pink; drain.

2. In a large saucepan or Dutch oven, combine water, carrots, celery, onion powder, oregano, garlic powder, basil, seasoning salt and pepper. Add lentils and rice. Bring to a boil. Reduce the heat; cover and simmer for 18-20 minutes or until the lentils and rice are tender.

3. Stir in tomato sauce; return to a boil. Add tortellini and sausage. Cook for 3-4 minutes or until tortellini are tender, stirring several times.

CASINGS REMOVED

To quickly remove casings from uncooked Italian sausage, make a lengthwise slit down the middle of the casing with a sharp knife. Then just peel the casing off.

PREP/TOTAL TIME
Prep: 5 min.
Cook: 30 min.
YIELD 13 servings

NUTRITION FACTS
One serving
(1-1/2 cups) equals:
- 270 calories
- 6 g fat
- 2 g saturated fat
- 27 mg cholesterol
- 651 mg sodium
- 36 g carbohydrate
- 11 g fiber
- 20 g protein

DIABETIC EXCHANGES
- 2 starch
- 2 lean meat

Steak Chili

PREP/TOTAL TIME
Prep: 20 min.
Cook: 2-1/2 hours
YIELD 6 servings

NUTRITION FACTS
One serving
(1 cup) equals:
185 calories
5 g fat
0 g saturated fat
56 mg cholesterol
90 mg sodium
12 g carbohydrate
0 g fiber
24 g protein

DIABETIC EXCHANGES
2-1/2 vegetable
2 lean meat

Why make ordinary ground beef chili when you can create this version featuring round steak? It's sure to earn you raves.

DeAnn Hill, Indianapolis, Indiana

- 1-1/2 pounds beef eye round roast, cut into 1-inch cubes
- 1 cup chopped onion
- 3 garlic cloves, minced
- 1 can (15 ounces) no-salt-added tomato sauce
- 1-1/4 cups water, *divided*
- 1-1/4 cups reduced-sodium V8 juice
- 1/2 teaspoon hot pepper sauce
- 1 tablespoon chili powder
- 1 tablespoon paprika
- 1-1/2 teaspoons ground cumin
- 1 teaspoon pepper
- 2 tablespoons all-purpose flour

1. In a large skillet, brown steak until meat is no longer pink. Drain, discarding all but 2 tablespoons drippings. Set meat aside.

2. In the same skillet, saute onion and garlic in drippings for 3 minutes or until crisp-tender. Return meat to pan. Add the tomato sauce, 1 cup water, V8 juice, hot pepper sauce and spices; bring to a boil. Reduce heat; cover and simmer 2-1/2 hours.

3. Combine flour with remaining water; whisk into chili. Bring to a boil; cook and stir for 2 minutes or until thickened. Cook 10 minutes longer or until heated through.

Ham and Lima Bean Soup

PREP/TOTAL TIME
Prep: 20 min. + standing
Cook: 1-1/4 hours
YIELD 5 servings

NUTRITION FACTS
One serving
(1-1/3 cups) equals:
263 calories
3 g fat
1 g saturated fat
13 mg cholesterol
932 mg sodium
39 g carbohydrate
12 g fiber
22 g protein

DIABETIC EXCHANGES
3 very lean meat
1 starch
1 vegetable

I trimmed down my recipe for bean soup and loved the results. If you'd like a thicker version, try adding some instant potato flakes to the soup after it boils.

Pam Felstein, Owings Mills, Maryland

- 8 ounces dried baby lima beans
- 2 cups chopped onions
- 2 garlic cloves, minced
- 2 cans (14-1/2 ounces *each*) reduced-sodium chicken broth
- 1-1/2 cups cubed fully cooked lean ham
- 1 cup sliced fresh carrots (1/4-inch slices)
- 1/2 cup water
- 1 jalapeno pepper, seeded and chopped
- 2 tablespoons minced fresh parsley
- 1/2 teaspoon pepper

1. Place lima beans in a Dutch oven or soup kettle; add water to cover by 2 in. Bring to a boil; boil for 2 minutes. Remove from the heat; cover and let stand for 1 to 4 hours or until beans are softened. Drain and rinse beans; discard liquid.

2. In a Dutch oven coated with cooking spray, cook onions and garlic until tender. Stir in the broth, ham, carrots, water, jalapeno, parsley, pepper and beans. Bring to a boil. Reduce heat; cover and simmer for 50 minutes or until beans are tender.

Editor's Note: When cutting hot peppers, disposable gloves are recommended. Avoid touching your face.

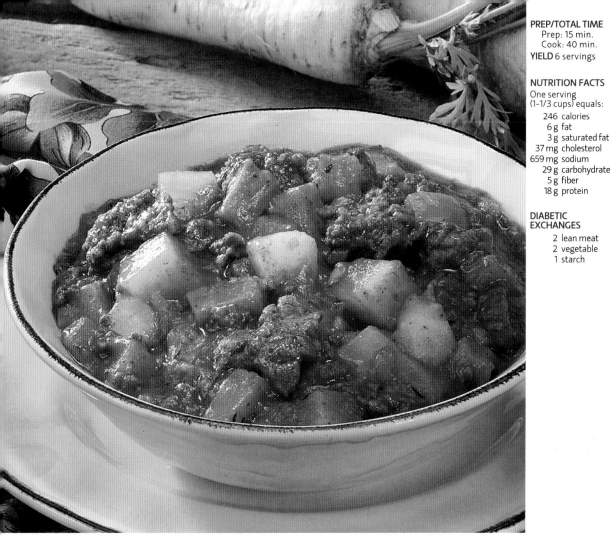

PREP/TOTAL TIME
Prep: 15 min.
Cook: 40 min.
YIELD 6 servings

NUTRITION FACTS
One serving
(1-1/3 cups) equals:
  246 calories
    6 g fat
    3 g saturated fat
   37 mg cholesterol
  659 mg sodium
   29 g carbohydrate
    5 g fiber
   18 g protein

DIABETIC EXCHANGES
  2 lean meat
  2 vegetable
  1 starch

Root Vegetable Beef Stew

I found this recipe a number of years ago. It's so satisfying on a cold fall or winter day.

Mary Rea, Orangeville, Ontario

  1 pound lean ground beef
  1 medium onion, chopped
  2 cans (14-1/2 ounces *each*) reduced-sodium beef broth
  1 medium sweet potato, peeled and cubed
  1 cup cubed carrots
  1 cup cubed peeled rutabaga
  1 cup cubed peeled parsnips
  1 cup cubed peeled potatoes
  2 tablespoons tomato paste
  1 teaspoon Worcestershire sauce

  1/2 teaspoon dried thyme
  1/4 teaspoon salt
  1/4 teaspoon pepper
  1 tablespoon cornstarch
  2 tablespoons water

1. In a Dutch oven or large kettle, cook beef and onion over medium heat until meat is no longer pink; drain. Add the broth, vegetables, tomato paste, Worcestershire sauce and seasonings. Bring to a boil. Reduce heat; cover and simmer for 30-40 minutes or until vegetables are tender.

2. In a small bowl, combine the cornstarch and water until smooth; stir into the stew. Bring to a boil; cook and stir for 2 minutes or until thickened.

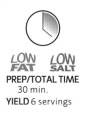

PREP/TOTAL TIME
30 min.
YIELD 6 servings

NUTRITION FACTS
One serving
(1 cup) equals:
108 calories
1 g fat
1 g saturated fat
3 mg cholesterol
224 mg sodium
19 g carbohydrate
3 g fiber
5 g protein

DIABETIC EXCHANGES
1 starch
1 vegetable

Italian Vegetable Soup

One night when my husband and I needed a quick supper, I threw together this satisfying soup using only the ingredients we had on hand. Now the recipe is one of our favorites.

Margaret Glassic, Easton, Pennsylvania

2 cans (14-1/2 ounces *each*) reduced-sodium chicken *or* vegetable broth
1 medium potato, peeled and cubed
1 medium onion, chopped
1 medium carrot, chopped
1 celery rib, chopped
1/2 cup frozen peas
1 bay leaf
1 teaspoon Italian seasoning
1/8 teaspoon pepper
1/2 cup small shell pasta, cooked and drained
1 can (14-1/2 ounces) diced tomatoes, undrained

1. In a large saucepan, combine the broth, vegetables, bay leaf, Italian seasoning and pepper. Bring to a boil. Reduce heat; cover and simmer for 15-20 minutes or until vegetables are crisp-tender.

2. Add the pasta and tomatoes; heat through. Discard bay leaf.

Cheesy Potato Soup

We like to eat steaming bowlfuls of this rich soup often throughout the winter. It really warms you up on a cold, windy day.

Doris Self, Greensboro, North Carolina

- 1 cup diced peeled potato
- 1/2 cup shredded carrot
- 1/4 cup chopped onion
- 1/4 cup chopped celery
- 1-3/4 cups reduced-sodium chicken broth
- 3 tablespoons cornstarch
- 1-3/4 cups fat-free evaporated milk
- 1 cup (4 ounces) finely shredded reduced-fat cheddar cheese

1. In a large saucepan, combine the potato, carrot, onion, celery and broth. Cover and simmer until potato is tender, about 12 minutes. Mash mixture with a potato masher.

2. Combine cornstarch and milk until smooth; gradually add to the vegetable mixture. Bring to a boil; cook and stir for 2 minutes or until thickened. And cheese; stir until melted.

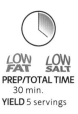

LOW FAT   **LOW SALT**

PREP/TOTAL TIME
30 min.
YIELD 5 servings

NUTRITION FACTS
One serving
(1 cup) equals:
199 calories
5 g fat
0 g saturated fat
20 mg cholesterol
153 mg sodium
24 g carbohydrate
0 g fiber
16 g protein

DIABETIC EXCHANGES
1 meat
1 fat-free milk
1/2 starch

Asian Shrimp Soup

I love this soup so much, I often double the recipe. In fact, I've nicknamed it the "House Specialty!" If I have leftover chicken or pork, I sometimes substitute it for the shrimp.

Michelle Smith, Sykesville, Maryland

- 1 ounce uncooked thin spaghetti, broken into 1-inch pieces
- 3 cups plus 1 tablespoon water, *divided*
- 3 teaspoons reduced-sodium chicken bouillon
- 1/2 teaspoon salt
- 1/2 cup sliced fresh mushrooms
- 1/2 cup fresh or frozen corn
- 1 teaspoon cornstarch
- 1-1/2 teaspoons reduced-sodium teriyaki sauce
- 1 cup thinly sliced romaine lettuce
- 1 can (6 ounces) small shrimp, rinsed and drained
- 2 tablespoons sliced green onion

1. Cook pasta according to package directions; drain. In a saucepan, combine 3 cups water, chicken bouillon and salt; bring to a boil. Stir in the mushrooms and corn. Reduce the heat; cook, uncovered, until vegetables are tender.

2. Combine cornstarch, teriyaki sauce and remaining water until smooth; stir into soup. Bring to a boil; cook and stir for 1-2 minutes or until slightly thickened. Reduce the heat; add the lettuce, shrimp, green onion and spaghetti; heat through.

LOW FAT

PREP/TOTAL TIME
20 min.
YIELD 4 servings

NUTRITION FACTS
One serving
(1 cup) equals:
111 calories
1 g fat
1 g saturated fat
74 mg cholesterol
725 mg sodium
13 g carbohydrate
1 g fiber
12 g protein

DIABETIC EXCHANGES
1 starch
1 very lean meat

LOW FAT

PREP/TOTAL TIME
30 min.
YIELD 10 servings

NUTRITION FACTS
One serving
(1 cup) equals:
179 calories
1 g fat
Trace saturated fat
0 mg cholesterol
491 mg sodium
37 g carbohydrate
10 g fiber
10 g protein

DIABETIC EXCHANGES
2 vegetable
1-1/2 starch
1 very lean meat

Three-Bean Chili

Lots of beans and zesty spices will make you forget that this chunky chili is on the lighter side. You'll never miss the meat!

Gail Rector-Evans, Hastings, Oklahoma

2-1/4 cups water
1 can (16 ounces) kidney beans, rinsed and drained
1 can (15-1/2 ounces) chili beans, undrained
1 can (15 ounces) pinto beans, rinsed and drained
1 can (15 ounces) tomato sauce
1 can (14-1/2 ounces) no-salt-added stewed tomatoes
1 can (6 ounces) tomato paste
1 tablespoon chili powder
1 teaspoon dried oregano
1 teaspoon minced garlic
1-1/2 cups fresh or frozen corn
1-1/2 cups coarsely chopped yellow summer squash

1. In a Dutch oven, combine the water, beans, tomato sauce, tomatoes, tomato paste and seasonings. Bring to a boil. Reduce heat; simmer, uncovered, for 10 minutes.

2. Add the corn and squash. Bring to a boil. Reduce heat; simmer 10 minutes longer or until the squash is tender.

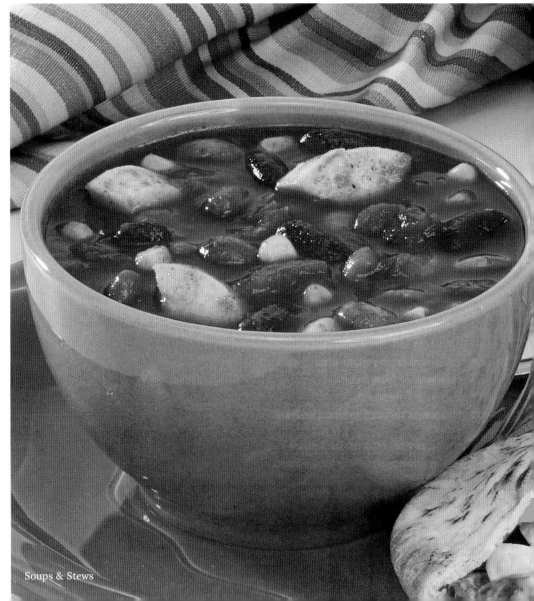

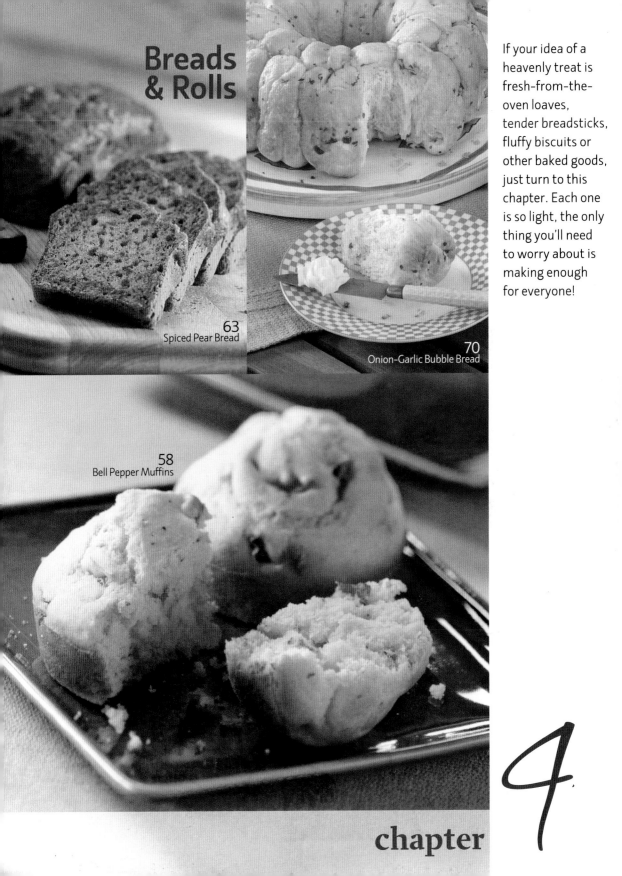

Breads & Rolls

If your idea of a heavenly treat is fresh-from-the-oven loaves, tender breadsticks, fluffy biscuits or other baked goods, just turn to this chapter. Each one is so light, the only thing you'll need to worry about is making enough for everyone!

63
Spiced Pear Bread

70
Onion-Garlic Bubble Bread

58
Bell Pepper Muffins

chapter 4.

PREP/TOTAL TIME
Prep: 35 min. +
rising
Bake: 15 min.
YIELD 2-1/2 dozen

NUTRITION FACTS
One serving
(1 roll) equals:
92 calories
1g fat
1g saturated fat
16 mg cholesterol
76 mg sodium
16 g carbohydrate
1g fiber
3 g protein

DIABETIC EXCHANGE
1 starch

Sweet Potato Yeast Rolls

Mashed sweet potatoes add a hint of color and flavor to these home-baked dinner rolls. The tempting knots have a tender texture, and they look lovely sprinkled with sesame seeds.

Taste of Home Test Kitchen

- 1 package (1/4 ounce) active dry yeast
- 1 cup warm fat-free milk (110° to 115°)
- 1 teaspoon plus 1/3 cup sugar, *divided*
- 1/3 cup cold mashed sweet potatoes
- 2 eggs, *separated*
- 2 tablespoons butter, softened
- 3/4 teaspoon salt
- 3-1/2 to 4 cups all-purpose flour
- 4 teaspoons cold water
- 1 tablespoon sesame seeds

1. In a large mixing bowl, dissolve yeast in warm milk. Add 1 teaspoon sugar; let stand for 5 minutes. Add the sweet potatoes, egg yolks, butter, salt, remaining sugar and 2 cups flour. Beat until smooth. Stir in enough remaining flour to form a soft dough.

2. Turn onto a floured surface; knead until smooth and elastic, about 6-8 minutes. Place in a bowl coated with cooking spray, turning once to coat top. Cover and let rise in a warm place until doubled, about 1-1/2 hours.

3. Punch dough down. Turn onto a lightly floured surface; divide into 30 balls. Roll each ball into a 10-in. rope; tie each rope into a loose knot. Place 2 in. apart on baking sheets coated with cooking spray. Cover and let rise until doubled, about 30 minutes.

4. In a small bowl, beat egg whites and cold water; brush over rolls. Sprinkle with sesame seeds. Bake at 350° for 15-17 minutes or until lightly browned. Remove from pans to cool on wire racks.

PREP/TOTAL TIME
Prep: 15 min.
Bake: 15 min.
YIELD 1 dozen

NUTRITION FACTS
One serving
(1 muffin) equals:
146 calories
7 g fat
4 g saturated fat
37 mg cholesterol
327 mg sodium
12 g carbohydrate
1g fiber
9 g protein

DIABETIC EXCHANGES
1 starch
1 lean meat
1/2 fat

Ham 'n' Cheese Muffins

As a grab-and-go breakfast or snack, these hearty ham muffins can't be beat. They're a real favorite with my three children.

Joy Cochran, Roy, Washington

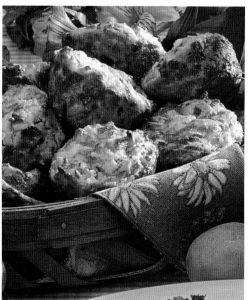

- 1/3 cup finely chopped onion
- 1 tablespoon butter
- 2 cups (8 ounces) shredded reduced-fat cheddar cheese
- 1-1/2 cups reduced-fat biscuit/baking mix
- 1/2 cup fat-free milk
- 1 egg, beaten
- 1 cup finely chopped fully cooked ham

1. In a nonstick skillet, saute the onion in butter until tender; set aside. In a bowl, combine the cheese and biscuit mix. Stir in the milk and egg just until moistened. Fold in the ham and onion.

2. Coat muffin cups with cooking spray or use paper liners; fill three-fourths full with batter. Bake at 425° for 13-15 minutes or until a toothpick comes out clean. Cool for 5 minutes before removing from pan to a wire rack. Serve warm.

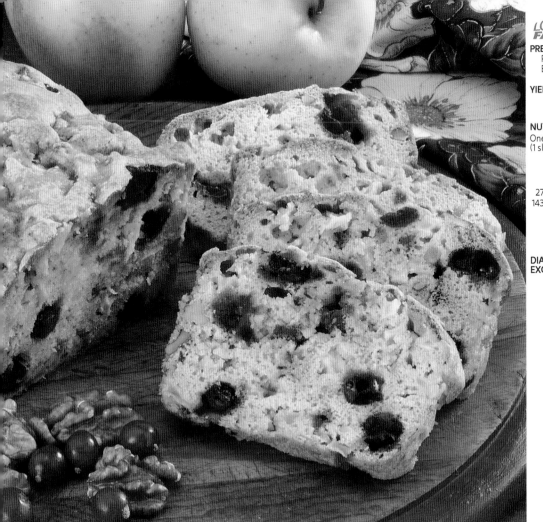

LOW FAT   LOW SALT

PREP/TOTAL TIME
Prep: 10 min.
Bake: 1 hour +
cooling
YIELD 1 loaf
(16 slices)

NUTRITION FACTS
One serving
(1 slice) equals:

140 calories
5 g fat
1 g saturated fat
27 mg cholesterol
143 mg sodium
22 g carbohydrate
1 g fiber
3 g protein

**DIABETIC
EXCHANGES**
1 starch
1 fat
1/2 fruit

Apple Cranberry Bread

Cranberries add a burst of tartness and bright color to this quick bread. Dotted with nuts, slices of the moist loaf are especially good for breakfast with a cup of coffee.

Phyllis Schmalz, Kansas City, Kansas

2	eggs
3/4	cup sugar
2	tablespoons canola oil
1-1/2	cups all-purpose flour
1-1/2	teaspoons baking powder
1	teaspoon ground cinnamon
1/2	teaspoon baking soda
1/2	teaspoon salt
2	cups chopped peeled tart apples
1	cup fresh or frozen cranberries
1/2	cup chopped walnuts

1. In a mixing bowl, beat the eggs, sugar and oil. Combine flour, baking powder, cinnamon, baking soda and salt; add to the egg mixture just until combined (batter will be very thick). Stir in the apples, cranberries and walnuts.

2. Transfer to an 8-in. x 4-in. x 2-in. loaf pan coated with cooking spray. Bake at 350° for 60-65 minutes or until a toothpick inserted near the center comes out clean. Cool for 10 minutes before removing from pan to a wire rack to cool completely.

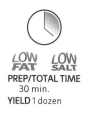

PREP/TOTAL TIME
30 min.
YIELD 1 dozen

NUTRITION FACTS
One serving
(1 muffin) equals:
119 calories
3 g fat
1 g saturated fat
23 mg cholesterol
228 mg sodium
20 g carbohydrate
1 g fiber
4 g protein

DIABETIC EXCHANGES
1 starch
1/2 fat

Bell Pepper Muffins

Featuring three types of peppers and a hint of basil, these tender muffins are especially good with chicken. I trimmed down the original recipe to cut the fat and cholesterol.

Karen Shipp, San Antonio, Texas

1/4 cup *each* chopped green pepper, sweet yellow pepper and sweet red pepper
2 tablespoons butter
2 cups all-purpose flour
2 tablespoons sugar
2-1/2 teaspoons baking powder
1/2 teaspoon salt
1/2 teaspoon dried basil
1 egg
1/4 cup egg substitute
1 cup fat-free milk

1. In a nonstick skillet, saute peppers in butter until tender; set aside. In a large bowl, combine the flour, sugar, baking powder, salt and basil. Combine the egg, egg substitute and milk; stir into dry ingredients just until moistened. Fold in the peppers.

2. Coat muffin cups with cooking spray; fill two-thirds full with batter. Bake at 400° for 15-18 minutes or until a toothpick comes out clean. Cool for 5 minutes before removing from pan to a wire rack.

Garlic Cheese Breadsticks

These slightly chewy breadsticks have plenty of garlic and cheese. Whenever I make some, my three daughters gobble them up.

Melinda Rhoads, Slippery Rock, Pennsylvania

1-3/4 to 2-1/2 cups all-purpose flour

1/4 cup toasted wheat germ

1 package (1/4 ounce) active dry yeast

1/2 teaspoon salt

1 cup water

1 tablespoon plus 2 teaspoons olive oil

1 tablespoon honey

2 tablespoons minced fresh parsley *or* 2 teaspoons dried parsley flakes

1 tablespoon minced fresh basil *or* 1 teaspoon dried basil

2 to 4 garlic cloves, minced

1/2 cup shredded part-skim mozzarella cheese

1/2 cup shredded Parmesan cheese

1. In a large bowl, combine 1-1/2 cups flour, wheat germ, yeast and salt. In a saucepan, heat the water, 1 tablespoon oil and honey to 120°-130°. Add to dry ingredients; stir just until moistened. Stir in enough remaining flour to form a soft dough.

2. Turn onto a lightly floured surface; knead until smooth and elastic, about 4-6 minutes. Cover and let rest for 10 minutes.

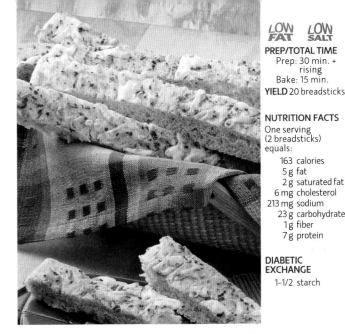

LOW FAT LOW SALT
PREP/TOTAL TIME
Prep: 30 min. + rising
Bake: 15 min.
YIELD 20 breadsticks

NUTRITION FACTS
One serving
(2 breadsticks) equals:
163 calories
5 g fat
2 g saturated fat
6 mg cholesterol
213 mg sodium
23 g carbohydrate
1 g fiber
7 g protein

DIABETIC EXCHANGE
1-1/2 starch

3. Roll into a 15-in. x 10-in. rectangle. Transfer to a greased 15-in. x 10-in. x 1-in. baking pan; press dough to edges of pan. Brush with remaining oil. Sprinkle with parsley, basil and garlic. Cover and let rise in a warm place until doubled, about 30 minutes.

4. Bake at 425° for 10 minutes. Sprinkle with cheeses. Bake 3-5 minutes longer or until cheese is melted and bread is golden brown. Cut into 20 breadsticks. Serve warm.

Orange Chocolate Chip Bread

When our orange tree was loaded with fruit, I was inspired to try this recipe. The bread makes a sweet homemade gift on holidays.

Misti Konsavage, Thonotosassa, Florida

1 cup fat-free milk

1/4 cup orange juice

1/3 cup sugar

1 egg

1 tablespoon finely grated orange peel

3 cups reduced-fat biscuit/baking mix

1/2 cup miniature semisweet chocolate chips

1. In a large bowl, combine the milk, orange juice, sugar, egg and orange peel. Stir in baking mix just until moistened. Stir in chocolate chips.

2. Pour into a 9-in. x 5-in. x 3-in. loaf pan coated with cooking spray. Bake at 350° for 45-50 minutes or until a toothpick inserted near the center comes out clean. Cool for 10 minutes before removing from pan to a wire rack.

LOW FAT LOW SALT
PREP/TOTAL TIME
Prep: 15 min.
Bake: 45 min.
YIELD 1 loaf
(16 slices)

NUTRITION FACTS
One serving
(1 slice) equals:
139 calories
3 g fat
1 g saturated fat
14 mg cholesterol
274 mg sodium
25 g carbohydrate
1 g fiber
3 g protein

DIABETIC EXCHANGES
1 starch
1 fruit

Italian Bread Wedges

These savory bread wedges aren't difficult to prepare, and they taste great. Try them with soups, salads or pasta dishes.

Danielle McIntyre, Medicine Hat, Alberta

- 3 teaspoons active dry yeast
- 1 cup warm water (110° to 115°), *divided*
- 1 teaspoon sugar
- 2 tablespoons canola oil
- 1 teaspoon salt
- 2-1/2 to 3 cups all-purpose flour

TOPPING:
- 1/3 cup fat-free Italian salad dressing
- 1/4 teaspoon garlic powder
- 1/4 teaspoon dried oregano
- 1/4 teaspoon dried thyme

Dash pepper
- 1 cup (4 ounces) shredded part-skim mozzarella cheese
- 1/4 cup grated Parmesan cheese

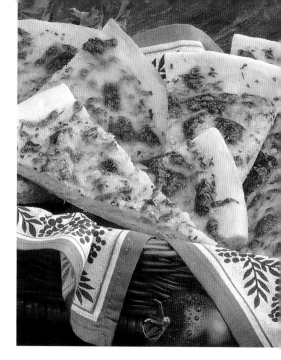

1. In a mixing bowl, dissolve yeast in 1/4 cup warm water. Add sugar; let stand for 5 minutes. Add oil, salt, remaining water and 2 cups flour; beat until smooth. Stir in enough remaining flour to form a soft dough.

2. Turn onto a floured surface; knead until smooth and elastic, about 6-8 minutes. Place in a bowl coated with cooking spray, turning once to grease top. Cover and let rise in a warm place until doubled, about 40 minutes.

3. Punch dough down. Turn onto a lightly floured surface. Pat dough flat; let rest for 5 minutes. Press into a greased 14-in. pizza pan. Spread with salad dressing. Combine the garlic powder, oregano, thyme and pepper; sprinkle over dough. Top with cheeses. Bake at 450° for 15-20 minutes or until golden brown. Cut into wedges; serve warm.

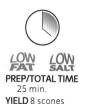

Peach Scones

As a special treat in the morning, I bake a batch of these light and fluffy scones. The dried peaches make them slightly sweet.

Molly Mochamer, Fort Wayne, Indiana

- 1-1/3 cups all-purpose flour
- 1/2 cup plus 2 teaspoons sugar, *divided*
- 1 teaspoon baking powder
- 1/2 teaspoon baking soda
- 1/2 teaspoon salt
- 2 tablespoons cold butter
- 1/2 cup plus 2 tablespoons reduced-fat sour cream
- 1/4 cup chopped dried peaches or apricots
- 1/2 teaspoon vanilla extract
- 1 teaspoon fat-free milk

1. In a bowl, combine the flour, 1/2 cup sugar, baking powder, baking soda and salt. Cut in butter until mixture resembles coarse crumbs. Add sour cream, peaches and vanilla; stir just until moistened.

2. Turn dough onto a floured surface; knead gently 4-5 times (dough will be sticky). Divide dough in half; gently pat each portion into an 8-in. circle on a baking sheet coated with cooking spray. Cut each into four wedges; separate wedges slightly.

3. Brush tops with milk; sprinkle with remaining sugar. Bake at 400° for 10-12 minutes or until golden brown.

Chive Garden Rolls

Everyone who's ever tried these rolls has found them impossible to resist. They go especially well with a salad or bowl of soup.

Joanie Elbourn, Gardner, Massachusetts

1 egg
1 cup (8 ounces) fat-free cottage cheese
1/4 cup vegetable oil
2 teaspoons honey
1 teaspoon salt
1 package (1/4 ounce) active dry yeast
1/2 cup warm water (110° to 115°)
1/4 cup toasted wheat germ
2-3/4 to 3-1/4 cups all-purpose flour
3 tablespoons minced chives

TOPPING:
1 egg, beaten
1 small onion, finely chopped

1. In a mixing bowl, combine the egg, cottage cheese, oil, honey and salt. Dissolve the yeast in warm water; add to egg mixture. Add the wheat germ and 1-1/2 cups flour. Mix on medium speed for 3 minutes. Add the chives and enough remaining flour to form a soft dough.

2. Turn onto a floured surface; knead until smooth and elastic, about 8-10 minutes. Place in a greased bowl, turning once to grease top. Cover and let rise in a warm place until doubled, about 1 hour.

3. Punch dough down; roll out to 3/4-in. thickness. Cut with a 3-in. round cutter. Place on baking sheets coated with cooking spray. Cover and let rise until doubled, about 45 minutes.

4. Brush tops with egg and sprinkle with onion. Bake at 350° for 15-20 minutes or until golden brown.

LOW SALT

PREP/TOTAL TIME
Prep: 35 min. + rising
Bake: 15 min.
YIELD about 1 dozen

NUTRITION FACTS
One serving
(1 roll) equals:
205 calories
6 g fat
0 g saturated fat
35 mg cholesterol
270 mg sodium
29 g carbohydrate
0 g fiber
8 g protein

DIABETIC EXCHANGES
2 starch
1 fat

Walnut Wheat Bread

My husband and I enjoy thick slices of this wholesome bread warm from the oven.

Rosadene Herold, Lakeville, Indiana

1-1/4 to 1-1/2 cups all-purpose flour
1-1/2 cups whole wheat flour
3/4 cup chopped walnuts
2 tablespoons brown sugar
1 package (1/4 ounce) active dry yeast
1 teaspoon salt
3/4 cup water
1/3 cup reduced-fat plain yogurt
2 tablespoons margarine

1. In a large mixing bowl, combine 3/4 cup all-purpose flour, whole wheat flour, walnuts, brown sugar, yeast and salt. In a saucepan, heat the water, yogurt and margarine to 120°-130°; stir into flour mixture. Add enough of the remaining all-purpose flour to form a soft dough.

2. Turn onto a floured surface; knead until smooth and elastic, about 6-8 minutes. Place in a bowl coated with cooking spray, turning once to grease top. Cover and let rise in a warm place until doubled, about 1 hour.

3. Punch dough down. Turn onto a lightly floured surface; divide into thirds. Shape each portion into a 15-in. rope. Place the ropes on a baking sheet coated with cooking spray and braid; pinch ends to seal and tuck under. Cover and let rise in a warm place until doubled, about 30 minutes. Bake at 375° for 23-28 minutes or until golden brown. Remove from pan to cool on a wire rack.

Hot Cross Buns

With their tender texture and pretty frosted crosses, these Easter buns are both yummy and attractive. A hint of orange in the icing adds a delicate, citrusy accent.

Dolores Skrout, Summerhill, Pennsylvania

4 to 5 cups all-purpose flour
1/3 cup sugar
1 package (1/4 ounce) active dry yeast
1-1/4 teaspoons ground cinnamon
1/2 teaspoon salt
1 cup fat-free milk
1/4 cup butter
2 eggs
3/4 cup raisins
1 egg yolk
2 tablespoons cold water

ICING:
1-1/2 cups confectioners' sugar
1/4 teaspoon grated orange peel
4 teaspoons orange juice

1. In a large mixing bowl, combine 2 cups flour, sugar, yeast, cinnamon and salt. In a saucepan, heat milk and butter to 120°-130°. Add to dry ingredients; beat just until moistened. Add eggs; beat until smooth. Stir in raisins and enough remaining flour to form a soft dough.

2. Turn onto a floured surface; knead until smooth and elastic, about 6-8 minutes. Place in a bowl coated with cooking spray, turning once to coat top. Cover and let rise in a warm place until doubled, about 1 hour.

3. Punch dough down; turn onto a lightly floured surface. Divide into 18 pieces; shape each into a ball. Place in two 9-in. round baking pans coated with cooking spray. Using a sharp knife, cut a cross on top of each roll. Cover and let rise in a warm place until doubled, about 30 minutes.

4. Beat egg yolk and water; brush over buns. Bake at 375° for 18-22 minutes or until golden brown. Remove from pans to wire racks to cool. Combine icing ingredients; pipe crosses on rolls.

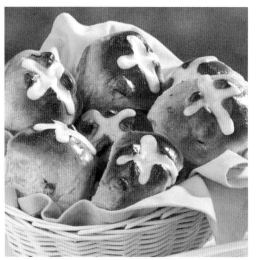

Spiced Pear Bread

My mom and I put up our own pears, so I always have plenty on hand when I want to make this wonderful bread. It's so moist and tasty, you'll want to have a second slice.

Rachael Barefoot, Linden, Michigan

- 3 cans (15-1/4 ounces *each*) sliced pears, drained and mashed
- 1 cup sugar
- 1/4 cup unsweetened applesauce
- 1/4 cup canola oil
- 3 eggs
- 3-1/4 cups all-purpose flour
- 3 teaspoons ground cinnamon
- 1 teaspoon baking soda
- 1 teaspoon baking powder
- 1 teaspoon ground cloves
- 1/2 teaspoon salt

1. In a large mixing bowl, combine the first five ingredients. Combine the flour, cinnamon, baking soda, baking powder, cloves and salt; gradually add to pear mixture and mix well.

2. Pour into four 5-3/4-in. x 3-in. x 2-in. loaf pans coated with cooking spray. Bake at 350° for 50-60 minutes or until a toothpick inserted near the center comes out clean. Cool for 10 minutes before removing from pans to wire racks.

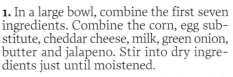

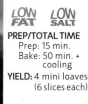

PREP/TOTAL TIME
Prep: 15 min.
Bake: 50 min. + cooling
YIELD: 4 mini loaves (6 slices each)

NUTRITION FACTS
One serving (1 slice) equals:
160 calories
3 g fat
Trace saturated fat
27 mg cholesterol
131 mg sodium
30 g carbohydrate
1 g fiber
3 g protein

DIABETIC EXCHANGE
2 starch

Jalapeno Corn Bread

This homemade corn bread that takes just minutes to bake is dressed up with plenty of jalapenos, green onion and cheddar cheese.

Angela Oelschlaeger, Tonganoxie, Kansas

- 1/2 cup cornmeal
- 1/2 cup all-purpose flour
- 1 teaspoon sugar
- 1/2 teaspoon salt
- 1/4 teaspoon baking powder
- 1/4 teaspoon baking soda
- 1/4 teaspoon garlic powder
- 1/2 cup cream-style corn
- 1/4 cup egg substitute
- 1/4 cup reduced-fat cheddar cheese
- 1/4 cup fat-free milk
- 2 tablespoons chopped green onion
- 1 tablespoon butter, melted
- 2 teaspoons chopped seeded jalapeno pepper

1. In a large bowl, combine the first seven ingredients. Combine the corn, egg substitute, cheddar cheese, milk, green onion, butter and jalapeno. Stir into dry ingredients just until moistened.

2. Pour into an 8-in. square baking dish coated with cooking spray. Bake at 425° for 12-14 minutes or until a toothpick inserted near the center comes out clean. Cut into squares; serve warm.

Editor's Note: When cutting hot peppers, disposable gloves are recommended. Avoid touching your face.

PREP/TOTAL TIME
30 min.
YIELD 9 servings

NUTRITION FACTS
One serving (1 square) equals:
94 calories
2 g fat
1 g saturated fat
5 mg cholesterol
261 mg sodium
15 g carbohydrate
1 g fiber
4 g protein

DIABETIC EXCHANGES
1 starch
1/2 fat

PREP/TOTAL TIME
Prep: 30 min. + rising
Bake: 35 min.
YIELD 4 loaves
(8 slices each)

NUTRITION FACTS
One serving
(1 slice) equals:
159 calories
4 g fat
1 g saturated fat
0 mg cholesterol
151 mg sodium
29 g carbohydrate
3 g fiber
3 g protein

DIABETIC EXCHANGES
1 starch
1 fruit
1/2 fat

Country Raisin Rye Bread

The recipe for this delicious bread came from my aunt. I made just a few changes to it, and it's been a favorite ever since. The dark loaves are moist and tender, with a delicate rye and sweet molasses flavor.

Carolyn Rose Sykora, Bloomer, Wisconsin

2	cups whole wheat flour
2	cups rye flour
1	tablespoon active dry yeast
1	teaspoon salt
2	cups water
1/2	cup plus 1 teaspoon olive oil, *divided*
1/2	cup molasses
1/2	cup honey
2-1/2	to 2-3/4 cups all-purpose flour
1	cup raisins

1. In a mixing bowl, combine 1 cup whole wheat flour, 1 cup rye flour, yeast and salt. In a saucepan, heat water, 1/2 cup oil, molasses and honey to 120°-130°. Add to dry ingredients; stir just until moistened. Stir in remaining whole wheat and rye flours and enough all-purpose flour to form a medium stiff dough.

2. Turn onto a floured surface; sprinkle with raisins. Knead until smooth and elastic, about 8-10 minutes. Grease a bowl with remaining oil. Place dough in bowl, turning once to grease top. Cover; let rise in a warm place until doubled, about 1-1/2 hours.

3. Punch dough down; turn onto a lightly floured surface. Divide into four pieces; shape each into a round loaf. Place 4 in. apart on two baking sheets coated with cooking spray. Cover and let rise until doubled, about 45 minutes. Bake at 325° for 35-40 minutes or until golden brown. Remove from pans to wire racks.

Three Grain Pan Rolls

The first time I made these rolls, I was a little worried that my husband wouldn't care for them...but he loved them! The seeds on top add extra flavor and a fun crunch.

Montserrat Wadsworth, Fallon, Nevada

   2 cups water
1/2 cup bulgur
   1 package (1/4 ounce) active dry yeast
   1 cup warm milk (110° to 115°)
1/2 cup quick-cooking oats
1/3 cup honey
   2 eggs
   2 teaspoons salt
3/4 teaspoon pepper
1-1/2 cups whole wheat flour
2-1/2 to 3-1/2 cups all-purpose flour
   2 tablespoons olive oil
   2 teaspoons *each* celery seed, fennel seed and sesame seeds
   1 teaspoon poppy seeds

1. In a saucepan, bring water to a boil. Stir in bulgur. Reduce heat; cover and simmer for 15 minutes or until tender. Drain. In a large mixing bowl, dissolve yeast in warm milk. Add the oats, honey, eggs, salt, pepper, cooked bulgur and whole wheat flour; beat until smooth. Stir in enough all-purpose flour to form a soft dough.

2. Turn onto a lightly floured surface; knead until elastic, about 6-8 minutes (mixture will be lumpy). Place in a bowl coated with cooking spray, turning once to coat top. Cover and let rise in a warm place until doubled, about 1-1/4 hours.

3. Punch dough down. Turn onto a lightly floured surface; divide into 22 pieces. Roll each into a ball. Brush two 9-in. round baking pans with some of the oil. Arrange 11 balls in each pan; brush the tops with the remaining oil.

4. Combine the celery seed, fennel seed, sesame seeds and poppy seeds; sprinkle over rolls. Cover and let rise in a warm place until doubled, about 40 minutes. Bake at 375° for 18-22 minutes or until golden brown. Remove from pans to wire racks.

Editor's Note: Look for bulgur in the cereal, rice or organic food aisle of your grocery store.

PREP/TOTAL TIME
Prep: 40 min. + rising
Bake: 20 min.
YIELD 22 rolls

NUTRITION FACTS
One serving
(1 roll) equals:

   157 calories
     3 g fat
     1 g saturated fat
   21 mg cholesterol
227 mg sodium
   29 g carbohydrate
     2 g fiber
     5 g protein

DIABETIC EXCHANGES
   2 starch
1/2 fat

Buttermilk Dill Bread

I use my bread machine to turn out this light, golden loaf with a mild dill flavor. It's one of my favorites to share with friends.

Billie Moss, El Sobrante, California

1-1/4 cups warm buttermilk (70° to 80°)
   2 tablespoons butter, softened
   2 tablespoons sugar
1-1/2 teaspoons dill weed
1/2 teaspoon salt
1/8 teaspoon white pepper
   3 cups bread flour
2-1/4 teaspoons active dry yeast

1. In bread machine pan, place all the ingredients in order suggested by manufacturer. Select basic bread setting. Choose crust color and loaf size if available. Bake according to bread machine directions (check dough after 5 minutes of mixing; add 1-2 tablespoons of water or flour if needed).

Editor's Note: If your bread machine has a time-delay feature, we recommend you do not use it for this recipe. Warmed buttermilk will appear curdled.

PREP/TOTAL TIME
Prep: 10 min.
Bake: 3-4 hours
YIELD 1 loaf (1-1/2 pounds and 16 slices)

NUTRITION FACTS
One serving
(1 slice) equals:

   104 calories
     2 g fat
     1 g saturated fat
     5 mg cholesterol
109 mg sodium
   19 g carbohydrate
     1 g fiber
     4 g protein

DIABETIC EXCHANGES
   1 starch
1/2 fat

Zucchini Bread

PREP/TOTAL TIME
Prep: 15 min.
Bake: 1 hour
YIELD 2 loaves
(16 slices each)

NUTRITION FACTS
One serving
(1 slice) equals:
160 calories
7 g fat
1 g saturated fat
20 mg cholesterol
109 mg sodium
23 g carbohydrate
1 g fiber
2 g protein

DIABETIC EXCHANGES
1 starch
1 fat
1/2 fruit

This easy-to-make quick bread is a delicious way to put garden zucchini to good use. The recipe yields two loaves, so you could share one with a neighbor or store it in the freezer.

Britt-Marie Knoblock, Lisle, Illinois

1/2 cup plus 2 tablespoons orange juice
1/2 cup canola oil
1/2 cup unsweetened applesauce
3 eggs, lightly beaten
2 teaspoons vanilla extract
3 cups all-purpose flour
2 cups sugar
4-1/2 teaspoons ground cinnamon
1-1/4 teaspoons baking powder
1 teaspoon salt
1/2 teaspoon baking soda
2 cups shredded zucchini
1 cup chopped pecans

1. In a bowl, combine the orange juice, oil, applesauce, eggs and vanilla. In a large bowl, combine the flour, sugar, cinnamon, baking powder, salt and baking soda; mix well. Add the orange juice mixture; stir just until combined. Fold in the zucchini and pecans.

2. Pour the batter into two 8-in. x 4-in. x 2-in. loaf pans coated with cooking spray. Bake at 350° for 60-65 minutes or until a toothpick inserted near the center comes out clean. Cool for 10 minutes before removing from the pans to wire racks to cool completely.

Ribbon Pumpkin Bread

PREP/TOTAL TIME
Prep: 15 min.
Bake: 40 min. + cooling
YIELD 2 loaves
(14 slices each)

NUTRITION FACTS
One serving
(2 slices) equals:
107 calories
3 g fat
1 g saturated fat
11 mg cholesterol
116 mg sodium
19 g carbohydrate
1 g fiber
3 g protein

DIABETIC EXCHANGES
1 starch
1/2 fat

No one will suspect they're eating lighter when you serve this pretty pumpkin bread with a ribbon of cream cheese inside.

Beth Ask, Ulster, Pennsylvania

6 ounces reduced-fat cream cheese
1/4 cup sugar
1 tablespoon all-purpose flour
2 egg whites

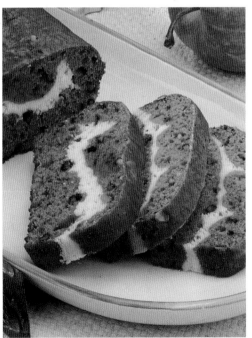

BATTER:

1 cup pumpkin
1/2 cup unsweetened applesauce
1 egg
2 egg whites
1 tablespoon canola oil
1-2/3 cups all-purpose flour
1-1/4 cups sugar
1 teaspoon baking soda
1/2 teaspoon salt
1/2 teaspoon ground cinnamon
1/2 teaspoon ground cloves
1/3 cup chopped walnuts

1. For filling, combine the cream cheese, sugar, flour and egg whites in a bowl; set aside. In a mixing bowl, beat the pumpkin, applesauce, egg, egg whites and oil. Combine the flour, sugar, baking soda, salt, cinnamon and cloves; add to the pumpkin mixture. Stir in the walnuts.

2. Divide half of the batter between two 8-in. x 4-in. x 2-in. loaf pans coated with cooking spray. Spread each with filling; top with remaining batter.

3. Bake at 350° for 40-45 minutes or until a toothpick inserted near the center comes out clean. Cool for 10 minutes before removing from pans to wire racks to cool completely. Refrigerate leftovers.

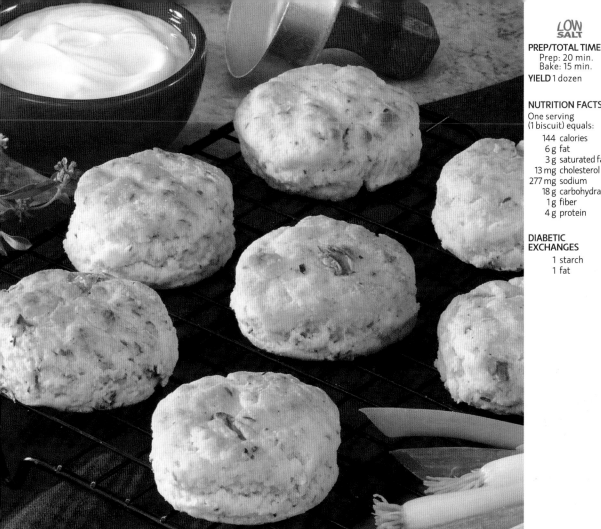

LOW
SALT

PREP/TOTAL TIME
Prep: 20 min.
Bake: 15 min.
YIELD 1 dozen

NUTRITION FACTS
One serving
(1 biscuit) equals:
144 calories
6 g fat
3 g saturated fat
13 mg cholesterol
277 mg sodium
18 g carbohydrate
1 g fiber
4 g protein

DIABETIC
EXCHANGES
1 starch
1 fat

Onion Herb Biscuits

These fluffy, well-seasoned biscuits are a pleasant way to round out almost any meal.

Taste of Home Test Kitchen

2 cups all-purpose flour

1 tablespoon baking powder

1 tablespoon minced fresh thyme
or 1 teaspoon dried thyme

1 teaspoon dried savory

1/2 teaspoon salt

1/4 teaspoon baking soda

1/4 teaspoon pepper

1-1/2 cups reduced-fat sour cream

2 tablespoons olive oil

1/4 cup thinly sliced green onions

1 tablespoon butter, melted

1. Combine the flour, baking powder, thyme, savory, salt, baking soda and pepper. Combine sour cream and oil. With a fork, stir sour cream mixture into dry ingredients just until blended and mixture holds together. Stir in green onions.

2. Turn onto a lightly floured surface; gently knead three or four times. Roll dough to 3/4-in. thickness; cut with a floured 2-1/2-in. biscuit cutter. Place 1 in. apart on ungreased baking sheet. Brush lightly with butter. Bake at 400° for 14-18 minutes or until lightly browned. Serve warm.

Maple Oat Bread

The first time I made this old-fashioned oat bread, my husband, two daughters and I quickly ate the entire loaf! We all agree that it's the best bread we've ever tasted.

Michele Odstrcilek, Lemont, Illinois

- 1 cup old-fashioned oats
- 1 cup boiling water
- 1 package (1/4 ounce) active dry yeast
- 1/3 cup warm water (110° to 115°)
- 1/2 cup maple syrup
- 2 teaspoons canola oil
- 1-1/2 teaspoons salt
- 3-1/2 to 4 cups all-purpose flour

TOPPING:

- 1 egg white, lightly beaten
- 2 tablespoons old-fashioned oats

1. Place 1 cup oats in a blender or food processor; cover and process for 6-7 seconds or until coarsely chopped. Transfer to a small bowl; add the boiling water. Let stand until mixture cools to 110°-115°.

2. In a large mixing bowl, dissolve yeast in the warm water; add maple syrup, oil, salt, oat mixture and 2 cups flour; beat until smooth. Stir in enough remaining flour to form a soft dough.

3. Turn onto a lightly floured surface; knead until smooth and elastic, about 6-8 minutes. Place in a greased bowl, turning once to grease top. Cover and let rise in a warm place until doubled, about 1 hour.

4. Punch dough down. Turn onto a lightly floured surface. Shape into a flattened 9-in. round loaf. Place in a greased 9-in. round baking dish. Cover and let rise until doubled, about 45 minutes.

5. Brush with egg white; sprinkle with oats. Bake at 350° for 30-35 minutes or until golden brown. Remove from pan to a wire rack to cool.

Superb Herb Bread

Caraway, poppy seeds, sage and nutmeg give this lovely bread its superb flavor. It received a blue ribbon at our fall festival.

Doris White, De Land, Illinois

1 cup warm fat-free milk (70° to 80°)

1 egg

2 tablespoons butter, softened, *divided*

2 tablespoons sugar

1 teaspoon salt

2 teaspoons caraway seeds

1-1/2 teaspoons poppy seeds

1-1/2 teaspoons dried minced onion

1 teaspoon rubbed sage

1/2 teaspoon ground nutmeg

2 cups bread flour

1 cup whole wheat flour

1-1/2 teaspoons active dry yeast

1. In bread machine pan, place the milk, egg, 1 tablespoon butter, sugar, salt, caraway seeds, poppy seeds, onion, sage, nutmeg, flours and yeast in the order suggested by manufacturer. Select dough setting (check dough after 5 minutes of mixing; add 1 to 2 tablespoons of water or flour if needed).

2. When the cycle is completed, turn dough onto a lightly floured surface.

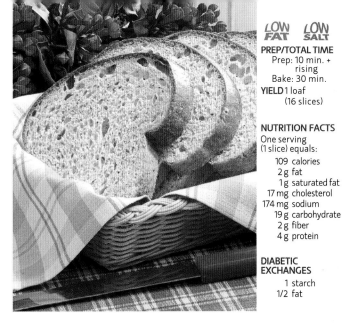

Punch down; shape into a loaf. Place in a 9-in. x 5-in. x 3-in. loaf pan coated with cooking spray. Cover and let rise in a warm place until doubled, about 45 minutes.

3. Bake at 350° for 30-35 minutes or until golden brown. Remove from pan to wire rack. Melt remaining butter; brush over loaf.

Editor's Note: If your bread machine has a time-delay feature, we recommend you do not use it for this recipe.

LOW FAT **LOW SALT**

PREP/TOTAL TIME
Prep: 10 min. + rising
Bake: 30 min.

YIELD 1 loaf
(16 slices)

NUTRITION FACTS
One serving
(1 slice) equals:
109 calories
2 g fat
1 g saturated fat
17 mg cholesterol
174 mg sodium
19 g carbohydrate
2 g fiber
4 g protein

DIABETIC EXCHANGES
1 starch
1/2 fat

Buttermilk Biscuits

I scribbled down this recipe when our family traveled to the Cooperstown Farm Museum many years ago. I must have gotten it right, because these biscuits always turn out great.

Patricia Kile, Greentown, Pennsylvania

2 cups all-purpose flour

3 teaspoons baking powder

1/2 teaspoon baking soda

1/4 teaspoon salt

3 tablespoons cold butter

3/4 to 1 cup buttermilk

1 tablespoon fat-free milk

1. In a bowl, combine the flour, baking powder, baking soda and salt; cut in butter until mixture resembles coarse crumbs. Stir in enough buttermilk just to moisten dough.

2. Turn onto a lightly floured surface; knead 3-4 times. Pat or roll to 3/4-in. thickness. Cut with a floured 2-1/2-in. biscuit cutter. Place on a baking sheet coated with cooking spray. Brush with milk. Bake at 450° for 12-15 minutes or until golden brown.

PREP/TOTAL TIME
Prep: 20 min.
Bake: 15 min.

YIELD 8 biscuits

NUTRITION FACTS
One serving
(1 biscuit) equals:
164 calories
5 g fat
3 g saturated fat
13 mg cholesterol
382 mg sodium
25 g carbohydrate
1 g fiber
4 g protein

DIABETIC EXCHANGES
1-1/2 starch
1 fat

Onion-Garlic Bubble Bread

PREP/TOTAL TIME
Prep: 10 min. + rising
Bake: 20 min.

YIELD 1 loaf
(24 pieces)

NUTRITION FACTS
One serving
(1 piece) equals:
87 calories
5 g fat
2 g saturated fat
10 mg cholesterol
169 mg sodium
10 g carbohydrate
1 g fiber
2 g protein

DIABETIC EXCHANGE
1 starch

I've relied on this bread recipe often over the years. Frozen dough hurries along the golden pull-apart loaf, which is wonderful with spaghetti and other Italian dishes.

Charlene Bzdok, Little Falls, Minnesota

1 loaf (1 pound) frozen bread dough, thawed

1/2 cup finely chopped sweet onion

1/2 cup butter, melted

2 garlic cloves, minced

1 teaspoon dried parsley flakes

1/4 teaspoon salt

1. Divide dough into 24 pieces. In a small bowl, combine the remaining ingredients. Dip each piece of dough into butter mixture; place in a 10-in. fluted tube pan coated with cooking spray.

2. Cover and let rise in a warm place until doubled, about 1 hour. Bake at 375° for 20-25 minutes or until golden brown. Serve warm.

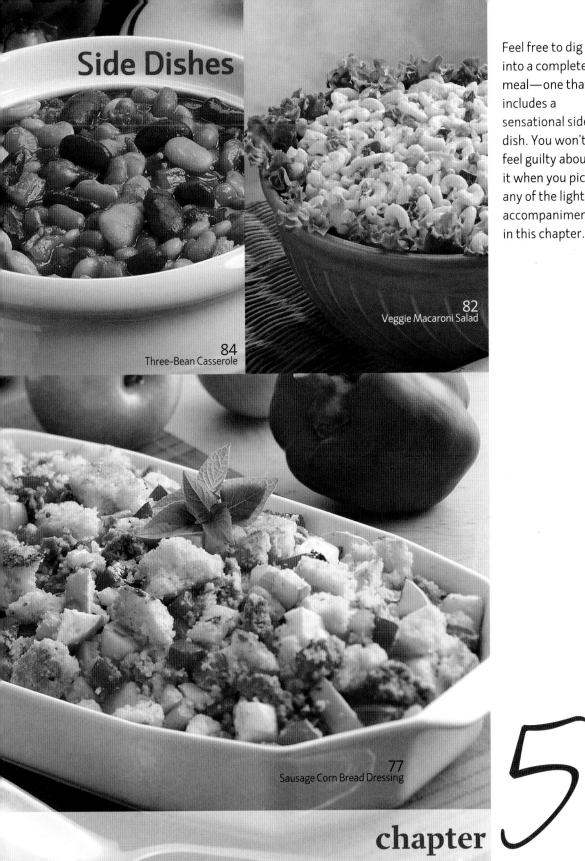

Side Dishes

Feel free to dig into a complete meal—one that includes a sensational side dish. You won't feel guilty about it when you pick any of the light accompaniments in this chapter.

82
Veggie Macaroni Salad

84
Three-Bean Casserole

77
Sausage Corn Bread Dressing

chapter 5

Sweet Potato Apple Scallop

PREP/TOTAL TIME
Prep: 30 min.
Bake: 25 min.
YIELD 7 servings

NUTRITION FACTS
One serving
(2/3 cup) equals:
221 calories
7 g fat
2 g saturated fat
9 mg cholesterol
48 mg sodium
41 g carbohydrate
4 g fiber
2 g protein

DIABETIC EXCHANGES
1-1/2 starch
1 fruit
1 fat

With apple slices and a topping of pecans, these sweet potatoes are ideal for holiday dinners. My cousin shared the recipe.

Sarah Joyce, Bedford, Texas

2	pounds sweet potatoes (about 3 medium)
2	medium apples, peeled and cored
1	tablespoon lemon juice
1/2	cup packed brown sugar
1/4	cup chopped pecans
1/2	teaspoon ground cinnamon
1/2	teaspoon pumpkin pie spice
1/2	teaspoon orange extract
2	tablespoons butter

1. Place sweet potatoes in a saucepan and cover with water. Bring to a boil; cook for 20-25 minutes or until tender. Drain and cool. Peel potatoes and cut into 1/4-in. slices. Place in a 13-in. x 9-in. x 2-in. baking dish coated with cooking spray. Cut apples into 1/4-in. rings; cut in half. Arrange over sweet potatoes. Sprinkle with lemon juice.

2. Combine the brown sugar, pecans, cinnamon, pumpkin pie spice and orange extract; sprinkle over apples. Dot with butter. Bake, uncovered, at 350° for 25-30 minutes or until apples are tender.

Baked Basil Fries

PREP/TOTAL TIME
Prep: 10 min.
Bake: 30 min.
YIELD 4 servings

NUTRITION FACTS
One serving equals:
162 calories
5 g fat
0 g saturated fat
5 mg cholesterol
117 mg sodium
27 g carbohydrate
3 g fiber
7 g protein

DIABETIC EXCHANGES
1-1/2 starch
1 fat

A Parmesan cheese and basil coating gives these "homegrown" fries their terrific flavor. They're a zippy alternative to high-fat fries.

Tammy Neubauer, Ida Grove, Iowa

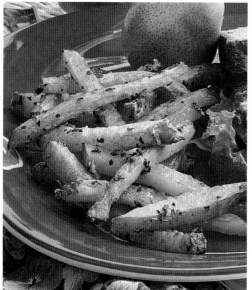

1/4	cup grated Parmesan cheese
1	tablespoon olive oil
1	tablespoon dried basil
1/4	teaspoon garlic powder
4	medium red potatoes

1. In a bowl, combine Parmesan cheese, oil, basil and garlic powder. Cut potatoes into 1/4-in. sticks. Add to cheese mixture; toss to coat.

2. Place in a 15-in. x 10-in. x 1-in. baking pan coated with cooking spray. Bake at 425° for 15 minutes; turn potatoes. Bake 15-20 minutes longer or until crisp and tender.

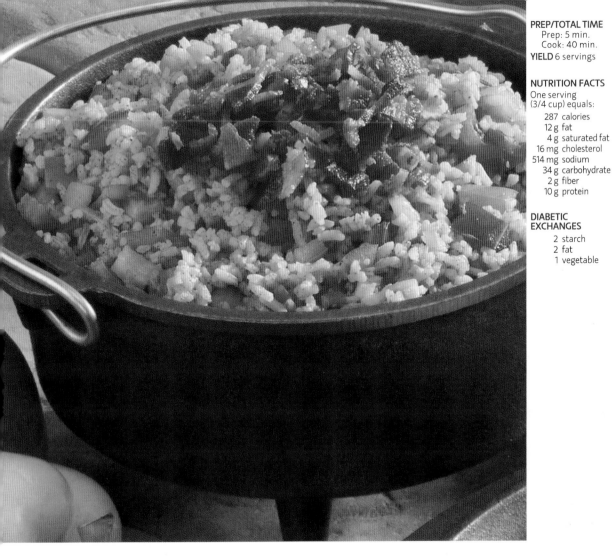

PREP/TOTAL TIME
Prep: 5 min.
Cook: 40 min.
YIELD 6 servings

NUTRITION FACTS
One serving
(3/4 cup) equals:
287 calories
12 g fat
4 g saturated fat
16 mg cholesterol
514 mg sodium
34 g carbohydrate
2 g fiber
10 g protein

DIABETIC EXCHANGES
2 starch
2 fat
1 vegetable

Spanish Rice with Bacon

I top off my Spanish Rice with Bacon for a hearty change of pace. A few jalapeno peppers give it an extra kick.

David Bias, Siloam Springs, Arkansas

- 6 bacon strips, diced
- 1 tablespoon canola oil
- 1 medium onion, chopped
- 1 cup uncooked long grain rice
- 1-3/4 cups water
- 2 large tomatoes, chopped
- 1 medium green pepper, chopped
- 2 jalapeno peppers, seeded and chopped
- 1 to 1-1/2 teaspoons chili powder
- 1/2 teaspoon salt

1. In a skillet, cook bacon over medium heat until crisp. Remove to paper towels. Add oil to the drippings; saute onion for 3 minutes. Add rice; cook and stir for 5 minutes or until golden brown. Stir in the remaining ingredients. Bring to a boil. Reduce heat; cover and simmer for 30 minutes or until rice is tender. Sprinkle with bacon.

Editor's Note: When cutting hot peppers, disposable gloves are recommended. Avoid touching your face.

Confetti Barley Pilaf

The slightly chewy texture of the barley, the tender vegetables and lively spices make this pilaf special enough for company.

Kris Erickson, Everett, Washington

PREP/TOTAL TIME
Prep: 10 min.
Cook: 55 min.
YIELD 6 servings

NUTRITION FACTS
One serving
(2/3 cup) equals:
169 calories
3 g fat
Trace saturated fat
0 mg cholesterol
507 mg sodium
32 g carbohydrate
7 g fiber
5 g protein

DIABETIC EXCHANGES
1-1/2 starch
1 vegetable
1/2 fat

1 large onion, finely chopped
1 garlic clove, minced
1 tablespoon canola oil
1 cup medium pearl barley
1 cup sliced fresh mushrooms
1/2 cup shredded carrot
1/2 cup coarsely shredded cabbage
1/2 cup chopped sweet red pepper
1 teaspoon dried basil
1 teaspoon dried oregano
2-1/2 cups chicken broth or vegetable broth

1. In a large nonstick skillet, saute the onion and garlic in oil until tender. Add the barley; saute for 3-5 minutes or until lightly browned. Add the mushrooms, carrot, cabbage, red pepper, basil and oregano. Cook and stir until the vegetables are crisp-tender, about 3 minutes.

2. Stir in broth; bring to a boil. Reduce heat; cover and simmer for 40-45 minutes or until liquid is absorbed and barley is tender.

Savory 'n' Saucy Baked Beans

This recipe dresses up canned baked beans in a jiffy using green pepper, tomatoes and celery. With just a hint of sweetness and a touch of garlic, this dish is a natural for summer picnics and patio meals.

A.G. Strickland, Marietta, Georgia

- 1/2 cup chopped onion
- 1/2 cup chopped green pepper
- 1/2 cup chopped celery
- 1 can (28 ounces) vegetarian baked beans
- 1 can (14-1/2 ounces) diced tomatoes, drained
- 1/2 teaspoon pepper
- 1/4 teaspoon salt
- 1/4 teaspoon garlic powder

1. In a large saucepan coated with cooking spray, cook the onion, green pepper and celery for 3 minutes or until tender. Stir in beans, tomatoes, pepper, salt and garlic powder. Bring to a boil. Reduce heat; simmer, uncovered, for 10-15 minutes.

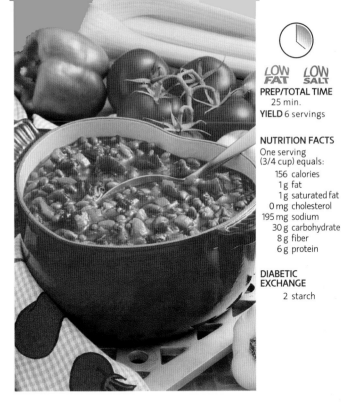

LOW FAT   LOW SALT

PREP/TOTAL TIME
25 min.
YIELD 6 servings

NUTRITION FACTS
One serving
(3/4 cup) equals:
- 156 calories
- 1 g fat
- 1 g saturated fat
- 0 mg cholesterol
- 195 mg sodium
- 30 g carbohydrate
- 8 g fiber
- 6 g protein

DIABETIC EXCHANGE
2 starch

Garlic-Chive Mashed Potatoes

Creamy and comforting, these savory spuds will complement many entrees. Stir in extra broth to get the texture you desire.

Leslie Cain, Starkville, Mississippi

- 3-1/2 pounds russet potatoes (about 5 large), peeled and quartered
- 3 garlic cloves, peeled
- 1/8 teaspoon paprika
- 1-1/2 cups (12 ounces) fat-free sour cream
- 1 cup reduced-sodium chicken broth, warmed
- 2 tablespoons minced chives
- 1 teaspoon salt
- 1/4 teaspoon pepper

1. Place the potatoes, garlic and paprika in a large saucepan or Dutch oven; cover with water. Bring to a boil. Reduce heat; cover and cook for 15-20 minutes or until potatoes are tender. Drain.

2. In a large mixing bowl, beat potatoes and garlic. Add the sour cream, broth, chives, salt and pepper; beat until smooth.

LIVELY CHIVES

An easy-to-grow perennial, chives lend a mild onion flavor to potatoes, eggs, fish and other dishes. To preserve your fresh chives, snip them into 1/4-inch lengths and freeze them in airtight storage containers.

LOW FAT

PREP/TOTAL TIME
30 min.
YIELD 10 servings

NUTRITION FACTS
One serving
(3/4 cup) equals:
- 152 calories
- 1 g fat
- 1 g saturated fat
- 0 mg cholesterol
- 354 mg sodium
- 33 g carbohydrate
- 2 g fiber
- 5 g protein

DIABETIC EXCHANGE
2 starch

Light Sweet Potato Casserole

You're bound to have sweet potato success when you whip up this casserole recipe. With its rich color, creamy texture and irresistible taste, it's sure to be a popular stop on your holiday table.

Taste of Home Test Kitchen

3 pounds sweet potatoes, peeled and cut into chunks

1/3 cup fat-free milk

1/4 cup egg substitute

2 tablespoons brown sugar

1/2 teaspoon salt

1/2 teaspoon vanilla extract

1/4 teaspoon ground cinnamon

1. Place sweet potatoes in a large saucepan or Dutch oven; cover with water. Bring to a boil. Reduce heat; cover and cook for 25-30 minutes or until tender. Drain.

2. In a large mixing bowl, beat the sweet potatoes, milk, egg substitute, brown sugar, salt and vanilla until smooth.

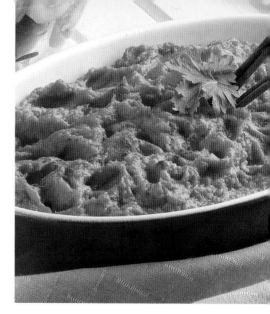

Transfer to a 1-1/2-qt. baking dish coated with cooking spray. Sprinkle with cinnamon. Bake, uncovered, at 350° for 25-30 minutes or until heated through.

Salsa Red Beans 'n' Rice

This skillet recipe is quick to prepare using canned kidney beans, brown rice and salsa. It's great with Mexican-style entrees but can also be served as a meatless main dish.

Diane Harrison, Mechanicsburg, Pennsylvania

1 medium green pepper, chopped

1/4 cup chopped red onion

3 green onions, finely chopped

4 garlic cloves, minced

1 tablespoon olive oil

5 cups cooked brown rice

1-1/4 cups salsa

1 can (16 ounces) kidney beans, rinsed and drained

1/2 teaspoon salt

1. In a large nonstick skillet, saute the green pepper, onions and garlic in oil until tender. Stir in the rice, salsa, beans and salt. Bring to a boil. Reduce the heat; simmer, uncovered, for 2-3 minutes or until heated through.

ABOUT BROWN RICE

Brown rice has the bran coating and the germ, which white rice does not. The bran is what makes brown rice a good source of fiber. Beside fiber, bran gives brown rice a nutty flavor and chewy texture and increases the cooking time. The germ is rich in oil, which over time will cause the rice to become rancid. Store brown rice in an airtight for up to six months. For longer storage refrigerate or freeze it.

Sausage Corn Bread Dressing

The phrases "holiday dinner" and "low-fat" are seldom used together...unless this corn bread stuffing is on the menu!

Rebecca Baird, Salt Lake City, Utah

- 1 cup all-purpose flour
- 1 cup cornmeal
- 1/4 cup sugar
- 3 teaspoons baking powder
- 1 teaspoon salt
- 1 cup buttermilk
- 1/4 cup unsweetened applesauce
- 2 egg whites

DRESSING:

- 1 pound turkey Italian sausage links, casings removed
- 4 celery ribs, chopped
- 1 medium onion, chopped
- 1 medium sweet red pepper, chopped
- 2 medium tart apples, chopped
- 1 cup chopped roasted or canned sweet chestnuts
- 3 tablespoons minced fresh parsley
- 2 garlic cloves, minced
- 1/2 teaspoon dried thyme
- 1/2 teaspoon pepper
- 1 cup reduced-sodium chicken broth
- 1 egg white

1. For corn bread, combine the first five ingredients in a large bowl. Combine the buttermilk, applesauce and egg whites; stir into dry ingredients just until moistened. Pour into an 8-in. square baking dish coated with cooking spray. Bake at 400° for 20-25 minutes or until a toothpick inserted near the center comes out clean. Cool on a wire rack.

2. In a large nonstick skillet, cook the sausage, celery, onion and red pepper over medium heat until meat is no longer pink; drain. Transfer to a large bowl. Crumble corn bread over mixture. Add apples, chestnuts, parsley, garlic, thyme and pepper. Stir in broth and egg white.

3. Transfer to a 13-in. x 9-in. x 2-in. baking dish coated with cooking spray. Cover and bake at 325° for 40 minutes. Uncover; bake 10 minutes longer or until lightly browned.

LOW FAT

PREP/TOTAL TIME
Prep: 30 min.
Bake: 50 min.

YIELD 16 servings

NUTRITION FACTS
One serving
(3/4 cup) equals:
- 164 calories
- 3 g fat
- 1 g saturated fat
- 16 mg cholesterol
- 473 mg sodium
- 25 g carbohydrate
- 2 g fiber
- 8 g protein

DIABETIC EXCHANGES
- 1-1/2 starch
- 1 vegetable

Mashed Potato Bake

PREP/TOTAL TIME
Prep: 35 min.
Bake: 35 min.
YIELD 12 servings

NUTRITION FACTS
One serving
(3/4 cup) equals:
185 calories
3 g fat
2 g saturated fat
13 mg cholesterol
507 mg sodium
37 g carbohydrate
2 g fiber
5 g protein

DIABETIC EXCHANGE
2-1/2 starch

I've made and shared this recipe so many times that my friends now refer to it as "Margie's Potatoes." It goes wonderfully with everything from beef to fish.

Margery Richmond, Fort Collins, Colorado

5 pounds potatoes, peeled and quartered

1 package (8 ounces) reduced-fat cream cheese, cubed

1 cup (8 ounces) reduced-fat sour cream

1/4 cup fat-free milk

1 teaspoon onion salt

1 teaspoon salt

Dash pepper

1. Place potatoes in a Dutch oven and cover with water. Bring to a boil. Reduce heat; cover and cook for 15-20 minutes or until tender. Drain.

2. In a large mixing bowl, mash the potatoes. Add the remaining ingredients; beat until blended. Transfer to a 13-in. x 9-in. x 2-in. baking dish coated with cooking spray. Bake, uncovered, at 350° for 30-35 minutes or until top is lightly browned.

Home-Style Coleslaw

PREP/TOTAL TIME
Prep: 20 min. + chilling
YIELD 7 servings

NUTRITION FACTS
One serving
(2/3 cup) equals:
88 calories
4 g fat
1 g saturated fat
5 mg cholesterol
292 mg sodium
12 g carbohydrate
3 g fiber
2 g protein

DIABETIC EXCHANGES
2 vegetable
1 fat

When chicken is on our table, this coleslaw usually makes an appearance, too. It's a mealtime staple at our house.

Joy Cochran, Roy, Washington

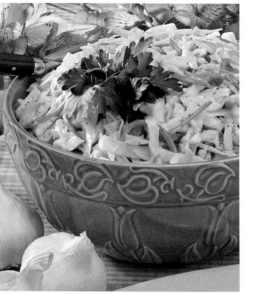

8 cups finely shredded cabbage

1/2 cup shredded carrot

DRESSING:

1/3 cup reduced-fat mayonnaise

1/3 cup fat-free sour cream

1 tablespoon sugar

2 teaspoons cider vinegar

1/2 teaspoon salt

1/4 teaspoon pepper

1. In a large bowl, combine cabbage and carrot. In a small bowl, combine the dressing ingredients. Pour over cabbage mixture; toss to coat. Cover and refrigerate for 6-8 hours or overnight.

Southwestern Hominy

Colorful and cheesy, this dish gets great flavor from green chilies and seasonings. It'll add pizzazz to most any meal.

Martha Holland, Reno, Nevada

- 1 cup chopped onion
- 2 garlic cloves, minced
- 2 cans (15-1/2 ounces *each*) yellow hominy, drained
- 2 cups chopped tomatoes
- 1 can (4 ounces) chopped green chilies
- 1 teaspoon chili powder
- 1/2 teaspoon ground cumin
- 1/4 teaspoon pepper
- 1/2 cup shredded reduced-fat cheddar cheese

1. In a large skillet coated with cooking spray, saute onion and garlic until tender. Add the hominy, tomatoes, chilies, chili powder, cumin and pepper; mix gently.

2. Transfer to a 2-qt. baking dish coated with cooking spray. Bake, uncovered, at 350° for 25 minutes. Sprinkle with cheese; bake 5 minutes longer or until the cheese is melted.

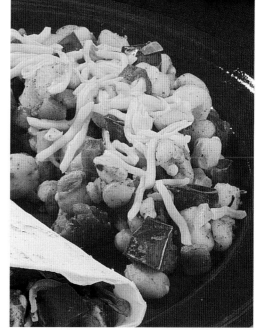

LOW FAT   LOW SALT

PREP/TOTAL TIME
Prep: 5 min.
Bake: 30 min.
YIELD 12 servings

NUTRITION FACTS
One serving
(1/2 cup) equals:
76 calories
1 g fat
0 g saturated fat
1 mg cholesterol
223 mg sodium
14 g carbohydrate
0 g fiber
3 g protein

DIABETIC EXCHANGE
1 starch

Maple-Glazed Parsnips and Carrots

There's a sweet hint of springtime in this veggie medley I drizzle with reduced-calorie syrup. It comes together quickly, too.

Bill Richards, Ironwood, Michigan

- 1 pound carrots, cut into 1/4-inch slices
- 1 pound parsnips, cut into 1/4-inch slices
- 4-1/2 teaspoons butter
- 1/4 cup plus 2 tablespoons reduced-calorie pancake syrup
- 1/4 cup orange juice
- 2 teaspoons grated orange peel
- 1/2 teaspoon salt
- 1 teaspoon minced fresh parsley

1. In a large skillet, cook and stir carrots and parsnips over medium heat in butter for 5 minutes. Combine the pancake syrup, orange juice, orange peel and salt; pour over carrot mixture. Cook over medium-high heat until mixture comes to a boil. Cover and cook for 6-7 minutes or until vegetables are crisp-tender.

2. Uncover; cook 1-2 minutes longer or until vegetables are tender and syrup mixture thickens and coats the vegetables. Sprinkle with parsley.

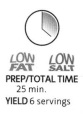

LOW FAT   LOW SALT

PREP/TOTAL TIME
25 min.
YIELD 6 servings

NUTRITION FACTS
One serving
(2/3 cup) equals:
144 calories
3 g fat
2 g saturated fat
8 mg cholesterol
279 mg sodium
29 g carbohydrate
4 g fiber
2 g protein

DIABETIC EXCHANGES
2 vegetable
1 starch
1/2 fat

NUTRITION FACTS
One serving
(1 cup) equals:
226 calories
7 g fat
5 g saturated fat
24 mg cholesterol
527 mg sodium
23 g carbohydrate
2 g fiber
19 g protein

**DIABETIC
EXCHANGES**
2 lean meat
1 starch
1 vegetable

Broccoli Rice Hot Dish

With broccoli, cheddar cheese and red peppers, this bountiful bake has plenty of appeal as a side dish or light entree.

Gretchen Widner, Sun City West, Arizona

2 cups hot cooked rice

3/4 cup shredded reduced-fat cheddar cheese

1/2 cup egg substitute

3/4 teaspoon garlic salt

FILLING:

1 package (10 ounces) frozen chopped broccoli, thawed

4 ounces chopped fresh mushrooms

1/2 cup chopped sweet red pepper

1/2 medium onion, chopped

1 cup egg substitute

1/2 cup fat-free milk

1/2 teaspoon onion salt

1/2 teaspoon pepper

1 cup (4 ounces) shredded reduced-fat cheddar cheese

1. In a large bowl, combine the rice, cheese, egg substitute and garlic salt. Press firmly into a 2-qt. baking dish coated with cooking spray. Bake at 375° for 10 minutes.

2. Meanwhile, place the broccoli, mushrooms, red pepper and onion in a steamer basket over 1 in. of boiling water in a saucepan. Bring to a boil; cover and steam for 5 minutes or until crisp-tender.

3. In a large bowl, combine the egg substitute, milk, onion salt and pepper; stir in vegetables. Pour over crust. Sprinkle with cheese. Bake, uncovered, at 375° for 25-30 minutes or until a knife inserted near the center comes out clean.

Salsa Potato Salad

Summer is a great time for potato salad, but fixing it with regular mayonnaise adds too much fat. Salsa perks up this version and disguises the fact that it's lighter.

Janet Lewis, Bangor, Pennsylvania

- 1/3 cup fat-free mayonnaise
- 2 tablespoons fat-free sour cream
- 1/4 cup salsa
- 1 tablespoon minced fresh parsley
- 3 cups cubed cooked unpeeled potatoes
- 1 celery rib, thinly sliced
- 1/4 cup chopped onion
- 1/2 cup shredded reduced-fat cheddar cheese

1. In a bowl, combine the mayonnaise, sour cream, salsa and parsley. In a large bowl, combine the potatoes, celery and onion. Add dressing and toss to coat. Stir in cheese. Cover and refrigerate for at least 1 hour before serving.

PREP/TOTAL TIME
Prep: 10 min. + chilling
YIELD 7 servings

NUTRITION FACTS
One serving
(1/2 cup) equals:
101 calories
2 g fat
1 g saturated fat
8 mg cholesterol
194 mg sodium
17 g carbohydrate
2 g fiber
4 g protein

DIABETIC EXCHANGE
1 starch

Crispy Baked Cauliflower

I prepare this simple side dish often. It's a tasty treatment for healthy cauliflower.

Elvera Dallman, Franklin, Nebraska

- 4 cups cauliflowerets
- 6 tablespoons all-purpose flour
- 1/4 teaspoon garlic powder
- 1/4 teaspoon paprika
- 1/4 teaspoon pepper
- 2-1/2 cups cornflakes, crushed
- 2 egg whites

1. Place cauliflower in a saucepan with a small amount of water. Cover and cook for 5-10 minutes or until crisp-tender; drain.

2. In a small resealable plastic bag, combine flour, garlic powder, paprika and pepper. Place cornflake crumbs in another resealable plastic bag. Lightly beat egg whites in a shallow bowl. Toss the cauliflowerets one at a time in flour mixture, then roll in egg whites and coat with crumbs. Place on a baking sheet coated with cooking spray. Bake at 425° for 15-20 minutes or until golden brown. Serve immediately.

THE POWER OF CAULIFLOWER

This low-calorie veggie packs a powerful nutrition punch. Cauliflower is an excellent source of vitamins C and K and a good source of vitamin B6 and folate. It also a good source of fiber.

PREP/TOTAL TIME
Prep: 20 min.
Bake: 15 min.
YIELD 6 servings

NUTRITION FACTS
One serving
(3/4 cup) equals:
92 calories
Trace fat
0 g saturated fat
0 mg cholesterol
145 mg sodium
19 g carbohydrate
0 g fiber
4 g protein

DIABETIC EXCHANGES
1 starch
1 vegetable

Tangy Onion Flowers

These flavorful baked onions are great with grilled meat. They aren't crispy like the fried "blooming onions" in restaurants, but we think they're equally delicious.

Karen Owen, Rising Sun, Indiana

PREP/TOTAL TIME
Prep: 25 min.
Bake: 30 min.
YIELD 8 servings

NUTRITION FACTS
One serving (1 half of an onion) equals:
48 calories
Trace fat
Trace saturated fat
0 mg cholesterol
203 mg sodium
11 g carbohydrate
1 g fiber
1 g protein

DIABETIC EXCHANGE
2 vegetable

    4 large sweet onions, peeled
  1/4 cup red wine vinegar
    1 tablespoon brown sugar
    1 teaspoon dried oregano
  1/2 teaspoon salt
  1/4 teaspoon pepper
  1/2 cup coarsely crushed fat-free salad croutons

1. Place the onions root end up on a microwave-safe plate. Microwave, uncovered, on high for 7-9 minutes or until crisp-tender. Invert onto a cutting board. Slice each onion into eight wedges to within 1/2 in. of bottom; fan out. Place each onion on a 12-in. square piece of foil coated with cooking spray.

2. In a small bowl, combine vinegar, brown sugar, oregano, salt and pepper. Brush some over onions; set remaining mixture aside. Fold foil around onions; seal tightly.

3. Place on a baking sheet. Bake at 425° for 30-35 minutes or until tender. Open foil carefully. Place onions on a serving platter. Drizzle with remaining vinegar mixture; sprinkle with croutons.

Editor's Note: This recipe was tested in a 1,100-watt microwave.

RED OR WHITE

Just like table wine, wine vinegar is made from red or white grapes. Red wine vinegar has a ruby red color and adds a pungent flavor to foods. It's used in vinaigrettes, sauces, marinades and meat dishes.

Veggie Macaroni Salad

When I bring this super salad to our church dinners, there's usually nothing left to take home. Toss in 2 or 3 cups of cooked turkey or chicken to create a filling main-dish.

Lynn Cole, Sagle, Idaho

PREP/TOTAL TIME
Prep: 35 min. + chilling
YIELD 10 servings

NUTRITION FACTS
One serving (3/4 cup) equals:
234 calories
8 g fat
2 g saturated fat
31 mg cholesterol
246 mg sodium
32 g carbohydrate
2 g fiber
8 g protein

DIABETIC EXCHANGES
2 starch
1-1/2 fat

    2 cups uncooked elbow macaroni
    1 large tomato, seeded and chopped
    1 cup frozen peas, thawed
  1/2 cup shredded reduced-fat cheddar cheese
  1/2 cup chopped celery
    1 hard-cooked egg, chopped
    2 green onions, sliced
DRESSING:
  3/4 cup reduced-fat mayonnaise
    1 cup fat-free plain yogurt
    2 tablespoons sugar
    1 tablespoon prepared mustard
  1/8 teaspoon celery seed

1. Cook macaroni according to package directions; drain and rinse in cold water. In a large bowl, combine the macaroni, tomato, peas, cheese, celery, egg and onions.

2. In a small bowl, combine the dressing ingredients. Pour over macaroni mixture and toss to coat. Refrigerate until serving.

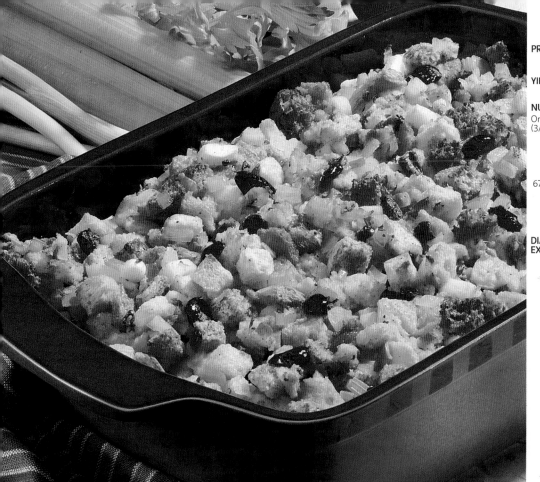

LOW FAT

PREP/TOTAL TIME
Prep: 20 min.
Bake: 30 min.
YIELD 12 servings

NUTRITION FACTS
One serving
(3/4 cup) equals:
183 calories
5 g fat
2 g saturated fat
5 mg cholesterol
671 mg sodium
31 g carbohydrate
2 g fiber
4 g protein

DIABETIC EXCHANGES
1 starch
1 fat
1/2 fruit

Sweet 'n' Savory Apple Stuffing

For Thanksgiving one year, I wanted a new stuffing recipe. With its bits of fruit and nuts, this one has become my favorite.

Karen Horne Staab, New Rochelle, New York

1 medium tart apple, peeled and chopped

2 celery ribs, chopped

1 medium onion, chopped

1/4 cup minced fresh parsley

3 green onions, thinly sliced

2 tablespoons chopped celery leaves

2 tablespoons butter

1/2 cup tropical medley dried fruit mix

1/4 cup dried cranberries

1/4 cup chopped pecans

1 teaspoon poultry seasoning

1/2 teaspoon salt

1/2 teaspoon rubbed sage

1/4 teaspoon pepper

1 can (14-1/2 ounces) reduced-sodium chicken broth

1-1/2 cups water

1 package (12 ounces) unseasoned stuffing croutons

1. In a skillet, cook the apple, celery, onion, parsley, green onions and celery leaves in butter until tender. Stir in the fruit mix, cranberries, pecans, poultry seasoning, salt, sage and pepper; mix well. Stir in broth, water and stuffing. Toss to coat evenly.

2. Transfer to a 13-in. x 9-in. x 2-in. baking dish coated with cooking spray. Cover and bake at 350° for 20 minutes. Uncover; bake 10-15 minutes longer or until heated through and lightly browned.

Three-Bean Casserole

This recipe came from a family reunion and is over 30 years old. I often take a big pot of these beans to large gatherings.

Jane Bone, Cape Coral, Florida

PREP/TOTAL TIME
Prep: 15 min.
Bake: 50 min.
YIELD 9 servings

NUTRITION FACTS
One serving
(3/4 cup) equals:
238 calories
3 g fat
1 g saturated fat
5 mg cholesterol
864 mg sodium
46 g carbohydrate
10 g fiber
10 g protein

DIABETIC EXCHANGES
2-1/2 starch
1 very lean meat

2 bacon strips, chopped
1 large green pepper, chopped
1 medium onion, chopped
1 can (28 ounces) pork and beans
1 can (16 ounces) kidney beans, rinsed and drained
1 can (15-1/4 ounces) lima beans, rinsed and drained
1/2 cup ketchup
1 jar (4 ounces) diced pimientos
1/4 cup packed brown sugar
1 tablespoon Worcestershire sauce
1 teaspoon ground mustard

1. In a large nonstick skillet, cook bacon over medium heat until crisp. Remove to paper towels; drain, reserving 1 tablespoon drippings. In the drippings, saute green pepper and onion until tender.

2. Combine the beans in a large bowl. Gently stir in the pepper mixture and bacon. Stir in the ketchup, pimientos, brown sugar, Worcestershire sauce and mustard until combined.

3. Transfer to a 2-qt. baking dish coated with cooking spray. Cover and bake at 350° for 50-60 minutes or until bubbly.

Fried Rice

I like to turn leftover rice into this tasty new side dish. With just four ingredients, it couldn't be easier to put together.

Suzanne McKinley, Lyons, Georgia

1/2	cup chopped green pepper

Egg substitute equivalent to 2 eggs

4	cups cooked rice
2	tablespoons reduced-sodium soy sauce

1. In a skillet coated with cooking spray, saute pepper until crisp-tender. Add egg substitute; cook and stir until egg is completely set. Chop egg into small pieces. Add rice and soy sauce; heat through.

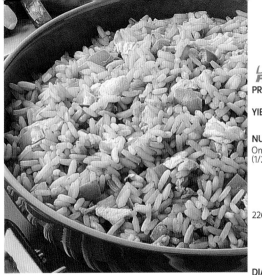

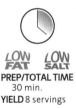

LOW FAT   LOW SALT

PREP/TOTAL TIME
15 min.
YIELD 9 servings

NUTRITION FACTS
One serving
(1/2 cup) equals:
105 calories
1 g fat
0 g saturated fat
1 mg cholesterol
226 mg sodium
20 g carbohydrate
0 g fiber
4 g protein

DIABETIC EXCHANGES
1 starch
1 vegetable

Confetti Potato Pancakes

My husband's family is Irish, and his mother makes potato pancakes quite often. Crispy on the outside and soft inside, these receive rave reviews, especially from my in-laws!

Betsy McDaniels, Colfax, Illinois

2	large potatoes (about 1-1/2 pounds)
2	medium zucchini
2	large carrots
1/2	cup finely chopped onion, *divided*
2	eggs, lightly beaten
1/2	cup all-purpose flour
1	to 2 garlic cloves, minced
1/2	teaspoon salt
1/2	teaspoon dried basil
1/4	teaspoon sugar
1	tablespoon canola oil

1. Coarsely shred the potatoes, zucchini and carrots; drain and pat dry. Place half of the shredded vegetables and 1/4 cup chopped onion in a food processor or blender; cover and process until finely chopped. Transfer to a bowl; add the eggs, flour, garlic, salt, basil, sugar and remaining onion and shredded vegetables.

2. In a large nonstick skillet, heat oil. Drop batter by 1/4 cupfuls into skillet; flatten to form patties. Fry until golden brown; turn and cook the second side.

LOW FAT   LOW SALT

PREP/TOTAL TIME
30 min.
YIELD 8 servings

NUTRITION FACTS
One serving
(2 pancakes) equals:
148 calories
3 g fat
1 g saturated fat
53 mg cholesterol
176 mg sodium
26 g carbohydrate
3 g fiber
5 g protein

DIABETIC EXCHANGES
1-1/2 starch
1 vegetable

LOW SALT

PREP/TOTAL TIME
15 min.
YIELD 8 servings

NUTRITION FACTS
One serving
(3/4 cup) equals:
135 calories
10 g fat
4 g saturated fat
19 mg cholesterol
198 mg sodium
7 g carbohydrate
2 g fiber
7 g protein

DIABETIC EXCHANGES
1 lean meat
1 vegetable
1 fat

Cheesy Zucchini Medley

When you have a bounty of garden-fresh zucchini, try this easy and delicious dish. It's wonderful to make on camping trips.

Ruth Ann Stelfox, Raymond, Alberta

4 medium zucchini, cut into 1/4-inch slices

1 large sweet onion, thinly sliced and separated into rings

1 medium sweet yellow pepper, julienned

1 medium green pepper, julienned

2 garlic cloves, minced

2 tablespoons canola oil

1/4 teaspoon salt

1/4 teaspoon pepper

1 cup (4 ounces) shredded cheddar cheese

1/2 cup shredded part-skim mozzarella cheese

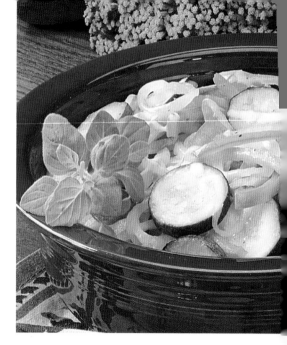

1. In a large skillet, saute the zucchini, onion, peppers and garlic in oil until crisp-tender. Sprinkle with salt and pepper; mix well. Sprinkle with cheeses. Remove from the heat. Let stand for 2-3 minutes or until cheese begins to melt.

LOW FAT **LOW SALT**

PREP/TOTAL TIME
15 min.
YIELD 16 servings

NUTRITION FACTS
One serving
(1/2 cup) equals:
96 calories
0 g fat
0 g saturated fat
0 mg cholesterol
100 mg sodium
22 g carbohydrate
2 g fiber
2 g protein

DIABETIC EXCHANGE
1-1/2 fruit

Creamy Fruit Salad

Four kinds of fruit combine with a smooth sauce in this yummy medley. I created it for my diabetic husband, and he loves it.

Loan Logan Lindley, Brackettville, Texas

1 can (20 ounces) unsweetened pineapple chunks, drained

1 can (15-1/4 ounces) sliced peaches in juice, drained

1 can (11 ounces) mandarin oranges, drained

4 medium tart apples, peeled and diced

1-1/2 cups cold fat-free milk

1/3 cup orange juice concentrate

1 package (1 ounce) sugar-free instant vanilla pudding mix

3/4 cup fat-free sour cream

1. In a large bowl, combine the fruit; set aside. In another bowl, whisk milk, orange juice concentrate and pudding mix for 2 minutes or until smooth. Add sour cream; mix well. Fold into fruit. Cover and refrigerate until serving.

Au Gratin Red Potatoes

I loved the potatoes my mother made when I was young, so I created this lightened-up version that goes well with any main course.

Kate Selner, St. Paul, Minnesota

- 2 pounds red potatoes, sliced
- 2 cups plus 2 tablespoons fat-free milk, *divided*
- 2 garlic cloves, minced
- 1 teaspoon dried basil
- 3/4 teaspoon salt
- 1/4 teaspoon pepper
- 3 tablespoons all-purpose flour
- 1/2 cup shredded cheddar cheese
- 1/4 cup shredded Parmesan cheese
- 2 tablespoons toasted wheat germ
- 1/2 teaspoon olive oil

1. In a large saucepan, combine the potatoes, 2 cups milk, garlic and seasonings. Bring to a boil. Reduce heat; simmer, uncovered, for 8-10 minutes or until potatoes are tender. With a slotted spoon, remove potatoes to a 1-1/2-qt. baking dish coated with cooking spray.

2. In a small bowl, combine flour and remaining milk until smooth; stir into hot milk mixture. Bring to a boil; cook and stir for 2 minutes until thickened. Reduce heat. Add cheddar cheese; stir until melted. Pour over potatoes; sprinkle with Parmesan. Combine wheat germ and oil; sprinkle over top.

3. Cover and bake at 375° for 20 minutes. Uncover; bake 5-10 minutes longer or until lightly browned and heated through. Let stand for 10 minutes before serving.

LOW FAT

PREP/TOTAL TIME
Prep: 20 min.
Bake: 25 min. + standing
YIELD 8 servings

NUTRITION FACTS
One serving
(1 cup) equals:
- 151 calories
- 4 g fat
- 2 g saturated fat
- 11 mg cholesterol
- 351 mg sodium
- 22 g carbohydrate
- 2 g fiber
- 8 g protein

DIABETIC EXCHANGES
1-1/2 starch
1/2 fat

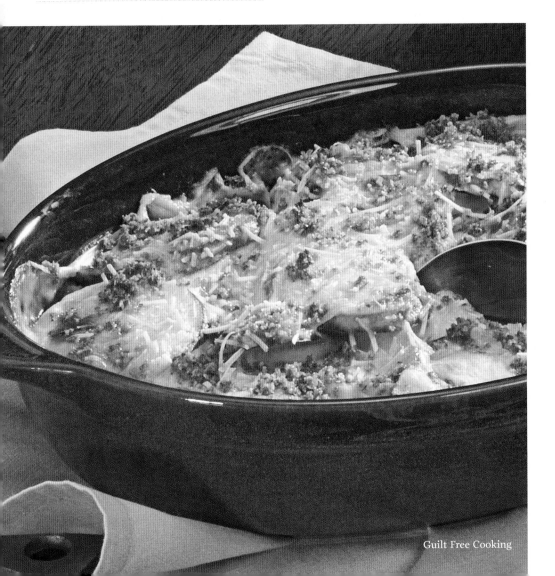

PREP/TOTAL TIME
Prep: 15 min. + chilling
YIELD 16 servings

NUTRITION FACTS
One serving
(1/2 cup) equals:
47 calories
1g fat
0g saturated fat
0mg cholesterol
46mg sodium
11g carbohydrate
0g fiber
2g protein

DIABETIC EXCHANGE
1 fruit

Molded Cranberry Fruit Salad

Cooking for someone on a restricted diet can be a real challenge, especially during the holidays when rich foods are prevalent. This cool and colorful salad appeals to everyone.

Virginia Rexroat, Jenks, Oklahoma

2 packages (.6 ounce *each*) sugar-free cherry gelatin

2 cups boiling water

1 package (12 ounces) fresh *or* frozen cranberries

1 large apple, peeled and chopped

1 large orange, peeled, chopped and seeded

1 piece of orange peel (1 inch)

1 can (20 ounces) crushed unsweetened pineapple, undrained

1. In a bowl, dissolve the gelatin in the boiling water. Stir in all remaining ingredients. Cool slightly.

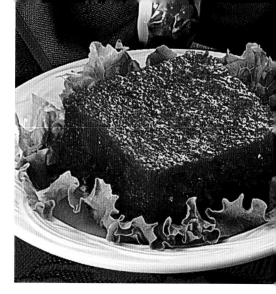

2. Process in small batches in a blender until coarsely chopped. Pour into a 13-in. x 9-in. x 2-in. dish or a 3-qt. serving bowl. Chill until set, about 2-3 hours.

PREP/TOTAL TIME
Prep: 5 min.
Bake: 30 min.
YIELD 7 servings

NUTRITION FACTS
One serving
(1 cup) equals:
81 calories
2g fat
0g saturated fat
4mg cholesterol
289mg sodium
11g carbohydrate
3g fiber
4g protein

DIABETIC EXCHANGES
1 vegetable
1/2 starch
1/2 fat

Creamy Broccoli Casserole

This saucy casserole won Grand Champion in the heart-healthy contest at a local fair. Folks always want to dig right in.

Rhonda Sells, Strafford, Missouri

2 packages (10 ounces *each*) frozen chopped broccoli, thawed and drained

1 can (10-3/4 ounces) reduced-fat reduced-sodium condensed cream of chicken soup, undiluted

2 teaspoons lemon juice

1/2 cup crushed seasoned stuffing

1 tablespoon reduced-fat margarine, melted

1/4 cup shredded reduced-fat cheddar cheese

1. Place broccoli in an 8-in. square baking dish coated with cooking spray. Combine soup and lemon juice; pour over broccoli. Toss stuffing and margarine; sprinkle over soup mixture.

2. Cover and bake at 350° for 25-30 minutes. Uncover; sprinkle with cheese. Bake 5 minutes longer or until cheese is melted.

CUTTING BUTTER

Margarine is a butter substitute made with vegetable oils. Both butter and regular margarine contain 80% fat (11 grams of fat per tablespoon). Using reduced-fat margarine in Creamy Broccoli Casserole makes this tasty dish lighter.

Cheese-Stuffed Potatoes

My husband and I often eat these as a main dish because they're so hearty.

Patricia Richardson, Bend, Oregon

- 4 medium baking potatoes (2 pounds)
- 1 cup chopped leeks (white portion only)
- 1 cup chopped onion
- 2 garlic cloves, minced
- 2 teaspoons olive oil
- 3/4 cup fresh or frozen corn
- 1/2 cup 2% cottage cheese
- 1/2 cup reduced-fat plain yogurt
- 1/2 teaspoon salt
- 1/4 teaspoon pepper

1. Wrap each potato in foil. Bake at 375° for 1 hour or until tender. Cool. Remove foil; cut potatoes in half lengthwise. Scoop out pulp, leaving a 1/4-in. shell; set shells aside. In a bowl, mash pulp until smooth.

2. In a skillet, saute the leeks, onion and garlic in oil. Add to mashed potatoes. Stir in the corn, cottage cheese, yogurt, salt and pepper. Spoon into potato shells.

3. Place on a baking sheet. Broil 6 in. from the heat for 3-5 minutes or until tops are golden brown.

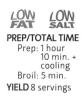

LOW FAT   LOW SALT

PREP/TOTAL TIME
Prep: 1 hour
10 min. +
cooling
Broil: 5 min.
YIELD 8 servings

NUTRITION FACTS
One serving
(1 potato half)
equals:
183 calories
2 g fat
1 g saturated fat
2 mg cholesterol
224 mg sodium
36 g carbohydrate
4 g fiber
6 g protein

DIABETIC EXCHANGES
2 starch
1 vegetable
1/2 fat

Green Bean Corn Casserole

This is a classic church-social dish and has become a family favorite. I reduced the fat in the recipe and find that it still has a very satisfying taste everyone loves.

Dawn Harvey, Danville, Pennsylvania

- 1 can (10-3/4 ounces) reduced-fat reduced-sodium condensed cream of celery soup, undiluted
- 1 cup (8 ounces) reduced-fat sour cream
- 1 cup (4 ounces) shredded reduced-fat cheddar cheese
- 1/2 cup finely chopped onion
- 1 package (16 ounces) frozen French-style green beans, thawed
- 2 cups frozen corn, thawed
- 1/4 cup crushed reduced-fat cheese crackers

Refrigerated butter-flavored spray

1. In a large bowl, combine the soup, sour cream, cheese and onion. Stir in the beans and corn. Transfer to a 2-qt. baking dish coated with cooking spray. Cover and bake at 350° for 25 minutes.

2. Uncover; sprinkle cracker crumbs around the edges. Spritz several times with butter-flavored spray. Bake 10-15 minutes longer or until heated through and edges are lightly browned.

PREP/TOTAL TIME
Prep: 10 min.
Bake: 35 min.
YIELD 7 servings

NUTRITION FACTS
One serving
(3/4 cup) equals:
178 calories
7 g fat
4 g saturated fat
18 mg cholesterol
454 mg sodium
22 g carbohydrate
3 g fiber
8 g protein

DIABETIC EXCHANGES
1 starch
1 lean meat
1 vegetable
1/2 fat

Dilly Potato Salad

Curry, dill and Dijon mustard provide the tangy flavor in this creamy potato salad.

Rosemarie Kondrk, Old Bridge, New Jersey

PREP/TOTAL TIME
Prep: 10 min.
Cook: 25 min.
YIELD 8 servings

NUTRITION FACTS
One serving
(2/3 cup) equals:
101 calories
Trace fat
0 g saturated fat
1 mg cholesterol
84 mg sodium
21 g carbohydrate
0 g fiber
4 g protein

DIABETIC EXCHANGE
1-1/2 starch

2 pounds red potatoes
1 cup fat-free plain yogurt
3 tablespoons fat-free mayonnaise
1/4 cup thinly sliced green onions
1 teaspoon Dijon mustard
1 teaspoon dill weed
1/2 teaspoon curry powder
1/8 teaspoon pepper

1. Place the potatoes in a large saucepan and cover with water; cover and bring to a boil. Cook until tender, about 25-30 minutes; drain.

2. In a large bowl, combine the remaining ingredients. Thinly slice potatoes; add to the yogurt mixture and toss gently until coated. Refrigerate until serving.

WITH OR WITHOUT THE SKIN

Potato salad...everyone has their favorite type. Generally, it's made without the skin. But for those who like to increase the amount of fiber in their diets leave the skin on. A serving of potatoes with the skin can have up to 3 grams of fiber. As an added bonus, you save kitchen time when you don't peel the spuds.

Broiled Parmesan Tomatoes

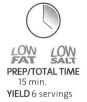

These tomatoes are a popular side dish in our home. Basil and garlic deliver plenty of flavor while a bread crumb topping gives a slight crunch to each serving.

Kara de la Vega, Somerset, California

PREP/TOTAL TIME
15 min.
YIELD 6 servings

NUTRITION FACTS
One serving
(1 tomato half)
equals:
55 calories
3 g fat
1 g saturated fat
1 mg cholesterol
64 mg sodium
6 g carbohydrate
1 g fiber
2 g protein

DIABETIC EXCHANGES
1 vegetable
1/2 fat

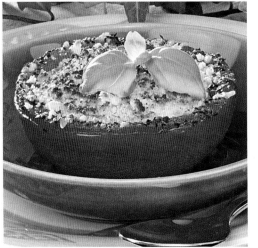

3 large tomatoes
1 tablespoon olive oil
1 garlic clove, minced
1/4 teaspoon coarsely ground pepper
1 tablespoon minced fresh basil *or* 1 teaspoon dried basil
3/4 cup soft bread crumbs
2 tablespoons grated Parmesan cheese

1. Slice tomatoes in half. Using a small spoon, remove seeds. Place tomato halves on a broiler pan coated with cooking spray. Combine the oil, garlic and pepper. Brush over tomatoes. Sprinkle with basil.

2. Broil about 6 in. from the heat for 3-4 minutes or until heated through. In a small bowl, combine bread crumbs and Parmesan cheese. Sprinkle over tomatoes. Broil 1-2 minutes longer or until crumbs are lightly browned. Serve immediately.

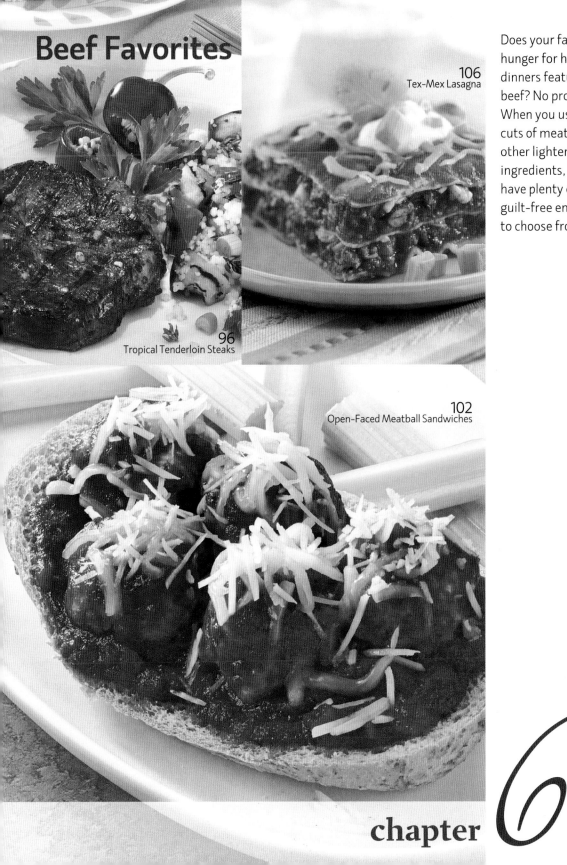

Beef Favorites

106
Tex-Mex Lasagna

96
Tropical Tenderloin Steaks

102
Open-Faced Meatball Sandwiches

Does your family hunger for hearty dinners featuring beef? No problem! When you use lean cuts of meat and other lightened-up ingredients, you'll have plenty of guilt-free entrees to choose from.

chapter 6

Mushroom Pizza Burgers

There's nothing better than a grilled burger at a picnic. This recipe fills the bill deliciously!

Harriet Stichter, Milford, Indiana

- 1/2 cup sliced fresh mushrooms
- 1/4 cup chopped onion
- 1 garlic clove, minced
- 1/2 teaspoon dried oregano
- 1 cup crushed tomatoes, undrained

BURGERS:

- 1-1/2 cups finely chopped fresh mushrooms
- 1/3 cup minced fresh basil
- 1 egg white, beaten
- 2 tablespoons grated Parmesan cheese
- 2 tablespoons dry bread crumbs
- 1/2 teaspoon salt
- 1/8 teaspoon pepper
- 1 pound lean ground beef
- 6 slices part-skim mozzarella cheese (3 ounces)
- 6 hamburger buns, split and toasted

1. In a small skillet coated with cooking spray, saute mushrooms and onion for 3 minutes. Add garlic and oregano; saute 1-2 minutes longer or until onion is tender. Stir in tomatoes. Cook, uncovered, over medium-low heat for 5 minutes, stirring occasionally. Set aside and keep warm.

2. In a large bowl, combine mushrooms, basil, egg white, Parmesan cheese, bread crumbs, salt and pepper. Crumble beef over mixture; mix well. Shape into six patties.

3. Coat grill rack with cooking spray before starting the grill. Grill patties, covered, over medium-hot heat for 4-5 minutes on each side or until meat juices run clear. Top patties with cheese and the tomato sauce. Serve over buns.

Steak Fajitas

I found this recipe and changed a few things to our liking. It's super Southwestern fare.

Jackie Hannahs, Fountain, Michigan

- 1 pound boneless beef sirloin steak, cut into thin 3-inch strips
- 2 teaspoons canola oil
- 1 medium green pepper, cut into thin strips
- 1 medium onion, quartered and thinly sliced
- 3 garlic cloves, minced
- 1/2 teaspoon chili powder
- 1/4 teaspoon dried oregano
- 1/4 teaspoon pepper
- 1 cup salsa *or* picante sauce
- 5 flour tortillas (8 inches), warmed

1. In a nonstick skillet, brown beef in oil; drain. Add the green pepper, onion, garlic, chili powder, oregano and pepper. Cook and stir for 5 minutes or until vegetables are crisp-tender. Add salsa; cook 3 minutes longer or until heated through.

2. Spoon 3/4 cup beef mixture down the center of each tortilla. Fold one side over filling and roll up. Serve immediately.

COLORFUL FAJITAS

To add color to these fajitas, try using a combination of sweet peppers. You can use a mixture of yellow, orange, green and even purple pepper strips. The leftover peppers can be added to salads or vegetable stir-fries. Store peppers in the refrigerator for up to 5 days or freeze for up to 12 months.

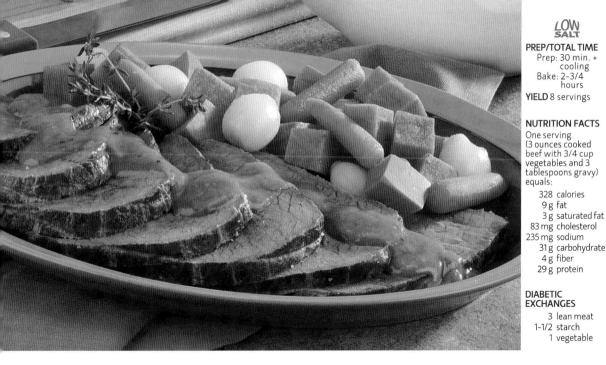

PREP/TOTAL TIME
Prep: 30 min. +
cooling
Bake: 2-3/4
hours
YIELD 8 servings

NUTRITION FACTS
One serving
(3 ounces cooked
beef with 3/4 cup
vegetables and 3
tablespoons gravy)
equals:

328 calories
9 g fat
3 g saturated fat
83 mg cholesterol
235 mg sodium
31 g carbohydrate
4 g fiber
29 g protein

DIABETIC EXCHANGES
3 lean meat
1-1/2 starch
1 vegetable

Autumn Pot Roast

This colorful dinner makes an excellent holiday meal. The cranberries mixed with horseradish give the beef fantastic taste.

Deby Kominski, Honesdale, Pennsylvania

1 boneless beef rump roast (about 3 pounds), tied
1/4 teaspoon salt
1/4 teaspoon pepper
2 teaspoons canola oil
3/4 cup fresh or frozen cranberries
1/2 cup water
1/4 cup sugar
1 cup reduced-sodium beef broth
1/3 cup prepared horseradish, drained
1 cinnamon stick (3 inches)
3 whole cloves
16 pearl onions
2 medium sweet potatoes (about 1-1/2 pounds), peeled and cut into 3/4-inch cubes
16 baby carrots
4 teaspoons cornstarch
2 tablespoons cold water

1. Sprinkle meat with salt and pepper. In a Dutch oven, brown meat in oil. Drain and remove from the heat. In a large saucepan, combine cranberries, water and sugar. Cook and stir over medium heat until cranberries pop and liquid is slightly thickened, about 8 minutes. Remove from the heat.

2. Add the broth and horseradish; pour over meat. Place cinnamon stick and cloves in a double thickness of cheesecloth; bring up corners of cloth and tie with kitchen string to form a bag. Add to Dutch oven. Cover and bake at 325° for 2 hours.

3. Meanwhile, in a large saucepan, bring 6 cups water to a boil. Add pearl onions; boil for 3 minutes. Drain and rinse in cold water; peel and set aside. Add sweet potatoes to Dutch oven. Cover and cook 15 minutes longer. Add carrots and onions; cover and cook 30-40 minutes more or until vegetables and meat are tender. Remove meat and vegetables; keep warm. Discard spice bag.

4. Cool pan juices for 10 minutes; transfer to a blender. Cover and process until smooth; return to pan. Combine cornstarch and cold water until smooth. Gradually whisk into pan juices. Bring to a boil; cook and stir for 1-2 minutes or until thickened. Serve with meat and vegetables.

Sirloin Veggie Kabobs

Planning a cookout menu is a breeze when you have this crowd-pleasing kabob recipe.

Trisha Ward, Atlanta, Georgia

PREP/TOTAL TIME
Prep: 30 min. +
     marinating
Grill: 10 min.
YIELD 4 servings

NUTRITION FACTS
One serving
(2 kabobs) equals:
    268 calories
    10 g fat
    2 g saturated fat
    63 mg cholesterol
    480 mg sodium
    20 g carbohydrate
    2 g fiber
    24 g protein

**DIABETIC
EXCHANGES**
    3 lean meat
    2 vegetable
    1/2 starch

2/3 cup chili sauce

1/2 cup dry red wine or beef broth

1/2 cup balsamic vinegar

2 tablespoons canola oil

4-1/2 teaspoons Worcestershire sauce

4-1/2 teaspoons dried minced onion

1 garlic clove, minced

1/2 teaspoon ground mustard

1/4 teaspoon salt

1 pound boneless beef sirloin steak, cut into 3/4-inch cubes

16 fresh baby portobello or large white mushrooms, halved

2 medium red onions, cut into wedges

1 medium sweet red pepper, cut into 3/4-inch pieces

1 medium sweet yellow pepper, cut into 3/4-inch pieces

1. In a small bowl, combine the first nine ingredients; mix well. Pour half into a large resealable plastic bag; add beef cubes. Seal bag and turn to coat. Pour the remaining marinade into another large resealable plastic bag; add mushrooms, onions and peppers. Seal bag and turn to coat. Refrigerate beef and vegetables for up to 4 hours.

2. If grilling the kabobs, coat the grill rack with cooking spray before starting the grill. Drain and discard the marinade from the beef. Drain the vegetables, reserving the marinade for basting. On eight metal or soaked wooden skewers, alternately thread beef and vegetables.

3. Grill, covered, over medium heat or broil 4-6 in. from the heat for 3-4 minutes on each side or until meat reaches desired doneness, turning three times and basting frequently with reserved marinade.

Down-Home Pot Roast

The aroma of my mom's pot roast made our mouths water. I've tried different variations, but this one is still my favorite.

Lenore Rein, Kelliher, Saskatchewan

- 1 boneless beef sirloin tip roast (3 pounds)
- 1 tablespoon canola oil
- 1 can (14-1/2 ounces) reduced-sodium beef broth
- 3 tablespoons cider vinegar
- 2 garlic cloves, minced
- 1/2 teaspoon dried basil
- 1/4 teaspoon dried thyme
- 1 small head cabbage, cut into wedges
- 4 medium potatoes, quartered
- 2 medium onions, cut into chunks
- 3 medium carrots, cut into chunks
- 1 medium sweet red pepper, cut into 1-inch pieces
- 1/2 teaspoon salt
- 1/2 teaspoon pepper
- 1/4 cup all-purpose flour
- 1/4 cup cold water

1. In a Dutch oven, brown roast on all sides in oil over medium-high heat; drain. Add broth. Pour vinegar over roast. Sprinkle with garlic, basil and thyme. Bring to a boil. Reduce heat; cover and simmer for 2 hours, turning roast occasionally. Add water if needed. Spoon off fat.

2. Add vegetables to pan. Sprinkle with salt and pepper. Cover and simmer for 35-45 minutes or until vegetables and meat are tender. Remove meat and vegetables to a serving platter and keep warm.

3. For gravy, pour drippings and loosened browned bits into a measuring cup. Skim fat, reserving 2 cups drippings. Return drippings to pan. Combine flour and cold water until smooth; gradually stir into drippings. Bring to a boil; cook and stir for 2 minutes or until thickened. Serve with meat and vegetables.

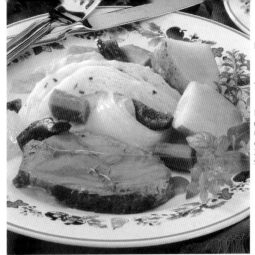

LOW SALT

PREP/TOTAL TIME
Prep: 15 min.
Cook: 2 hours 35 min.

YIELD 12 servings

NUTRITION FACTS
One serving (3 ounces cooked beef with 2 tablespoons sauce) equals:
258 calories
7 g fat
2 g saturated fat
61 mg cholesterol
235 mg sodium
25 g carbohydrate
4 g fiber
25 g protein

DIABETIC EXCHANGES
3 lean meat
2 vegetable
1/2 starch

Zippy Burgers

Lean ground beef is enhanced with onion powder, chili powder and red pepper flakes. These satisfying burgers are sure to sizzle at any summer meal.

Taste of Home Test Kitchen

- 1/4 cup beer *or* beef broth
- 2 tablespoons Worcestershire sauce
- 2 teaspoons chili powder
- 1 teaspoon onion powder
- 1/2 teaspoon crushed red pepper flakes
- 1/4 teaspoon salt
- 1/4 teaspoon pepper
- 1 pound lean ground beef
- 4 hamburger buns, split

1. In a bowl, combine the first seven ingredients. Crumble beef over mixture and mix well. Shape into four patties.

2. If grilling the hamburgers, coat grill rack with cooking spray before starting the grill. Grill hamburgers, covered, over medium heat or broil 4 in. from the heat for 6-8 minutes on each side or until a meat thermometer reads 160°. Serve on buns.

PREP/TOTAL TIME
20 min.

YIELD 4 servings

NUTRITION FACTS
One serving (1 burger) equals:
314 calories
12 g fat
4 g saturated fat
70 mg cholesterol
557 mg sodium
25 g carbohydrate
2 g fiber
25 g protein

DIABETIC EXCHANGES
3 lean meat
1-1/2 starch

Tropical Tenderloin Steaks

Marinated in citrus juices, ginger and rum extract, these out-of-the-ordinary steaks deliver unbelievable flavor in every bite.

Mitzi Sentiff, Alexandria, Virginia

PREP/TOTAL TIME
Prep: 10 min. + marinating
Grill: 20 min.
YIELD 8 servings

NUTRITION FACTS
One serving
(3 ounces cooked beef) equals:
223 calories
11g fat
4 g saturated fat
72 mg cholesterol
142 mg sodium
6 g carbohydrate
Trace fiber
23 g protein

DIABETIC EXCHANGES
3 lean meat
1/2 starch

1 cup reduced-sodium chicken broth
3/4 cup orange juice
1/4 cup ketchup
1/4 cup unsweetened pineapple juice
3 tablespoons packed brown sugar
3 tablespoons lime juice
2 garlic cloves, minced
1 tablespoon minced fresh gingerroot
1/4 teaspoon vanilla extract
1/4 teaspoon rum extract
1/4 teaspoon ground cloves
1/4 teaspoon dried thyme
1/4 teaspoon cayenne pepper
1 beef tenderloin (2 pounds), cut into 8 pieces

1. In a small bowl, combine the first 13 ingredients. Pour 2 cups into a large resealable plastic bag; add the beef. Seal bag and turn to coat; refrigerate for 3 hours. Cover and refrigerate remaining marinade for basting.

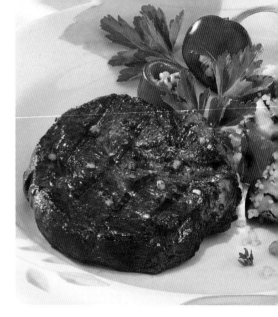

2. If grilling the steaks, coat grill rack with cooking spray before starting the grill. Drain and discard marinade from steaks. Grill, covered, over medium heat or broil 4-6 in. from the heat for 8-10 minutes on each side or until meat reaches desired doneness (for medium-rare, a meat thermometer should read 145°; medium, 160°; well-done, 170°), brushing occasionally with reserved marinade.

Salisbury Steak with Gravy

This easy recipe was shared at a weight-loss meeting I attended. My whole family really enjoys these ground beef patties.

Danelle Weiher, Verndale, Minnesota

PREP/TOTAL TIME
Prep: 15 min.
Bake: 50 min.
YIELD 4 servings

NUTRITION FACTS
One serving
(1 patty) equals:
266 calories
9 g fat
4 g saturated fat
77 mg cholesterol
727 mg sodium
21 g carbohydrate
1 g fiber
24 g protein

DIABETIC EXCHANGES
3 lean meat
1-1/2 starch

1/2 cup fat-free milk
14 fat-free saltines, crushed
2 tablespoons dried minced onion
2 teaspoons dried parsley flakes
1 pound lean ground beef
1 jar (12 ounces) fat-free beef gravy
2 tablespoons ketchup
2 teaspoons Worcestershire sauce
1/4 teaspoon pepper

1. In a large bowl, combine the milk, saltines, onion and parsley. Crumble beef over mixture and mix well. Shape into four patties. Place in an 8-in. square baking dish coated with cooking spray.

2. In a small bowl, combine gravy, ketchup, Worcestershire and pepper; pour over patties. Bake, uncovered, at 350° for 50-55 minutes or until meat is no longer pink.

Cabbage Rolls

This is an excellent recipe for traditional cabbage rolls. In summer when tomatoes are plentiful, I use peeled fresh tomatoes in place of the canned diced ones.

Dolly Mullen, Langley, Washington

1	medium head cabbage
3/4	pound lean ground beef
1/2	cup chopped onion
1	can (14-1/2 ounces) diced tomatoes, undrained
1/2	cup water
1/3	cup instant brown rice
1	can (15 ounces) tomato sauce
1	tablespoon Worcestershire sauce
1/2	teaspoon dried basil
1/2	teaspoon dried thyme
1/2	teaspoon sugar
1/2	cup shredded part-skim mozzarella cheese

1. Cook cabbage in boiling water just until leaves fall off head. Set aside 8 large leaves for rolls. (Refrigerate remaining cabbage for another use.) Cut out the thick vein from the bottom of each reserved leaf, making a V-shaped cut. Set aside.

2. In a large nonstick skillet, cook the ground beef and onion over medium heat until meat is no longer pink; drain. Stir in tomatoes and water; bring to a boil. Stir in rice; return to a boil. Reduce heat; cover and simmer for 5 minutes.

3. Place about 1/3 cup beef mixture on each reserved cabbage leaf; overlap cut ends of leaf. Fold in sides, beginning from the cut end. Roll up completely to enclose filling.

4. In a bowl, combine the tomato sauce, Worcestershire sauce, basil, thyme and sugar. Spread half on the bottom of an 11-in. x 7-in. x 2-in. baking dish coated with cooking spray. Top with cabbage rolls and remaining tomato sauce mixture.

5. Cover and bake at 350° for 30 minutes. Uncover; sprinkle with cheese. Bake 5-10 minutes longer or until bubbly and cheese is melted.

PREP/TOTAL TIME
Prep: 35 min.
Bake: 35 min.
YIELD 4 servings

NUTRITION FACTS
One serving
(2 cabbage rolls)
equals:

281 calories
9 g fat
4 g saturated fat
50 mg cholesterol
897 mg sodium
24 g carbohydrate
4 g fiber
24 g protein

DIABETIC EXCHANGES
3 lean meat
3 vegetable
1/2 starch

PREP/TOTAL TIME
30 min.
YIELD 6 servings

NUTRITION FACTS
One serving
(1 piece) equals:
250 calories
9 g fat
4 g saturated fat
28 mg cholesterol
439 mg sodium
22 g carbohydrate
1 g fiber
19 g protein

DIABETIC EXCHANGES
2 lean meat
1-1/2 starch
1/2 fat

Tortilla Pie

My husband and two daughters just can't get enough of this fun, not-too-spicy supper.

Lisa King, Caledonia, Michigan

1/2 pound lean ground beef
1/4 cup chopped onion
1 garlic clove, minced
1 can (14-1/2 ounces) Italian *or* Mexican diced tomatoes, drained
1/2 teaspoon chili powder
1/4 teaspoon ground cumin
3/4 cup part-skim ricotta cheese
1/4 cup shredded part-skim mozzarella cheese
3 tablespoons minced fresh cilantro, *divided*
4 flour tortillas (8 inches)
1/2 cup shredded reduced-fat cheddar cheese

1. In a large nonstick skillet, cook the beef, onion and garlic over medium heat until meat is no longer pink; drain. Stir in the tomatoes, chili powder and cumin. Bring to a boil; remove from the heat. In a small bowl, combine the ricotta cheese, mozzarella cheese and 2 tablespoons cilantro.

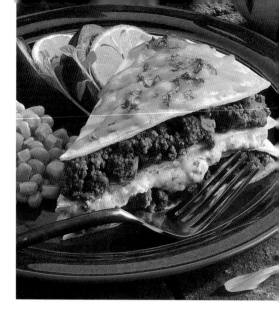

2. Place one tortilla in a 9-in. round baking pan coated with cooking spray. Layer with half of the meat sauce, one tortilla, all of the ricotta mixture, another tortilla and the remaining meat sauce. Top with remaining tortilla; sprinkle with cheddar cheese and remaining cilantro. Cover and bake at 400° for 15 minutes or until heated through and cheese is melted.

PREP/TOTAL TIME
25 min.
YIELD 4 servings

NUTRITION FACTS
One serving equals:
268 calories
8 g fat
3 g saturated fat
43 mg cholesterol
236 mg sodium
16 g carbohydrate
2 g fiber
32 g protein

DIABETIC EXCHANGES
3 lean meat
1 starch
1 vegetable

Skillet Ole

While this pleasantly spiced dish is cooking, I fix ranch-style beans and a green salad so the whole meal is ready in about 30 minutes.

Lillie Glass, Dripping Springs, Texas

1/2 pound lean ground beef
1/2 pound lean ground turkey
1 small onion, chopped
1/4 cup chopped green pepper
1 can (8 ounces) no-salt-added tomato sauce
1 cup cooked rice
1 to 1-1/2 teaspoons chili powder
3/4 cup shredded reduced-fat cheddar cheese

1. In a large skillet, cook beef, turkey, onion and green pepper over medium heat until meat is no longer pink; drain.

2. Stir in tomato sauce, rice and chili powder. Cook for 10 minutes; sprinkle with the cheese. Cover and cook for 2 minutes or until cheese is melted.

SODIUM INTAKE

If sodium intake is not a factor in your diet, feel free to use regular tomato sauce in this no-fuss skillet dish.

Brisket with Gravy

Served with a slightly sweet gravy and topped with onions, this robust beef brisket looks and tastes special enough for guests.

Pat Patty, Spring, Texas

- 1 fresh beef brisket (about 4 pounds)
- 1/2 teaspoon pepper
- 1 large onion, thinly sliced and separated into rings
- 1 can (12 ounces) beer *or* nonalcoholic beer
- 1/2 cup chili sauce
- 3 tablespoons brown sugar
- 2 garlic cloves, minced
- 2 tablespoons cornstarch
- 1/4 cup cold water

1. Place beef in a roasting pan. Sprinkle with pepper and top with onion. Combine the beer, chili sauce, brown sugar and garlic; stir until sugar is dissolved. Pour over meat.

2. Cover and bake at 325° for 3-1/2 hours. Uncover; bake 15-30 minutes longer or until onions are lightly browned and meat is tender. Remove meat and onions to a serving platter and keep warm.

3. Pour drippings and loosened browned bits into a saucepan. Skim fat. Combine cornstarch and water until smooth. Gradually stir into pan drippings. Bring to a boil; cook and stir for 2 minutes or until thickened. Slice meat thinly across the grain. Serve with gravy.

Editor's Note: This is a fresh beef brisket, not corned beef.

PREP/TOTAL TIME
Prep: 10 min.
Bake: 3-1/2 hours
YIELD 12 servings

NUTRITION FACTS
One serving
(3 ounces cooked beef) equals:

- 270 calories
- 12 g fat
- 4 g saturated fat
- 88 mg cholesterol
- 389 mg sodium
- 9 g carbohydrate
- 1 g fiber
- 28 g protein

DIABETIC EXCHANGES
- 3 lean meat
- 1 fat
- 1/2 starch

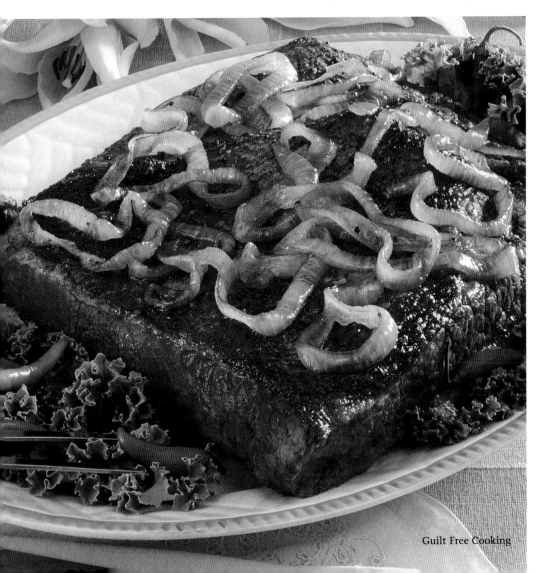

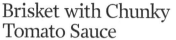

Mediterranean Beef Toss

This dish is a great way to use ground beef. Whenever I make it, I get many compliments.

Phyllis Stewart, Goodwood, Ontario

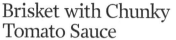

1/2 pound lean ground beef

4 garlic cloves, minced

3/4 teaspoon salt, *divided*

1/4 teaspoon pepper

3 teaspoons olive oil, *divided*

1 medium red onion, sliced

2 medium zucchini, sliced

1 medium green pepper, cut into 1-inch pieces

1 can (28 ounces) diced tomatoes, undrained

1 teaspoon red wine vinegar

1 teaspoon dried basil

1 teaspoon dried thyme

Hot cooked spaghetti, optional

1. In a nonstick skillet, cook the beef, garlic, 1/4 teaspoon salt and pepper in 1 teaspoon oil over medium heat until meat is no longer pink; drain. Remove and keep warm. In the same skillet, saute onion in remaining oil for 2 minutes. Add zucchini and green pepper; cook and stir for 4-6 minutes or until vegetables are crisp-tender.

2. Stir in the tomatoes, vinegar, basil, thyme and remaining salt. Add the beef mixture; heat through. Serve over the spaghetti if desired.

PREP/TOTAL TIME
25 min.
YIELD 4 servings

NUTRITION FACTS
One serving (1-1/2 cups calculated without spaghetti) equals:
204 calories
9 g fat
3 g saturated fat
21 mg cholesterol
739 mg sodium
18 g carbohydrate
6 g fiber
15 g protein

DIABETIC EXCHANGES
2 lean meat
1 starch
1/2 fat

Brisket with Chunky Tomato Sauce

When I treat dinner guests to this impressive brisket, they all say the same thing–it's the best beef they've ever tasted.

Linda Blaska, Atlanta, Georgia

1 fresh beef brisket (4-1/2 pounds)

1 teaspoon salt

1/4 to 1/2 teaspoon pepper

1 tablespoon olive oil

3 large onions, chopped

2 garlic cloves, minced

1 cup dry red wine *or* beef broth

1 can (14-1/2 ounces) diced tomatoes, undrained

2 celery ribs with leaves, chopped

1/2 teaspoon dried thyme

1/2 teaspoon dried rosemary, crushed

1 bay leaf

1 pound carrots, cut into 1/2-inch slices

1. Season brisket with salt and pepper. In a Dutch oven, brown brisket in oil over medium-high heat. Remove and keep warm. In the same pan, saute onions and garlic until tender. Place brisket over onions. Add the wine or broth, tomatoes, celery, thyme, rosemary and bay leaf.

2. Cover and bake at 325° for 2 hours, basting occasionally. Add carrots; bake 1 hour longer or until meat is tender. Discard bay leaf. Cool for 1 hour; cover and refrigerate overnight.

3. Trim visible fat from brisket and skim fat from tomato mixture. Thinly slice beef across the grain. In a saucepan, warm tomato mixture; transfer to a shallow roasting pan. Top with sliced beef. Cover and bake at 325° for 30 minutes or until heated through. Serve sauce over beef.

Editor's Note: This is a fresh beef brisket, not corned beef.

PREP/TOTAL TIME
Prep: 15 min.
Bake: 3 hours 30 min. + chilling
YIELD 12 servings

NUTRITION FACTS
One serving (6 ounces cooked beef) equals:
316 calories
12 g fat
4 g saturated fat
100 mg cholesterol
394 mg sodium
10 g carbohydrate
2 g fiber
38 g protein

DIABETIC EXCHANGES
4 lean meat
2 fat

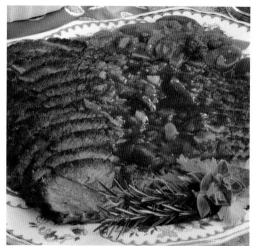

Beef Fillets with Portobello Sauce

These tasty steaks seem special but are fast enough for everyday dinners. We enjoy the fillets with crusty French bread and salad.

Christel Stein, Tampa, Florida

- 2 beef tenderloin steaks (4 ounces *each*)
- 1/2 cup dry red wine *or* reduced-sodium beef broth
- 1 teaspoon all-purpose flour
- 1/2 cup reduced-sodium beef broth
- 1 teaspoon *each* steak sauce, Worcestershire sauce and ketchup
- 1/2 teaspoon ground mustard
- 4 ounces fresh baby portobello mushrooms, sliced
- 1/4 teaspoon pepper
- 1/8 teaspoon salt
- 1 tablespoon minced chives, optional

1. In a nonstick skillet coated with cooking spray, brown steaks on both sides over medium-high heat. Remove and keep warm.

2. Reduce heat to medium. Add wine or broth to pan, stirring to loosen browned bits; cook for 2-3 minutes or until liquid is reduced by half. Combine flour and broth until smooth; whisk into the pan juices. Add steak sauce, Worcestershire sauce, ketchup and mustard. Bring to a boil.

3. Return steaks to the skillet; add mushrooms. Cook for 4-5 minutes on each side or until meat reaches desired doneness (for medium-rare, a meat thermometer should read 145°; medium, 160°; well-done, 170°). Sprinkle with the pepper, salt and minced chives if desired.

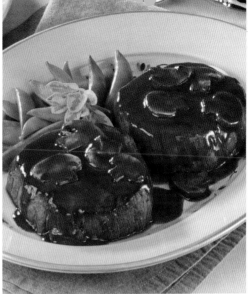

PREP/TOTAL TIME
30 min.
YIELD 2 servings

NUTRITION FACTS
One serving (1 steak with 1/3 cup sauce) equals:

  255 calories
  8 g fat
  3 g saturated fat
  72 mg cholesterol
422 mg sodium
  7 g carbohydrate
  1 g fiber
26 g protein

DIABETIC EXCHANGES
  3 lean meat
  1 starch

Gingered Beef Stir-Fry

This tempting entree features tender beef and veggies that keep a bit of their crunch.

Grace Nicholson, Willow Grove, Pennsylvania

- 1 egg white
- 1 tablespoon cornstarch
- 1/2 teaspoon sugar
- 1/4 teaspoon ground ginger
- 1/4 teaspoon pepper
- 1 beef flank steak (1 pound), cut into thin strips
- 1 tablespoon canola oil
- 1/2 cup chopped green onions
- 2 tablespoons reduced-sodium soy sauce
- 2 medium carrots, thinly sliced
- 1 medium zucchini, thinly sliced
- 1/4 pound fresh *or* frozen snow peas, thawed

Hot cooked rice

1. In a large bowl, whisk egg white, cornstarch, sugar, ginger and pepper until smooth. Add beef and toss to coat; set aside.

2. In a large nonstick skillet, heat oil. Saute onions for 1 minute or until crisp-tender. Add beef; stir-fry for 6-7 minutes or until meat is browned and no longer pink. Stir in soy sauce. Add carrots, zucchini and peas; stir-fry for 4-5 minutes or until all vegetables are crisp-tender. Serve over rice.

TOP PICK

To choose the freshest zucchini, look for a firm heavy squash with a moist stem end and a shiny skin. Smaller squash are generally sweeter and more tender.

LOW SALT
PREP/TOTAL TIME
20 min.
YIELD 5 servings

NUTRITION FACTS
One serving (1 cup calculated without rice) equals:

  240 calories
  10 g fat
  0 g saturated fat
  47 mg cholesterol
246 mg sodium
  14 g carbohydrate
  0 g fiber
23 g protein

DIABETIC EXCHANGES
  3 lean meat
  1 vegetable
  1/2 starch

PREP/TOTAL TIME
Prep: 30 min.
Cook: 10 min.
YIELD 8 servings

NUTRITION FACTS
One serving
(1 sandwich) equals:
277 calories
10 g fat
4 g saturated fat
47 mg cholesterol
506 mg sodium
28 g carbohydrate
3 g fiber
20 g protein

DIABETIC EXCHANGES
2 lean meat
1-1/2 starch
1 vegetable
1/2 fat

Open-Faced Meatball Sandwiches

My husband and I love meatball subs, so I came up with this easy-to-fix recipe that's perfect after a long, busy day.

Karen Barthel, North Canton, Ohio

1/4   cup egg substitute

1/2   cup soft bread crumbs

1/4   cup finely chopped onion

2   garlic cloves, minced

1/2   teaspoon onion powder

1/2   teaspoon dried oregano

1/2   teaspoon dried basil

1/4   teaspoon pepper

Dash salt

1-1/4   pounds lean ground beef

2   cups garden-style pasta sauce

4   hoagie buns, split

2   tablespoons shredded part-skim mozzarella cheese

Shredded Parmesan cheese, optional

1. In a large bowl, combine the first nine ingredients. Crumble beef over mixture and mix well. Shape into 40 meatballs, 1 in. each. In a large skillet coated with cooking spray, brown meatballs in batches; drain.

2. Place meatballs in a large saucepan. Add the pasta sauce; bring to a boil. Reduce heat; cover and simmer for 10-15 minutes or until meat is no longer pink. Spoon meatballs and sauce onto bun halves; sprinkle with mozzarella and Parmesan if desired.

Stuffed Flank Steak

This recipe came with my first slow cooker.
I'm now on my fourth, and I still love this dish!

Kathy Clark, Byron, Minnesota

- 1 beef flank steak (2 pounds)
- 1 medium onion, chopped
- 1 garlic clove, minced
- 1 tablespoon butter
- 1-1/2 cups soft bread crumbs (about 3 slices)
- 1/2 cup chopped fresh mushrooms
- 1/4 cup minced fresh parsley
- 1/4 cup egg substitute
- 3/4 teaspoon poultry seasoning
- 1/2 teaspoon salt
- 1/8 teaspoon pepper
- 1/2 cup beef broth
- 2 teaspoons cornstarch
- 4 teaspoons water

1. Flatten steak to 1/2-in. thickness; set aside. In a nonstick skillet, saute onion and garlic in butter until tender. Add the crumbs, mushrooms, parsley, egg substitute, seasoning, salt and pepper; mix well. Spread over steak to within 1 in. of edge. Roll up jelly-roll style, starting with a long side; tie with kitchen string. Place in a 5-qt. slow cooker; add broth. Cover; cook on low for 8-10 hours.

2. Remove meat to a serving platter and keep warm. Skim fat from cooking juices; pour into a small saucepan. Combine cornstarch and water until smooth; stir into juices. Bring to a boil; cook and stir for 1-2 minutes or until thickened. Remove string before slicing steak; serve with gravy.

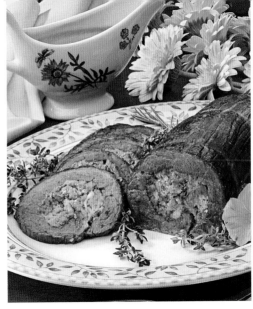

PREP/TOTAL TIME
Prep: 20 min.
Cook: 8 hours
YIELD 8 servings

NUTRITION FACTS
One serving
(1 slice) equals:

- 230 calories
- 11 g fat
- 5 g saturated fat
- 62 mg cholesterol
- 348 mg sodium
- 6 g carbohydrate
- 1 g fiber
- 26 g protein

DIABETIC EXCHANGES
- 3 lean meat
- 1/2 starch
- 1/2 fat

Chicken-Fried Steak

We raise cattle, so beef is a mainstay at our house.
I adapted this traditional main dish to leave a lot of the fat behind.

Carol Dale, Greenville, Texas

- 3/4 cup all-purpose flour
- 1/4 teaspoon pepper
- 1 pound boneless beef round steak, cut into serving-size pieces
- 1/2 cup fat-free milk
- 2 tablespoons canola oil

GRAVY:
- 2 tablespoons water
- 4-1/2 teaspoons all-purpose flour
- 3/4 cup fat-free milk
- 1/8 teaspoon pepper

1. In a shallow bowl, combine flour and pepper. Add beef; turn to coat. Remove meat and pound with a mallet to tenderize. Pour milk into another shallow bowl. Heat oil in a skillet. Dip meat in milk, then coat again in flour mixture; add to skillet. Cover; cook over low heat for 10 minutes. Turn; cook 10 minutes longer. Remove and keep warm.

2. For gravy, add the water to skillet; stir to loosen browned bits from pan. In a small bowl, combine flour, milk and pepper until smooth. Stir into skillet. Bring to a boil; cook and stir for 1-2 minutes or until thickened. Serve with steak.

LOW SALT

PREP/TOTAL TIME
30 min.
YIELD 4 servings

NUTRITION FACTS
One serving
(calculated without gravy) equals:

- 307 calories
- 11 g fat
- 0 g saturated fat
- 71 mg cholesterol
- 67 mg sodium
- 19 g carbohydrate
- 1 g fiber
- 30 g protein

DIABETIC EXCHANGES
- 4 meat
- 1-1/2 starch

Shredded Beef Barbecue

PREP/TOTAL TIME
Prep: 10 min.
Cook: 8 hours
YIELD 12 servings

NUTRITION FACTS
One serving
(1 sandwich) equals:
313 calories
9 g fat
2 g saturated fat
59 mg cholesterol
688 mg sodium
33 g carbohydrate
2 g fiber
26 g protein

DIABETIC
EXCHANGES
3 lean meat
2 starch

After simmering for hours in a homemade barbecue sauce, this roast is very tender and shreds easily. The mixture freezes well, too.

Lori Bergquist, Wilton, North Dakota

1 boneless beef sirloin tip roast (2-1/2 pounds)

1/2 teaspoon salt

1/4 teaspoon pepper

1 tablespoon canola oil

1 cup *each* ketchup and water

1/2 cup chopped onion

1/3 cup packed brown sugar

3 tablespoons Worcestershire sauce

2 tablespoons lemon juice

2 tablespoons cider vinegar

2 tablespoons Dijon mustard

2 teaspoons celery seed

2 teaspoons chili powder

12 kaiser rolls, split

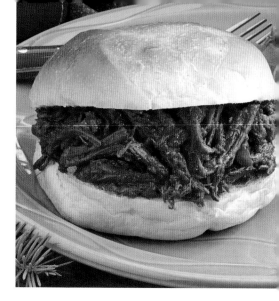

1. Sprinkle roast with salt and pepper. In a nonstick skillet, brown roast in oil on all sides over medium-high heat; drain. Transfer to a 5-qt. slow cooker. Combine ketchup, water, onion, sugar, Worcestershire, lemon juice, vinegar, mustard, celery seed and chili powder; pour over roast.

2. Cover and cook on low for 8-10 hours or until meat is tender. Remove meat; shred with two forks and return to slow cooker. Spoon 1/2 cup meat mixture onto each roll.

Oven Swiss Steak

LOW SALT

PREP/TOTAL TIME
Prep: 10 min.
Bake: 1 hour
30 min.
YIELD 8 servings

NUTRITION FACTS
One serving
(calculated without
noodles) equals:
209 calories
10 g fat
0 g saturated fat
68 mg cholesterol
112 mg sodium
4 g carbohydrate
0 g fiber
26 g protein

DIABETIC
EXCHANGES
3 lean meat
1 vegetable

This fork-tender entree gets in the oven fast and has lots of sauce left over for dipping.

Sue Call, Beech Grove, Indiana

2 pounds boneless beef round steak (1/2 inch thick)

1/4 teaspoon pepper

1 medium onion, thinly sliced

1 can (4 ounces) mushroom stems and pieces, drained

1 can (8 ounces) no-salt-added tomato sauce

Hot cooked noodles

1. Trim beef; cut into serving-size pieces. Place in a greased 13-in. x 9-in. x 2-in. baking dish. Sprinkle with pepper. Top with the onion, mushrooms and tomato sauce.

2. Cover and bake at 325° for 1-3/4 to 2 hours or until meat is tender. Serve over noodles.

TENDERIZING STEAK

Round steak is an economical and lean cut of beef, but it can also be chewy. The low oven temperature and long cooking time in Oven Swiss Steak make a perfect cooking technique to tenderize this beef cut.

Zucchini Beef Lasagna

This fresh-tasting and mildly seasoned Italian entree is a real crowd-pleaser.

Brenda Tumasone, Newhall, California

- 1 pound lean ground beef
- 2 garlic cloves, minced
- 2 cans (8 ounces *each*) no-salt-added tomato sauce
- 1/2 cup water
- 1 can (6 ounces) tomato paste
- 2 bay leaves
- 1 teaspoon minced fresh parsley
- 1 teaspoon Italian seasoning
- 1 package (16 ounces) lasagna noodles, cooked, rinsed and drained
- 1 cup fat-free cottage cheese
- 1 small zucchini, sliced and cooked
- 1 cup (8 ounces) reduced-fat sour cream

1. In a skillet, cook beef and garlic over medium heat until meat is no longer pink; drain. Add tomato sauce, water, tomato paste, bay leaves, parsley and Italian seasoning; mix well. Bring to a boil; reduce heat. Simmer, uncovered, for 30-40 minutes. Discard the bay leaves.

2. Spread 1/2 cup meat sauce in a 13-in. x 9-in. x 2-in. baking dish coated with cooking spray. Arrange five noodles over sauce, cutting to fit. Spread with cottage cheese. Cover with five noodles, half of the meat sauce and the zucchini. Cover with five noodles and sour cream. Top with remaining noodles and meat sauce.

3. Bake, uncovered, at 350° for 30-35 minutes or until heated through. Let stand for 15 minutes before cutting.

LOW SALT

PREP/TOTAL TIME
Prep: 50 min.
Bake: 30 min. + standing
YIELD 12 servings

NUTRITION FACTS
One serving
(1 piece) equals:
187 calories
8 g fat
0 g saturated fat
21 mg cholesterol
270 mg sodium
19 g carbohydrate
2 g fiber
14 g protein

DIABETIC EXCHANGES
1 starch
1 lean meat
1 vegetable
1/2 fat

Beef Noodle Casserole

This is truly an old standby that's been in my family for years. It can be assembled the night before and baked the next day.

Karen Mathis, Penfield, New York

- 4-1/2 cups uncooked yolk-free noodles
- 1 pound lean ground beef
- 1 small onion, chopped
- 1/2 cup chopped green pepper
- 1 can (10-3/4 ounces) reduced-fat reduced-sodium condensed cream of mushroom soup, undiluted
- 1/4 cup grated Parmesan cheese
- 1 can (4 ounces) mushroom stems and pieces, drained
- 1 jar (2 ounces) diced pimientos, drained
- 1 tablespoon butter, melted
- 1 teaspoon dried thyme
- 1/4 teaspoon salt

1. Cook noodles according to package directions; drain. In a nonstick skillet, cook the beef, onion and green pepper over medium heat until meat is no longer pink; drain. In a large bowl, combine the soup, Parmesan cheese, mushrooms, pimientos, butter, thyme and salt; mix well. Stir in the noodles and beef mixture.

2. Transfer to a 2-qt. baking dish coated with cooking spray. Cover and bake at 350° for 25-30 minutes or until casserole is heated through.

PREP/TOTAL TIME
Prep: 15 min.
Bake: 25 min.
YIELD 6 servings

NUTRITION FACTS
One serving
(1 cup) equals:
295 calories
11 g fat
5 g saturated fat
46 mg cholesterol
527 mg sodium
27 g carbohydrate
3 g fiber
21 g protein

DIABETIC EXCHANGES
2 lean meat
1-1/2 starch
1 vegetable
1 fat

Tex-Mex Lasagna

This recipe combines my love of lasagna with my love of Mexican food. I tried to make the recipe healthier by using extra-lean ground beef and I increased the fiber by adding beans.

Athena Russell, Florence, South Carolina

PREP/TOTAL TIME
Prep: 20 min.
Bake: 45 min. + standing
YIELD 12 servings

NUTRITION FACTS
One serving
(1 piece) equals:
381 calories
13 g fat
7 g saturated fat
47 mg cholesterol
1,170 mg sodium
39 g carbohydrate
5 g fiber
25 g protein

DIABETIC EXCHANGES
3 lean meat
2 starch
1 vegetable

1	pound lean ground beef
1	can (16 ounces) refried black beans
1	can (15 ounces) black beans, rinsed and drained
1/2	cup frozen corn, thawed
1	jalapeno pepper, seeded and chopped
1	envelope taco seasoning
1	can (15 ounces) tomato sauce, *divided*
2-1/2	cups salsa
12	no-cook lasagna noodles
1-1/2	cups (6 ounces) shredded reduced-fat Monterey Jack cheese *or* Mexican cheese blend
1-1/2	cups (6 ounces) shredded reduced-fat cheddar cheese
1	cup (8 ounces) fat-free sour cream
1	medium ripe avocado, peeled and cubed
4	green onions, thinly sliced

1. In a large nonstick skillet, cook beef over medium heat until no longer pink; drain. Stir in the beans, corn, jalapeno, taco seasoning and 3/4 cup tomato sauce.

2. Combine salsa and remaining tomato sauce. Spread 1/4 cup into a 13-in. x 9-in. x 2-in. baking dish coated with cooking spray. Layer with four noodles (noodles will overlap slightly), half of the meat sauce, 1 cup salsa mixture, 1/2 cup Monterey Jack cheese and 1/2 cup cheddar cheese. Repeat layers. Top with the remaining noodles, salsa mixture and cheeses.

3. Cover and bake at 350° for 45-50 minutes or until edges are bubbly and cheese is melted. Let stand for 10 minutes before cutting. Serve with sour cream, avocado and onions.

Editor's Note: When cutting hot peppers, disposable gloves are recommended. Avoid touching your face.

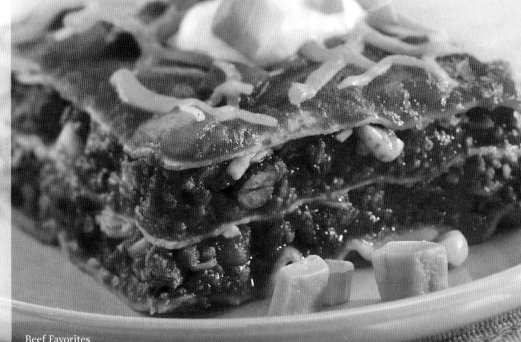

Flavorful Meat Loaf

I can't have much salt, so I created this meat loaf that's really tasty without it.

Lillian Wittler, Norfolk, Nebraska

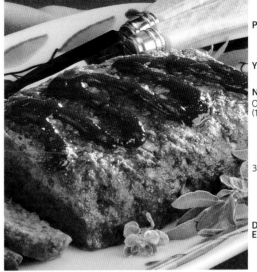

- 2 egg whites
- 1/2 cup 1% milk
- 3 slices whole wheat bread, torn into pieces
- 1/4 cup finely chopped onion
- 1 teaspoon Worcestershire sauce
- 1/4 teaspoon onion powder
- 1/4 teaspoon garlic powder
- 1/4 teaspoon ground mustard
- 1/4 teaspoon rubbed sage
- 1/4 teaspoon pepper
- 1 pound lean ground beef
- 3 tablespoons ketchup

1. In a large bowl, beat egg whites. Add milk and bread; let stand for 5 minutes. Stir in the onion, Worcestershire sauce and seasonings. Crumble beef over mixture; mix well. Shape into a loaf in an 11-in. x 7-in. x 2-in. baking pan coated with cooking spray. Bake, uncovered, at 350° for 35 minutes; drain.

2. Spoon the ketchup over meat loaf. Bake 10-20 minutes longer or until a meat thermometer reads 160°. Let stand for 10 minutes before slicing.

PREP/TOTAL TIME
Prep: 15 min.
Bake: 45 min. + standing
YIELD 5 servings

NUTRITION FACTS
One serving
(1 slice) equals:
228 calories
9 g fat
4 g saturated fat
35 mg cholesterol
307 mg sodium
13 g carbohydrate
1 g fiber
23 g protein

DIABETIC EXCHANGES
3 lean meat
1 starch

Onion Beef Stroganoff

If you like classic Stroganoff, you'll love this lightened-up version featuring tender strips of beef, onion and sliced mushrooms.

Beth Bries, Farley, Iowa

- 1 tablespoon cornstarch
- 1 envelope onion mushroom soup mix
- 1/4 teaspoon salt
- 1/4 teaspoon pepper
- 1 cup fat-free evaporated milk
- 1 pound boneless beef sirloin steak, cut into thin strips
- 2 teaspoons canola oil
- 1/2 medium onion, sliced and separated into rings
- 1 garlic clove, minced
- 1-1/2 cups sliced fresh mushrooms
- 1 cup (8 ounces) fat-free plain yogurt
- Hot cooked noodles
- 1 tablespoon minced fresh parsley

1. In a saucepan, combine the cornstarch, soup mix, salt and pepper. Gradually stir in the milk until blended. Bring to a boil; cook and stir 2 minutes or until thickened. Remove from the heat; keep warm.

2. In a nonstick skillet, brown beef in oil. Add the onion and garlic; cook and stir for 2 minutes. Add mushrooms; cook 1 minute longer or until mushrooms are tender. Reduce heat to low; stir in yogurt and reserved sauce. Cook and stir for 3-5 minutes on low until heated through. Serve over noodles; sprinkle with parsley.

PREP/TOTAL TIME
30 min.
YIELD 4 servings

NUTRITION FACTS
One serving (3/4 cup calculated without noodles) equals:
303 calories
9 g fat
2 g saturated fat
75 mg cholesterol
755 mg sodium
21 g carbohydrate
1 g fiber
34 g protein

DIABETIC EXCHANGES
3 lean meat
1 fat-free milk
1/2 starch

Slow Cooker Beef Au Jus

It's easy to fix this roast, which has terrific onion flavor. Sometimes I also add cubed potatoes and baby carrots to the slow cooker to make a full meal plus leftovers.

Carol Hille, Grand Junction, Colorado

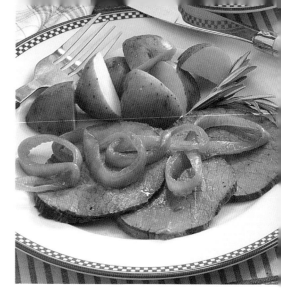

NUTRITION FACTS

One serving
(3 ounces cooked
beef with 1/4 cup
pan juices) equals:

188 calories
7 g fat
2 g saturated fat
82 mg cholesterol
471 mg sodium
3 g carbohydrate
Trace fiber
28 g protein

DIABETIC EXCHANGE

3 lean meat

1 boneless beef rump roast
(3 pounds)
1 large onion, sliced
3/4 cup reduced-sodium beef broth
1 envelope (1 ounce) au jus gravy mix
2 garlic cloves, halved
1/4 teaspoon pepper

1. Cut roast in half. In a large nonstick skillet coated with cooking spray, brown meat on all sides over medium-high heat.

2. Place onion in a 5-qt. slow cooker. Top with meat. Combine the broth, gravy mix, garlic and pepper; pour over meat. Cover and cook on low for 6-7 hours or until meat and onion are tender.

3. Remove the meat to a cutting board. Let stand for 10 minutes. Thinly slice meat and return to the slow cooker; serve with pan juices and onion.

Easy Beef Goulash

I found the recipe for this stovetop goulash years ago in an old cookbook. If you ask me, it really hits the spot with a slice of warm, home-baked bread and a dish of applesauce.

Phyllis Pollock, Erie, Pennsylvania

NUTRITION FACTS

One serving
(1 cup) equals:

272 calories
7 g fat
2 g saturated fat
45 mg cholesterol
371 mg sodium
29 g carbohydrate
2 g fiber
22 g protein

DIABETIC EXCHANGES

2 starch
2 lean meat

1-1/2 cups uncooked spiral pasta
1 pound boneless beef sirloin steak, cut into 1/8-inch-thick strips
1 tablespoon canola oil
1 medium onion, chopped
1 medium green pepper, chopped
1 can (14-1/2 ounces) diced tomatoes, undrained
1-1/2 cups water
1 cup reduced-sodium beef broth
1-1/2 teaspoons red wine vinegar
1 to 2 teaspoons paprika
1 teaspoon sugar
1/2 teaspoon salt
1/4 teaspoon caraway seeds
1/4 teaspoon pepper
2 tablespoons all-purpose flour
1/4 cup cold water

1. Cook pasta according to package directions. Meanwhile, in a large nonstick skillet, stir-fry beef in oil for 4-5 minutes or until meat is no longer pink. Add onion and green pepper; cook and stir for 2 minutes. Stir in tomatoes, water, broth, vinegar and seasonings. Bring to a boil. Reduce heat; cover and simmer for 15 minutes.

2. In a small bowl, combine flour and cold water until smooth. Add to skillet. Bring to a boil; cook and stir for 2 minutes or until thickened. Drain the pasta; stir into beef mixture.

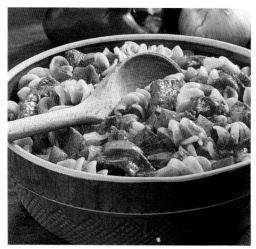

Spaghetti with Italian Meatballs

This hearty spaghetti dinner is one of my family's all-time favorite recipes.

Sharon Crider, St. Robert, Missouri

- 3/4 cup chopped onion
- 1 garlic clove, minced
- 1 tablespoon olive oil
- 1 can (28 ounces) Italian crushed tomatoes, undrained
- 1 can (6 ounces) tomato paste
- 1 cup water
- 1-1/2 teaspoons dried oregano
- 1/2 teaspoon salt
- 1/2 teaspoon pepper

MEATBALLS:

- 4 slices white bread, torn
- 1/2 cup water
- 2 eggs, lightly beaten
- 1/2 cup grated Parmesan cheese
- 1 garlic clove, minced
- 1 teaspoon dried basil
- 1 teaspoon dried parsley flakes
- 1/2 teaspoon salt
- 1 pound lean ground beef
- 2 teaspoons olive oil
- 1 package (16 ounces) spaghetti

1. In a large saucepan coated with cooking spray, cook onion and garlic in oil until tender. Stir in the tomatoes, tomato paste, water, oregano, salt and pepper. Bring to a boil. Reduce heat; cover and simmer for 30 minutes.

2. Meanwhile, in a small bowl, soak bread in water for 5 minutes. Squeeze out excess liquid. In a large bowl, combine the eggs, Parmesan cheese, garlic, basil, parsley, salt and bread. Crumble beef over mixture and mix well. Shape into 1-in. balls.

3. In a large nonstick skillet coated with cooking spray, brown meatballs in batches in oil over medium heat. Add meatballs to sauce; return to a boil. Reduce heat; simmer, uncovered, for 30 minutes or until meatballs are no longer pink.

4. Cook spaghetti according to package directions; drain. Serve spaghetti with meatballs and sauce.

PREP/TOTAL TIME
Prep: 20 min.
Cook: 1-1/4 hours
YIELD 10 servings

NUTRITION FACTS
One serving
(3 meatballs and 1/2 cup sauce with 2/3 cup spaghetti) equals:
- 368 calories
- 9 g fat
- 3 g saturated fat
- 73 mg cholesterol
- 661 mg sodium
- 50 g carbohydrate
- 3 g fiber
- 20 g protein

DIABETIC EXCHANGES
- 2-1/2 starch
- 2 lean meat
- 2 vegetable
- 1/2 fat

Italian Shepherd's Pie

You just can't beat the convenience of this one-dish dinner. I often prepare this pie the night before so that the next day, I can serve my family a satisfying supper in no time.

Rosanne Reynolds, Kissimmee, Florida

PREP/TOTAL TIME
Prep: 30 min.
Bake: 45 min.
YIELD 6 servings

NUTRITION FACTS
One serving equals:
398 calories
11 g fat
0 g saturated fat
80 mg cholesterol
976 mg sodium
43 g carbohydrate
0 g fiber
34 g protein

DIABETIC EXCHANGES
3-1/2 lean meat
2-1/2 starch
1 vegetable

- 1 cup Italian bread crumbs
- 1 cup cold water
- 4 medium potatoes, peeled
- 1-1/4 pounds ground beef
- 1/2 cup finely chopped onion
- 1/2 cup finely chopped celery
- 1 can (8 ounces) tomato sauce
- 1 can (4 ounces) mushrooms, drained and finely chopped
- 1 garlic clove, minced
- 1/4 teaspoon pepper
- 1-1/2 cups frozen peas and carrots
- 1/2 cup shredded part-skim mozzarella cheese

1. Combine crumbs and water; let stand for 5 minutes. Cook potatoes in boiling water until tender. Combine beef, onion, celery, tomato sauce, mushrooms, garlic and pepper. Stir in crumb mixture.

2. Spread into an ungreased 11-in. x 7-in. x 2-in. baking dish. Top with peas and carrots. Drain the potatoes; mash with cheese. Spread over vegetables, sealing to pan. Bake at 375° for 45-60 minutes or until meat is no longer pink.

BREAD CRUMB BASICS

Unless a recipe specifically calls for soft bread crumbs, use dry bread crumbs. For Italian Shepherd's Pie, look for Italian bread crumbs at your grocery store.

Chuck Wagon Wraps

If you're a fan of beans, you'll savor these robust wraps. I combine baked beans, beef and corn, then roll it all up in tortillas.

Wendy Conger, Winfield, Illinois

PREP/TOTAL TIME
25 min.
YIELD 12 servings

NUTRITION FACTS
One serving
(1 wrap) equals:
373 calories
11 g fat
4 g saturated fat
27 mg cholesterol
605 mg sodium
50 g carbohydrate
4 g fiber
20 g protein

DIABETIC EXCHANGES
3 starch
2 lean meat
1/2 fat

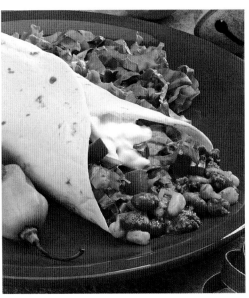

- 1 pound lean ground beef
- 1 can (28 ounces) barbecue-flavored baked beans
- 2 cups frozen corn, thawed
- 4-1/2 teaspoons Worcestershire sauce
- 1 cup (4 ounces) shredded reduced-fat cheddar cheese
- 12 flour tortillas (8 inches), warmed
- 3 cups shredded lettuce
- 1-1/2 cups chopped fresh tomatoes
- 3/4 cup reduced-fat sour cream

1. In a large nonstick skillet, cook beef over medium heat until no longer pink; drain. Stir in beans, corn and Worcestershire sauce; mix well. Bring to a boil. Reduce heat; simmer, uncovered, for 4-5 minutes or until heated through. Sprinkle with cheese; cook 1-2 minutes longer.

2. Spoon about 1/2 cup off-center on each tortilla; top with lettuce, tomatoes and sour cream. Roll up.

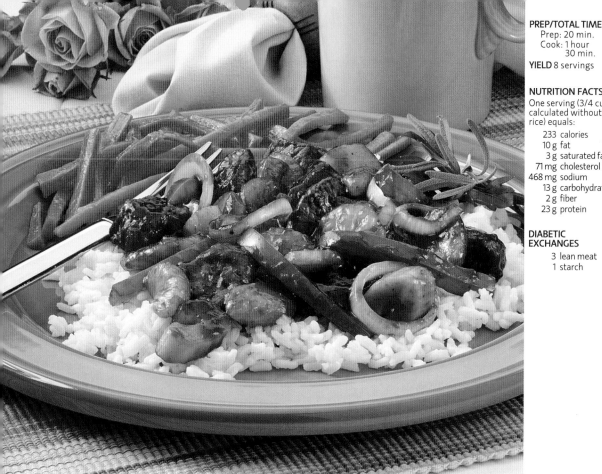

PREP/TOTAL TIME
Prep: 20 min.
Cook: 1 hour
30 min.
YIELD 8 servings

NUTRITION FACTS
One serving (3/4 cup
calculated without
rice) equals:

233 calories
10 g fat
3 g saturated fat
71 mg cholesterol
468 mg sodium
13 g carbohydrate
2 g fiber
23 g protein

DIABETIC
EXCHANGES
3 lean meat
1 starch

Cantonese Beef

When you're craving oriental food, try this saucy main dish served on rice. It's a great alternative to high-calorie takeout.

Michelle Harvey, Noblesville, Indiana

1 can (11 ounces) mandarin oranges

2 pounds beef stew meat, cut into 1-inch cubes

1 small onion, sliced

1 tablespoon canola oil

1-1/2 cups water

1/3 cup reduced-sodium soy sauce

1/2 teaspoon ground ginger

4 celery ribs, sliced

1 small green pepper, julienned

1 can (8 ounces) sliced water chestnuts, drained

3 tablespoons cornstarch

3 tablespoons cold water

Hot cooked rice

1. Drain oranges, reserving juice; set oranges aside. In a Dutch oven, brown beef and onion in oil; drain. Stir in the water, soy sauce, ginger and reserved juice. Bring to a boil. Reduce heat; cover and simmer for 1 to 1-1/2 hours or until beef is tender.

2. Add the celery, green pepper and water chestnuts. Cover and cook for 20-30 minutes or until vegetables are tender. Combine cornstarch and cold water until smooth; stir into beef mixture. Bring to a boil; cook and stir for 2 minutes or until thickened. Stir in reserved oranges. Serve with rice.

PREP/TOTAL TIME
Prep: 10 min. +
   marinating
Grill: 15 min.
YIELD 4 servings

NUTRITION FACTS
One serving
(1/4 of steak with
2 tablespoons
sauce) equals:

   225 calories
   10 g fat
   5 g saturated fat
   51 mg cholesterol
   353 mg sodium
   5 g carbohydrate
   Trace fiber
   26 g protein

**DIABETIC
EXCHANGE**
   4 lean meat

Flank Steak with Horseradish Sauce

This overnight marinade performs double duty; it gently flavors and tenderizes the lean cut of beef.

Taste of Home Test Kitchen

1   beef flank steak (1 pound)
3   tablespoons lemon juice
2   tablespoons Dijon mustard
2   tablespoons Worcestershire sauce
2   garlic cloves, minced
1/8 teaspoon hot pepper sauce

HORSERADISH SAUCE:

1/4 cup fat-free mayonnaise
1/4 cup reduced-fat sour cream
1   tablespoon Dijon mustard
2   green onions, finely chopped
2   teaspoons prepared horseradish

1. Score the surface of the steak with shallow diagonal cuts at 1-in. intervals, making diamond shapes. Repeat on other side.

2. In a large resealable plastic bag, combine the next five ingredients. Add steak. Seal bag and turn to coat; refrigerate for 8 hours

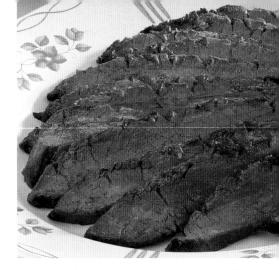

or overnight. Combine the sauce ingredients; cover and refrigerate.

3. Drain and discard marinade from steak. Grill steak, covered, over medium-hot heat for 7-9 minutes on each side or until meat reaches desired doneness (for medium-rare, a meat thermometer should read 145°; medium, 160°; well done, 170°). Thinly slice steak across the grain; serve with sauce.

Old-World Sauerbraten

Crushed gingersnaps, lemon and vinegar give this marinated, slow-cooked roast and gravy their appetizing sweet-sour flavor.

Susan Garoutte, Georgetown, Texas

1-1/2 cups water, *divided*
1-1/4 cups cider vinegar, *divided*
2   large onions, sliced, *divided*
1   medium lemon, sliced
15 whole cloves, *divided*

6   bay leaves, *divided*
6   whole peppercorns
2   tablespoons sugar
2   teaspoons salt
1   boneless beef sirloin tip roast
    (3 pounds), cut in half
1/4 teaspoon pepper
12 gingersnap cookies, crumbled

1. In a large resealable plastic bag, combine 1 cup water, 1 cup vinegar, half of the onions, lemon, 10 cloves, four bay leaves, peppercorns, sugar and salt; mix well. Add roast. Seal the bag and turn to coat; refrigerate overnight, turning occasionally.

2. Drain and discard marinade. Place roast in a 5-qt. slow cooker; add pepper and remaining water, vinegar, onions, cloves and bay leaves. Cover and cook on low for 6-8 hours or until meat is tender.

3. Remove roast and keep warm. Discard bay leaves and cloves. Stir in gingersnaps. Cover and cook on high for 10-15 minutes or until gravy is thickened. Slice roast; serve with gravy.

PREP/TOTAL TIME
Prep: 10 min. +
   marinating
Cook: 6 hours
   10 min.
YIELD 12 servings

NUTRITION FACTS
One serving
(3 ounces cooked
beef with 1/4 cup
gravy) equals:

   214 calories
   7 g fat
   2 g saturated fat
   71 mg cholesterol
   495 mg sodium
   12 g carbohydrate
   1 g fiber
   26 g protein

**DIABETIC
EXCHANGES**
   3 lean meat
   1/2 starch

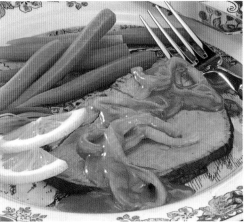

Hearty Taco Casserole

Instead of preparing homemade tortillas for dinner one night, I used the dough to make the crust of this dish. It was an instant hit.

Krista Frank, Rhododendron, Oregon

- 2/3 cup uncooked brown rice
- 1-1/3 cups plus 4 to 5 tablespoons water, *divided*
- 3/4 cup all-purpose flour
- 3/4 teaspoon baking powder
- 1/8 teaspoon salt
- 2 tablespoons cold butter

FILLING:

- 1/2 pound lean ground beef
- 1/2 cup chopped onion
- 1/2 cup chopped green pepper
- 2 garlic cloves, minced
- 1 cup water
- 1 envelope taco seasoning
- 2 eggs, lightly beaten
- 1/4 cup minced fresh cilantro
- 1 cup (4 ounces) shredded reduced-fat cheddar cheese
- 2 cups shredded lettuce
- 2 medium tomatoes, chopped
- 3/4 cup salsa
- 1/2 cup fat-free sour cream

1. In a small saucepan, bring rice and 1-1/3 cups water to a boil. Reduce heat; cover and simmer for 30-35 minutes or until rice is tender and water is absorbed.

2. Meanwhile, in a large bowl, combine flour, baking powder and salt; cut in butter until crumbly. Stir in enough remaining water to form a soft dough. On a floured surface, roll dough into a 12-in. x 8-in. rectangle. Press into a 13-in. x 9-in. x 2-in. baking dish coated with cooking spray. Bake at 400° for 13-15 minutes or until very lightly browned.

3. For filling, in a large nonstick skillet, cook the beef, onion, green pepper and garlic over medium heat until meat is no longer pink; drain. Add water, taco seasoning and cooked rice. Bring to a boil. Reduce heat; simmer, uncovered, for 2-3 minutes or until thickened. Remove from the heat. Stir in eggs and cilantro. Spread over crust.

4. Cover and bake for 15-17 minutes or until filling is set. Cut into squares. Top with cheese, lettuce and tomatoes. Serve with salsa and sour cream.

PREP/TOTAL TIME
Prep: 30 min.
Bake: 35 min.
YIELD 8 servings

NUTRITION FACTS
One serving
(1 piece) equals:
284 calories
10 g fat
5 g saturated fat
87 mg cholesterol
764 mg sodium
33 g carbohydrate
3 g fiber
15 g protein

DIABETIC EXCHANGES
2 starch
1 lean meat
1 vegetable
1 fat

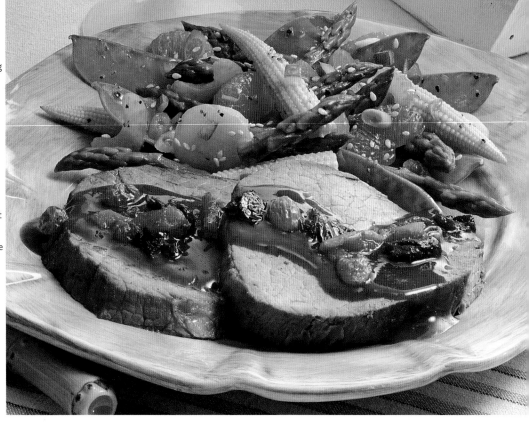

PREP/TOTAL TIME
Prep: 25 min. +
marinating
Bake: 2-1/4
hours +
standing
YIELD 8 servings

NUTRITION FACTS
One serving
(3 ounces cooked
beef with 2
tablespoons
gravy) equals:
317 calories
6 g fat
2 g saturated fat
71 mg cholesterol
285 mg sodium
38 g carbohydrate
4 g fiber
26 g protein

DIABETIC EXCHANGES
3 lean meat
1-1/2 fruit
1 starch

Spiced Beef Roast

In the South, this tangy roast is traditionally served cold or at room temperature, but we like it piping hot. It's perfect for special occasions, and the leftovers are great.

Barb Bredthauer, Omaha, Nebraska

1 medium onion, thinly sliced
1 cup white vinegar
1/2 cup beef broth
1/2 cup packed brown sugar
1 bay leaf
1 teaspoon ground ginger
3/4 teaspoon salt
1/2 teaspoon *each* ground allspice, cinnamon and nutmeg
1/2 teaspoon pepper
1/8 teaspoon cayenne pepper
1 boneless beef sirloin tip roast *or* round roast (2 pounds)
3/4 cup *each* chopped dried plums and apricots
1/4 cup golden raisins
1 teaspoon cornstarch
2 tablespoons cold water

1. For marinade, combine the onion, vinegar, broth, brown sugar, bay leaf and seasonings in a small saucepan. Cook and stir over medium heat until sugar is dissolved. Cool to room temperature.

2. Pierce roast several times with a meat fork; place in a large resealable plastic bag. Add cooled marinade. Seal bag and turn to coat; refrigerate for 8 hours or overnight.

3. Place the meat and the marinade in an ungreased 11-in. x 7-in. x 2-in. baking dish. Bake, uncovered, at 325° for 1-1/2 hours. Stir in dried fruit and raisins. Bake 45-55 minutes longer or until meat and fruit are tender. Discard bay leaf. Remove roast to a platter; let stand for 10 minutes before slicing.

4. For gravy, combine cornstarch and water until smooth. Pour the pan juices into a saucepan; gradually stir in cornstarch mixture. Bring to a boil; cook and stir for 2 minutes or until thickened. Serve with beef.

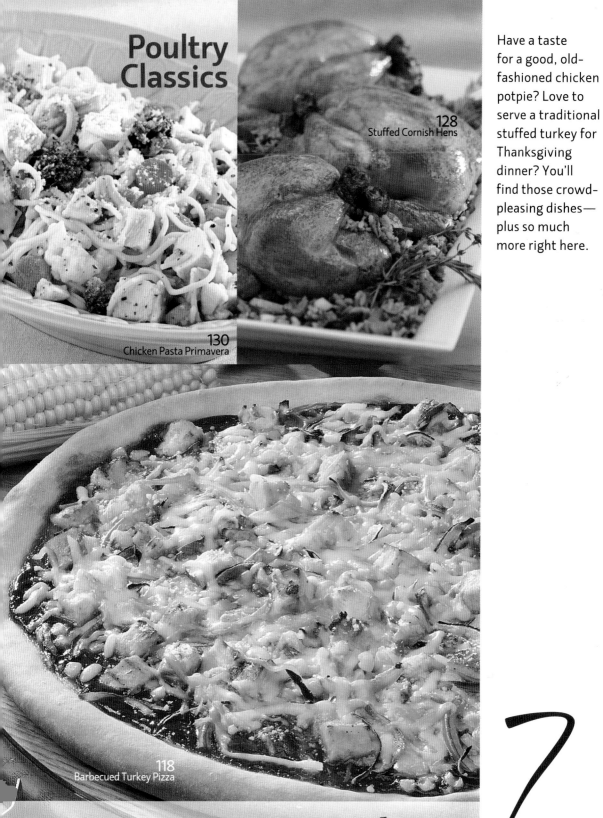

Poultry Classics

128
Stuffed Cornish Hens

130
Chicken Pasta Primavera

118
Barbecued Turkey Pizza

Have a taste for a good, old-fashioned chicken potpie? Love to serve a traditional stuffed turkey for Thanksgiving dinner? You'll find those crowd-pleasing dishes—plus so much more right here.

chapter 7

Horseradish-Crusted Turkey Tenderloins

PREP/TOTAL TIME
Prep: 10 min.
Bake: 25 min.
YIELD 4 servings

Looking for a lighter entree that's ideal for company? Consider this saucy specialty.

Ellen Cross, Hubbardsville, New York

NUTRITION FACTS
One serving
(3 ounces cooked
turkey with 3
tablespoons
sauce) equals:
  237 calories
  9 g fat
  2 g saturated fat
85 mg cholesterol
404 mg sodium
  8 g carbohydrate
  1 g fiber
  29 g protein

**DIABETIC
EXCHANGES**
  3 very lean
    meat
  2 fat
  1/2 starch

- 2 tablespoons reduced-fat mayonnaise
- 2 tablespoons prepared horseradish
- 1 pound turkey tenderloins
- 1/2 cup soft bread crumbs
- 2 tablespoons minced fresh parsley
- 2 tablespoons chopped green onion

SAUCE:

- 1/4 cup reduced-fat mayonnaise
- 1/4 cup fat-free plain yogurt
- 2 tablespoons fat-free milk
- 1 tablespoon prepared horseradish
- 1 tablespoon Dijon mustard
- 1/4 teaspoon paprika

1. Combine mayonnaise and horseradish; spread over turkey. In a shallow dish, combine the bread crumbs, parsley and onion. Roll turkey in crumb mixture to coat.

2. Place in an 11-in. x 7-in. x 2-in. baking dish coated with cooking spray. Bake, uncovered, at 425° for 25-30 minutes or until a meat thermometer reads 170°.

3. In a small bowl, combine the sauce ingredients. Slice turkey; serve with sauce.

CRUMB CLUE

To make fresh bread crumbs, tear slices of fresh white, French or whole wheat bread into 2-in. pieces. Place in a food processor or blender; cover and pulse several times to make coarse crumbs. One slice of bread yields about 1/2 cup crumbs.

Savory Roasted Chicken

LOW SALT

PREP/TOTAL TIME
Prep: 10 min.
Bake: 1-1/2 hours
    + standing
YIELD 10 servings

When you want an impressive centerpiece for Sunday dinner or a special-occasion meal, you can't go wrong with this golden chicken. The moist, tender meat is enhanced with a delicious hint of orange, savory and thyme.

Taste of Home Test Kitchen

NUTRITION FACTS
One serving
(4 ounces cooked
chicken, skin
removed, calculated
without gravy)
equals:
  197 calories
  8 g fat
  2 g saturated fat
86 mg cholesterol
267 mg sodium
  Trace carbohydrate
  Trace fiber
  29 g protein

**DIABETIC
EXCHANGE**
  4 lean meat

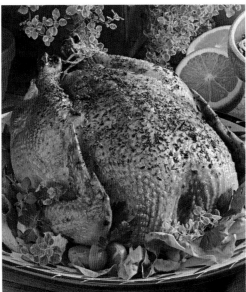

- 1 roasting chicken (6 to 7 pounds)
- 1 teaspoon onion salt
- 1/2 teaspoon dried thyme
- 1/2 teaspoon dried savory
- 1/4 teaspoon grated orange peel
- 1/4 teaspoon pepper
- 1 teaspoon canola oil

1. Place chicken on a rack in a shallow roasting pan. Carefully loosen the skin above the breast meat. Combine the onion salt, thyme, savory, orange peel and pepper; rub half of the herb mixture under the loosened skin. Rub chicken skin with oil; sprinkle with remaining herb mixture.

2. Bake at 375° for 1-1/2 to 2 hours or until a meat thermometer reads 180°. Let stand for 10-15 minutes. Remove skin before carving. Skim fat and thicken pan juices for gravy if desired.

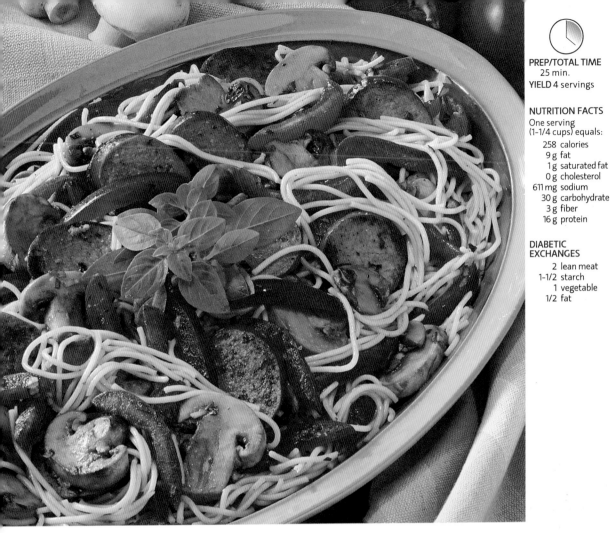

PREP/TOTAL TIME
25 min.
YIELD 4 servings

NUTRITION FACTS
One serving
(1-1/4 cups) equals:
  258 calories
  9 g fat
  1 g saturated fat
  0 g cholesterol
611 mg sodium
  30 g carbohydrate
  3 g fiber
  16 g protein

DIABETIC
EXCHANGES
  2 lean meat
1-1/2 starch
  1 vegetable
  1/2 fat

Smoked Sausage with Pasta

Chock-full of sausage, mushrooms, basil and tomatoes, this quick recipe satisfies even the toughest critics. It's one of my husband's favorites, and he has no idea it's light.

Ruth Ann Ruddell, Shelby, Michigan

4	ounces uncooked angel hair pasta
1/2	pound reduced-fat smoked turkey sausage, cut into 1/2-inch slices
2	cups sliced fresh mushrooms
2	garlic cloves, minced
4-1/2	teaspoons minced fresh basil *or* 1-1/2 teaspoons dried basil
1	tablespoon olive oil
2	cups julienned seeded plum tomatoes
1/8	teaspoon salt
1/8	teaspoon pepper

1. Cook the pasta according to the package directions. Meanwhile, in a large nonstick skillet, saute the sausage, mushrooms, garlic and basil in oil until the mushrooms are tender.

2. Drain the pasta; add to the sausage mixture. Add the tomatoes, salt and pepper; toss gently. Heat through.

SEEDING TOMATOES

To quickly seed plum tomatoes, cut in half lengthwise—a serrated knife works great for cutting tomatoes. Then scoop the seeds out with a metal spoon. You'll have seedless tomatoes ready in a jiffy for chopping or cutting into julienne strips.

PREP/TOTAL TIME
Prep: 20 min.
+ standing
Bake: 25 min.
YIELD 8 servings

NUTRITION FACTS
One serving
(1 slice) equals:
366 calories
9 g fat
4 g saturated fat
38 mg cholesterol
663 mg sodium
52 g carbohydrate
2 g fiber
20 g protein

DIABETIC
EXCHANGES
3 starch
2 lean meat
1/2 fat

Barbecued Turkey Pizza

My bread machine makes the crust for this mouthwatering pizza. The barbecue sauce, turkey, vegetables and cheese deliver so much flavor, even your biggest pizza fans won't believe it's on the lighter side.

Krista Frank, Rhododendron, Oregon

1 cup water (70° to 80°)
2 tablespoons olive oil
1 tablespoon sugar
1 teaspoon salt
3 cups all-purpose flour
2 teaspoons active dry yeast
3/4 cup barbecue sauce
1-1/2 cups cubed cooked turkey breast
1/2 cup fresh or frozen corn, thawed
1 small red onion, julienned
1 small green pepper, julienned
1 garlic clove, minced
1 cup (4 ounces) shredded part-skim mozzarella cheese
1/2 cup shredded reduced-fat cheddar cheese
1/4 cup grated Parmesan cheese

1. In bread machine pan, place the first six ingredients in order suggested by manufacturer. Select dough setting (check dough after 5 minutes of mixing; add 1 to 2 tablespoons of water or flour if needed).

2. When cycle is complete, turn dough onto a lightly floured surface. Punch down; cover and let stand for 10 minutes. Roll dough into a 14-in. circle. Transfer to a 14-in. pizza pan coated with cooking spray; build up edges slightly.

3. Spread barbecue sauce over crust. Layer with half of the turkey, corn, onion, green pepper, garlic and cheese. Repeat layers. Bake at 400° for 25-30 minutes or until the crust is golden brown.

Salsa Chicken Skillet

Diced chicken and veggies are stirred with spicy salsa to create this satisfying dinner.

LaDonna Reed, Ponca City, Oklahoma

- 1 pound boneless skinless chicken breasts, cut into 1/2-inch pieces
- 2 teaspoons canola oil
- 1/2 pound fresh mushrooms, sliced
- 1 medium green pepper, chopped
- 3/4 cup chopped onion
- 1/2 cup chopped celery
- 1/2 cup frozen corn, thawed
- 1 garlic clove, minced
- 2 cups salsa
- 2 cups hot cooked rice
- 1/4 cup shredded reduced-fat cheddar cheese
- 1/2 cup reduced-fat sour cream

1. In a large skillet, saute chicken in oil until no longer pink; drain and set aside. Coat skillet with cooking spray. Saute mushrooms, green pepper, onion, celery, corn and garlic for 6-8 minutes or until vegetables are tender. Add salsa and reserved chicken; heat through. Serve over rice. Top with cheese and sour cream.

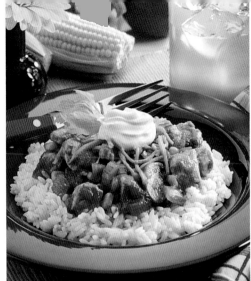

PREP/TOTAL TIME
25 min.
YIELD 4 servings

NUTRITION FACTS
One serving (1-1/4 cups over 1/2 cup cooked rice with 1 tablespoon sour cream) equals:

355 calories
7 g fat
2 g saturated fat
66 mg cholesterol
649 mg sodium
39 g carbohydrate
7 g fiber
29 g protein

DIABETIC EXCHANGES
3 lean meat
2 starch
2 vegetable

Brown Rice 'n' Apple Stuffed Turkey

The distinctive flavors of autumn abound in this lovely stuffing. Apple bits and raisins add fruitiness to the brown rice.

Taste of Home Test Kitchen

- 1 can (14-1/2 ounces) reduced-sodium chicken broth
- 1/2 cup unsweetened apple juice, *divided*
- 1/2 teaspoon salt, *divided*
- 1 cup uncooked long grain brown rice
- 1/3 cup raisins
- 1/2 cup chopped celery
- 1/2 cup chopped onion
- 1 tablespoon butter
- 1 cup chopped tart apple
- 1 teaspoon poultry seasoning
- 1/4 teaspoon pepper
- 1 turkey (10 to 12 pounds)

1. In a saucepan, combine the broth, 1/3 cup apple juice and 1/4 teaspoon salt. Bring to a boil. Stir in the rice and raisins. Return to a boil. Reduce heat; cover and simmer for 40-50 minutes or until the rice is tender.

2. Meanwhile, in a nonstick skillet, cook celery and onion in butter for 2 minutes. Add apple; cook and stir for 3 minutes or until vegetables are tender. Combine the rice mixture, apple mixture, poultry seasoning, pepper and remaining apple juice and salt.

3. Just before baking, loosely stuff turkey. Skewer turkey openings; tie drumsticks together. Place breast side up on a rack in a roasting pan. Bake, uncovered, at 325° for 2-3/4 to 3 hours or until a meat thermometer reads 180° for the turkey and 165° for the stuffing. (Cover loosely with foil if turkey browns too quickly.)

4. Cover turkey and let stand for 20 minutes. Remove stuffing and carve turkey, discarding skin. If desired, thicken pan drippings for gravy.

Editor's Note: Stuffing may be prepared as directed and baked separately in a 1-1/2-qt. baking dish coated with cooking spray. Cover and bake at 325° for 25 minutes. Uncover; bake 10-15 minutes longer or until heated through.

PREP/TOTAL TIME
Prep: 1 hour
Bake: 2-3/4 hours + standing
YIELD 6 servings with leftovers

NUTRITION FACTS
One serving (3 ounces cooked turkey with 3/4 cup stuffing, calculated without gravy) equals:

286 calories
8 g fat
3 g saturated fat
51 mg cholesterol
443 mg sodium
37 g carbohydrate
3 g fiber
17 g protein

DIABETIC EXCHANGES
2-1/2 starch
1 lean meat

Seasoned Turkey Burgers

This fun mixture of turkey and dressing tastes almost like Thanksgiving on a bun. The moist burgers are great alone, but my family likes them best with lettuce, onion, tomato and a dab of mayonnaise.

Viki Engelhardt, Grand Rapids, Michigan

1/2 cup herb-seasoned stuffing croutons

1 pound ground turkey breast

1 small onion, finely chopped

5 hamburger buns, split

Lettuce leaves, onion, tomato slices and fat-free mayonnaise, optional

1. Crush or process stuffing croutons into fine crumbs. In a bowl, combine crumbs, turkey and onion. Shape into five patties.

2. Broil or grill over medium-hot heat for 8-10 minutes, turning once. Serve on buns with lettuce, onion, tomato and mayonnaise if desired.

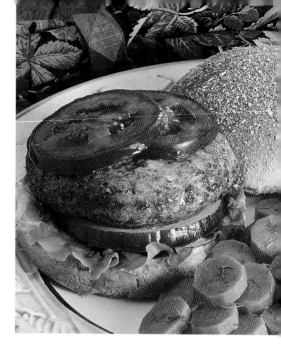

Nostalgic Chicken and Dumplings

You'll have old-fashioned goodness without all the fuss when you fix this slow-cooked supper. It features tender chicken, light dumplings and a full-flavored sauce.

Brenda Edwards, Hereford, Arizona

6 bone-in chicken breast halves (10 ounces *each*), skin removed

2 whole cloves

12 pearl onions, *divided*

1 bay leaf

1 garlic clove, minced

1/2 teaspoon salt

1/2 teaspoon dried thyme

1/2 teaspoon dried marjoram

1/4 teaspoon pepper

1/2 cup reduced-sodium chicken broth

1/2 cup white wine *or* additional chicken broth

3 tablespoons cornstarch

1/4 cup cold water

1/2 teaspoon browning sauce, optional

1 cup reduced-fat biscuit/baking mix

6 tablespoons fat-free milk

1 tablespoon minced fresh parsley

1. Place the chicken in a 5-qt. slow cooker. Insert cloves into one onion; add to slow cooker. Add bay leaf and remaining onions. Sprinkle chicken with garlic, salt, thyme, marjoram and pepper. Pour broth and wine or additional broth over chicken mixture. Cover and cook on low for 4-1/2 to 5 hours or until chicken juices run clear and a meat thermometer reads 170°.

2. Remove chicken to a platter and keep warm. Discard cloves and bay leaf. Increase temperature to high. In a small bowl, combine the cornstarch, water and browning sauce if desired until smooth. Stir into slow cooker.

3. In another small bowl, combine biscuit mix, milk and parsley. Drop by tablespoonfuls onto simmering liquid. Cover and cook on low for 20-25 minutes or until a toothpick inserted into dumplings comes out clean (do not lift cover while simmering). Serve dumplings and gravy with chicken.

Light Chicken Cordon Bleu

I simply love chicken cordon bleu, but because I am watching my cholesterol, I could not afford to indulge in it very often. Then I trimmed down a recipe I received in my high school home economics class years ago. The creamy sauce makes this dish even more special.

Shannon Strate, Salt Lake City, Utah

- 8 boneless skinless chicken breast halves (4 ounces *each*)
- 1/2 teaspoon pepper
- 8 slices (1 ounce *each*) lean deli ham
- 1-1/2 cups (6 ounces) shredded part-skim mozzarella cheese
- 2/3 cup fat-free milk
- 1 cup crushed cornflakes
- 1 teaspoon paprika
- 1/2 teaspoon garlic powder
- 1/4 teaspoon salt

SAUCE:

- 1 can (10-3/4 ounces) reduced-fat reduced-sodium condensed cream of chicken soup, undiluted
- 1/2 cup fat-free sour cream
- 1 teaspoon lemon juice

1. Flatten chicken to 1/4-in. thickness. Sprinkle with pepper; place a ham slice and 3 tablespoons of cheese down the center of each piece. Roll up and tuck in ends; secure with toothpicks. Pour milk into a shallow bowl. In another bowl, combine the cornflakes, paprika, garlic powder and salt. Dip chicken in milk, then roll in crumbs.

2. Place in a 13-in. x 9-in. x 2-in. baking dish coated with cooking spray. Bake, uncovered, at 350° for 25-30 minutes or until juices run clear.

3. Meanwhile, in a small saucepan, whisk the soup, sour cream and lemon juice until blended; heat through. Discard toothpicks from chicken; serve with sauce.

PREP/TOTAL TIME
Prep: 20 min.
Bake: 25 min.
YIELD 8 servings

NUTRITION FACTS
One serving
(1 chicken
breast half with
2 tablespoons
sauce) equals:

- 306 calories
- 7 g fat
- 3 g saturated fat
- 91 mg cholesterol
- 990 mg sodium
- 16 g carbohydrate
- Trace fiber
- 41 g protein

DIABETIC EXCHANGES
- 3 lean meat
- 1 starch
- 1 fat

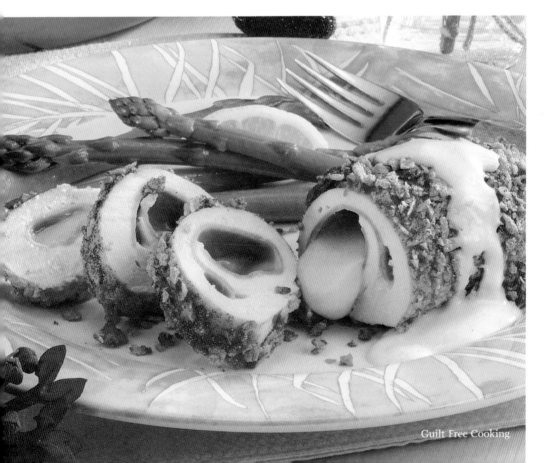

Herbed Stuffed Green Peppers

PREP/TOTAL TIME
Prep: 25 min.
Bake: 30 min.
YIELD 6 servings

NUTRITION FACTS
One serving
(1 stuffed pepper)
equals:
267 calories
10 g fat
0 g saturated fat
51 mg cholesterol
483 mg sodium
29 g carbohydrate
0 g fiber
21 g protein

DIABETIC
EXCHANGES
2 meat
2 vegetable
1 starch

This main dish is loaded with taste. The blend of dried herbs adds an abundance of flavor—there's no need for salt.

Bea Taus, Fremont, California

- 6 green peppers, tops and seeds removed
- 1 pound ground turkey
- 1 can (28 ounces) crushed tomatoes
- 1 medium onion, chopped
- 2 celery ribs, chopped
- 2 garlic cloves, minced
- 1 teaspoon dried oregano
- 1/2 teaspoon dried thyme
- 1/2 teaspoon dried rosemary
- 1/2 teaspoon dried basil
- 1/2 teaspoon rubbed sage
- 1/8 teaspoon pepper
- 1-1/2 cups cooked rice
- 1/3 cup shredded part-skim mozzarella cheese

1. In a large kettle, blanch peppers in boiling water for 3 minutes. Drain and rinse in cold water. Set aside. In a large nonstick skillet, brown the turkey over medium heat. Remove and set aside.

2. In the same skillet, combine tomato liquid, onion, celery, garlic and herbs. Simmer until vegetables are tender and the mixture has begun to thicken. Stir in tomatoes, turkey and rice.

3. Stuff into peppers and place in a baking pan. Bake, uncovered, at 350° for 30 minutes. Top each pepper with about 1 tablespoon cheese. Bake 3 minutes longer or until the cheese is melted.

Chicken Jambalaya

LOW FAT

PREP/TOTAL TIME
Prep: 20 min.
Cook: 1 hour
YIELD 6 servings

NUTRITION FACTS
One serving
(1 cup) equals:
302 calories
4 g fat
1 g saturated fat
43 mg cholesterol
452 mg sodium
45 g carbohydrate
3 g fiber
21 g protein

DIABETIC
EXCHANGES
2-1/2 starch
1-1/2 lean meat
1 vegetable

I think this jambalaya is just as good as, if not better than, the higher-fat version. I often put this recipe on my party menus.

Lynn Desjardins, Atkinson, New Hampshire

- 3/4 pound boneless skinless chicken breasts, cubed
- 3 cups reduced-sodium chicken broth

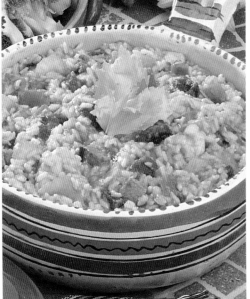

- 1-1/2 cups uncooked brown rice
- 4 ounces reduced-fat smoked turkey sausage, diced
- 1/2 cup thinly sliced celery with leaves
- 1/2 cup chopped onion
- 1/2 cup chopped green pepper
- 2 to 3 teaspoons Cajun *or* Creole seasoning
- 1 to 2 garlic cloves, minced
- 1/8 teaspoon hot pepper sauce
- 1 bay leaf
- 1 can (14-1/2 ounces) no-salt-added diced tomatoes, undrained

1. In a large nonstick skillet lightly coated with cooking spray, saute chicken for 2-3 minutes. Stir in the next 10 ingredients. Bring to a boil. Reduce heat; cover and simmer for 50-60 minutes.

2. Stir in tomatoes; cover and simmer 10 minutes longer or until liquid is absorbed and rice is tender. Remove from the heat; let stand for 5 minutes. Discard bay leaf.

Editor's Note: The following spices may be substituted for the Creole seasoning: 1/2 teaspoon *each* paprika and the garlic powder, and a pinch *each* cayenne pepper, dried thyme and ground cumin.

Chicken Noodle Casserole

I have to be creative at mealtimes to fix something quick, delicious and nutritious. This homey dish fits all of my requirements!

Lori Gleason, Minneapolis, Minnesota

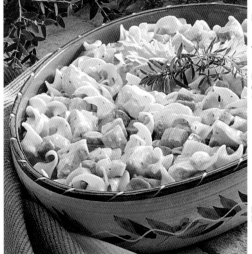

- 2/3 cup chopped onion
- 1 garlic clove, minced
- 1 tablespoon olive oil
- 1-1/2 pounds boneless skinless chicken breasts, cut into 3/4-inch cubes
- 1 can (14-1/2 ounces) chicken broth
- 1-1/2 cups chopped carrots
- 3 celery ribs, chopped
- 1/2 teaspoon dried savory
- 3 tablespoons butter
- 3 tablespoons all-purpose flour
- 3/4 teaspoon salt
- 1/8 teaspoon white pepper
- 1-1/2 cups 2% milk
- 1-1/4 cups shredded reduced-fat cheddar cheese
- 8 ounces wide egg noodles, cooked and drained

1. In a large nonstick skillet, saute onion and garlic in oil until tender. Add chicken; cook and stir until no longer pink. Add the broth, carrots, celery and savory. Bring to a boil. Reduce heat; cover and simmer for 10-15 minutes or until vegetables are tender.

2. In a saucepan, melt butter. Stir in the flour, salt and pepper until smooth. Gradually add milk. Bring to a boil; cook and stir for 2 minutes or until thickened. Remove from the heat; stir in cheese until melted. Pour over chicken mixture. Add noodles; mix well.

3. Transfer to a 3-qt. baking dish coated with cooking spray. Bake, uncovered, at 350° for 15-20 minutes or until bubbly.

PREP/TOTAL TIME
Prep: 20 min.
Bake: 15 min.
YIELD 8 servings

NUTRITION FACTS
One serving
(1 cup) equals:
- 343 calories
- 11 g fat
- 5 g saturated fat
- 95 mg cholesterol
- 681 mg sodium
- 30 g carbohydrate
- 2 g fiber
- 31 g protein

DIABETIC EXCHANGES
- 3 lean meat
- 2 starch
- 1 fat

Spanish Chicken and Rice

Using cooked chicken, this meaty tomato and rice meal-in-one bakes quickly.

Patricia Rutherford, Winchester, Illinois

- 2/3 cup finely chopped onion
- 1/4 cup sliced fresh mushrooms
- 1-1/4 cups cubed cooked chicken breast
- 2 plum tomatoes, peeled and chopped
- 1/2 cup cooked long grain rice
- 1/2 cup reduced-sodium tomato juice
- 1/2 cup reduced-sodium chicken broth
- 1/3 cup frozen peas
- 1 tablespoon chopped pimientos
- 1/8 teaspoon dried tarragon
- 1/8 teaspoon dried savory

Pinch pepper

1. In a skillet coated with cooking spray, saute onion and mushrooms for 4 minutes or until tender. Place in an ungreased 1-qt. baking dish. Stir in the remaining ingredients. Cover and bake at 375° for 5-20 minutes or until liquid is absorbed.

LIVELY LEFTOVERS

Spanish Chicken and Rice is a great way to use up leftover chicken. Cooked chicken may be stored in the refrigerator for up to 4 days. Or, keep the extra chicken in your freezer for up to 4 months.

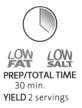

LOW FAT   LOW SALT
PREP/TOTAL TIME
30 min.
YIELD 2 servings

NUTRITION FACTS
One serving
(1-1/2 cups) equals:
- 207 calories
- 4 g fat
- 0 g saturated fat
- 54 mg cholesterol
- 108 mg sodium
- 25 g carbohydrate
- 0 g fiber
- 19 g protein

DIABETIC EXCHANGES
- 2 very lean meat
- 1 vegetable
- 1/2 fat

PREP/TOTAL TIME
25 min.
YIELD 4 servings

NUTRITION FACTS
One serving
(1 cup) equals:
  285 calories
  8 g fat
  2 g saturated fat
39 mg cholesterol
908 mg sodium
  34 g carbohydrate
  3 g fiber
  19 g protein

**DIABETIC
EXCHANGES**
  2 lean meat
  2 vegetable
1-1/2 starch

Fettuccine Italiana

I perk up a platter of fettuccine with spicy sausage and delicately flavored asparagus and mushrooms. This special-looking entree is easy enough for an everyday meal.

Janet Quigley, Galveston, Texas

  8 ounces uncooked fettuccine

  1 package (14 ounces) reduced-fat smoked turkey sausage, thinly sliced

  2 cups cut fresh asparagus (1-1/2-inch pieces)

  1 cup sliced fresh mushrooms

1/4 cup chopped onion

  1 garlic clove, minced

1/2 teaspoon dried thyme

  1 tablespoon olive oil

  1 tablespoon cornstarch

  1 cup reduced-sodium chicken broth

1/4 cup shredded Parmesan *or* Romano cheese

1. Cook fettuccine according to package directions. Meanwhile, in a large saucepan, saute turkey sausage, asparagus, mushrooms, onion, garlic and thyme in oil until vegetables are tender.

2. Combine cornstarch and chicken broth until smooth; stir into sausage mixture. Bring to a boil; cook and stir for 1-2 minutes or until thickened. Drain fettuccine. Add to sausage mixture; toss to coat. Sprinkle with Parmesan cheese.

Chicken Lasagna

This lightened-up lasagna is a satisfying alternative to the ground beef variety.

Marilynn Hieronymus, Sedalia, Missouri

- 1 medium onion, chopped
- 1/2 cup chopped green pepper
- 3 tablespoons butter, melted
- 6 ounces fresh mushrooms, sliced
- 1 can (10-3/4 ounces) condensed reduced-fat reduced-sodium cream of mushroom soup, undiluted
- 1/3 cup fat-free milk
- 1 jar (2 ounces) diced pimientos, drained
- 1/2 teaspoon dried basil
- 2-1/2 cups cubed cooked chicken
- 8 ounces reduced-fat process cheese (Velveeta), cubed
- 1-1/2 cups fat-free cream-style cottage cheese
- 1/2 cup grated Parmesan cheese, *divided*
- 9 lasagna noodles, cooked and drained
- 2 teaspoons minced fresh parsley

1. In a saucepan, saute onion and green pepper in butter until tender. Add mushrooms; cook until tender. Remove from the heat; stir in soup, milk, pimientos and basil. In a bowl, combine the chicken, process cheese, cottage cheese and 1/4 cup Parmesan cheese.

2. Spread a fourth of the mushroom sauce in a 13-in. x 9-in. x 2-in. baking dish coated with cooking spray. Top with three cooked noodles, half of the chicken mixture and a fourth of the mushroom sauce. Repeat layers of noodles, chicken mixture and mushroom sauce. Top with the remaining noodles and mushroom sauce.

3. Sprinkle with parsley and remaining Parmesan. Cover and bake at 350° for 30 minutes. Uncover; bake 15-20 minutes longer or until hot and bubbly. Let stand for 15 minutes before cutting.

PREP/TOTAL TIME
Prep: 20 min.
Bake: 30 min. + standing
YIELD 12 servings

NUTRITION FACTS
One serving
(1 piece) equals:
196 calories
7 g fat
3 g saturated fat
31 mg cholesterol
696 mg sodium
130 g carbohydrate
7 g fiber
9 g protein

DIABETIC EXCHANGES
2 lean meat
1-1/2 fat
1 starch
1 vegetable

Oven-Fried Chicken

Tarragon, ginger and cayenne pepper flavor the cornmeal coating on my "fried" chicken.

Daucia Brooks, Westmoreland, Tennessee

- 1/2 cup cornmeal
- 1/2 cup dry bread crumbs
- 1 teaspoon dried tarragon
- 1 teaspoon ground ginger
- 1/2 teaspoon salt
- 1/4 teaspoon cayenne pepper
- 1/4 teaspoon pepper
- 3 egg whites
- 2 tablespoons fat-free milk
- 1/2 cup all-purpose flour
- 6 bone-in chicken breast halves (6 ounces *each*)

Refrigerated butter-flavored spray

1. In a shallow bowl, combine the first seven ingredients. In another shallow bowl, combine egg whites and milk. Place flour in a third shallow bowl. Coat chicken with flour; dip in the egg white mixture, then roll in cornmeal mixture.

2. Place in a 15-in. x 10-in. x 2-in. baking pan coated with cooking spray. Bake, uncovered, at 350° for 40 minutes. Spritz with butter-flavored spray. Bake 10-15 minutes longer or until juices run clear.

LOW FAT

PREP/TOTAL TIME
Prep: 10 min.
Bake: 40 min.
YIELD 6 servings

NUTRITION FACTS
One serving
(1 chicken breast half) equals:
248 calories
2 g fat
1 g saturated fat
63 mg cholesterol
375 mg sodium
24 g carbohydrate
1 g fiber
30 g protein

DIABETIC EXCHANGES
4 very lean meat
1-1/2 starch

PREP/TOTAL TIME
25 min.
YIELD 6 servings

NUTRITION FACTS
One serving
(1 sandwich) equals:
340 calories
8 g fat
3 g saturated fat
56 mg cholesterol
637 mg sodium
39 g carbohydrate
2 g fiber
27 g protein

DIABETIC EXCHANGES
3 lean meat
2-1/2 starch

Barbecued Turkey Sandwiches

These tangy sandwiches are a welcome break from beef barbecue and sloppy joes. The turkey cooks in a lip-smacking sauce.

Barbara Smith, Columbus, Ohio

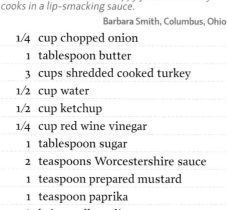

1/4	cup chopped onion
1	tablespoon butter
3	cups shredded cooked turkey
1/2	cup water
1/2	cup ketchup
1/4	cup red wine vinegar
1	tablespoon sugar
2	teaspoons Worcestershire sauce
1	teaspoon prepared mustard
1	teaspoon paprika
6	kaiser rolls, split

1. In a large nonstick skillet, saute the onion in butter until tender. Add the turkey, water, ketchup, vinegar, sugar, Worcestershire sauce, mustard and paprika. Bring to a boil. Reduce the heat; simmer, uncovered, for 15 minutes or until the sauce is thickened. Serve on rolls.

PREP/TOTAL TIME
20 min.
YIELD 4 servings

NUTRITION FACTS
One serving (1 cup calculated without spaghetti) equals:
251 calories
6 g fat
1 g saturated fat
68 mg cholesterol
745 mg sodium
17 g carbohydrate
4 g fiber
30 g protein

DIABETIC EXCHANGES
3 lean meat
3 vegetable

Stir-Fried Chicken Marinara

This hearty dish is chock-full of chicken and vegetables. It's a dinnertime favorite.

Bonnie Buckley, Kansas City, Missouri

1	can (14-1/2 ounces) diced tomatoes, undrained
1	tablespoon cornstarch
1	can (8 ounces) tomato sauce
1/4	cup reduced-sodium chicken broth
1/4	cup dry red wine *or* additional chicken broth
1/2	teaspoon *each* dried basil and thyme
1/4	teaspoon salt
1	pound boneless skinless chicken breasts, cut into 2-inch strips
2	garlic cloves, minced
1	tablespoon olive oil
1	small onion
1	medium green *or* sweet yellow pepper, julienned
1	small eggplant, peeled and cut into 3/4-inch cubes (about 3 cups)

Hot cooked spaghetti

2	tablespoons grated Parmesan cheese

1. Drain tomatoes, reserving juice. Set the tomatoes aside. In a bowl, combine the cornstarch, tomato sauce, chicken broth, wine or additional broth, seasonings and reserved juice until smooth. Set aside.

2. In a large nonstick skillet or wok, stir-fry chicken and garlic in hot oil until no longer pink. Remove and keep warm. In same skillet, stir-fry onion and pepper for 4 minutes. Add eggplant; stir-fry for 4-5 minutes or until tender.

3. Stir sauce; add to the pan. Bring to a boil; cook and stir for 2 minutes or until thickened. Add the chicken and tomatoes; heat through. Serve over pasta. Top with cheese.

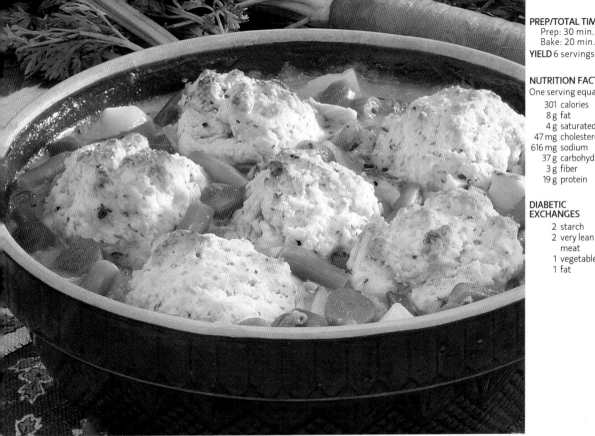

PREP/TOTAL TIME
Prep: 30 min.
Bake: 20 min.
YIELD 6 servings

NUTRITION FACTS
One serving equals:
301 calories
8 g fat
4 g saturated fat
47 mg cholesterol
616 mg sodium
37 g carbohydrate
3 g fiber
19 g protein

DIABETIC EXCHANGES
2 starch
2 very lean meat
1 vegetable
1 fat

Turkey Biscuit Potpie

This comforting dish is loaded with chunks of turkey, potatoes, carrots and beans.

Shirley Francey, St. Catharines, Ontario

1	large onion, chopped
1	garlic clove, minced
1-1/2	cups cubed peeled potatoes
1-1/2	cups sliced carrots
1	cup frozen cut green beans, thawed
1	cup reduced-sodium chicken broth
4-1/2	teaspoons all-purpose flour
1	can (10-3/4 ounces) reduced-fat condensed cream of mushroom soup, undiluted
2	cups cubed cooked turkey
2	tablespoons minced fresh parsley
1/2	teaspoon dried basil
1/2	teaspoon dried thyme
1/4	teaspoon pepper

BISCUITS:

1	cup all-purpose flour
2	teaspoons baking powder
1/2	teaspoon dried oregano
2	tablespoons butter
7	tablespoons 1% milk

1. In a large saucepan coated with cooking spray, cook onion and garlic over medium heat until tender. Add potatoes, carrots, beans and broth; bring to a boil. Reduce heat; cover and simmer for 15-20 minutes or until potatoes are tender.

2. Remove from the heat. Combine the flour and mushroom soup; stir into vegetable mixture. Add the turkey and seasonings. Transfer to a 2-qt. baking dish coated with cooking spray.

3. In a large bowl, combine the flour, baking powder and oregano. Cut in the butter until evenly distributed. Stir in milk. Drop batter in six mounds onto hot turkey mixture. Bake, uncovered, at 400° for 20-25 minutes or until a toothpick inserted in center of biscuits comes out clean and biscuits are golden brown.

Stuffed Cornish Hens

With a succulent stuffing of cranberries, rice and mushrooms, these golden hens are sure to become a favorite for special occasions in your home. They're a nice change of pace from the traditional holiday turkey.

Nancy Horsburgh, Everett, Ontario

NUTRITION FACTS
One serving (1 hen half with 1/3 cup stuffing calculated without skin) equals:

257 calories
7 g fat
3 g saturated fat
123 mg cholesterol
564 mg sodium
20 g carbohydrate
1 g fiber
29 g protein

DIABETIC EXCHANGES
4 very lean meat
1-1/2 starch
1/2 fat

1/2 cup chopped celery

1/4 cup sliced fresh mushrooms

2 tablespoons butter

1 package (6 ounces) fast-cooking long grain and wild rice mix

1 can (14-1/2 ounces) reduced-sodium chicken broth

1/4 cup water

2/3 cup sliced water chestnuts, chopped

1/2 cup dried cranberries

1/2 cup chopped green onions

2 tablespoons reduced-sodium soy sauce

5 Cornish game hens (20 ounces *each*)

1. In a large saucepan coated with cooking spray, cook celery and mushrooms in butter until tender. Stir in rice; cook 1 minute longer. Stir in the contents of the rice seasoning packet, broth and water. Bring to a boil. Reduce heat; cover and simmer for 5-6 minutes or until rice is tender. Stir in the water chestnuts, cranberries, onions and soy sauce. Stuff into hens.

2. Place on a rack in a shallow roasting pan. Bake at 375° for 50-60 minutes or until juices run clear and a meat thermometer inserted into stuffing reads 165°. Cut each hen in half lengthwise to serve.

Sweet-and-Sour Chicken

When I went on a restricted diet, I revamped my old sweet-and-sour chicken recipe. No one could even tell the difference!

Eva Marie Collins, Bolivar, Missouri

- 1/2 pound boneless skinless chicken breasts, cut into strips
- 1 medium carrot, sliced
- 1/4 cup chopped onion
- 1-1/2 teaspoons canola oil
- 1 small zucchini, sliced
- 1 cup snow peas, thawed
- 1/2 medium sweet red *or* green pepper, cut into strips
- 3 tablespoons sugar
- 2 tablespoons cornstarch
- 1/8 teaspoon pepper
- 1 can (6 ounces) pineapple juice
- 3 tablespoons ketchup
- 2 tablespoons lemon juice
- 2 tablespoons reduced-sodium soy sauce
- 1 can (8 ounces) unsweetened pineapple chunks, drained
- 2 cups hot cooked rice

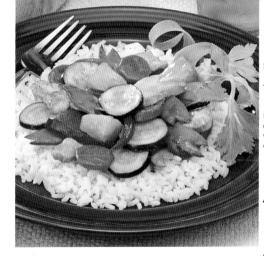

LOW FAT

PREP/TOTAL TIME
25 min.
YIELD 4 servings

NUTRITION FACTS
One serving (1 cup with 1/2 cup rice) equals:
307 calories
3 g fat
Trace saturated fat
33 mg cholesterol
400 mg sodium
52 g carbohydrate
4 g fiber
18 g protein

DIABETIC EXCHANGES
2 starch
2 very lean meat
1 vegetable
1 fruit

1. In a nonstick skillet, cook the chicken, carrot and onion in oil until chicken is browned. Add the zucchini, peas and red pepper; cook and stir until vegetables are crisp-tender.

2. In a bowl, combine sugar, cornstarch, pepper and pineapple juice until smooth. Stir in the ketchup, lemon juice and soy sauce. Pour over the chicken mixture. Add the pineapple. Bring to a boil; cook and stir for 2 minutes or until thickened. Serve over rice.

Turkey Sloppy Joes

This tangy sandwich filling is so easy to prepare in the slow cooker, and it goes over big at events. When I take it to potlucks, I'm always asked for my secret ingredient.

Marylou LaRue, Freeland, Michigan

- 1 pound ground turkey breast
- 1 small onion, chopped
- 1/2 cup chopped celery
- 1/4 cup chopped green pepper
- 1 can (10-3/4 ounces) reduced-fat reduced-sodium condensed tomato soup, undiluted
- 1/2 cup ketchup
- 1 tablespoon brown sugar
- 2 tablespoons prepared mustard
- 1/4 teaspoon pepper
- 8 hamburger buns, split

1. In a large saucepan coated with cooking spray, cook the turkey, onion, celery and green pepper over medium heat until meat is no longer pink; drain if necessary. Stir in the soup, ketchup, brown sugar, mustard and pepper.

2. Transfer to a 3-qt. slow cooker. Cover and cook on low for 4 hours. Serve on buns.

PREP/TOTAL TIME
Prep: 15 min.
Cook: 4 hours
YIELD 8 servings

NUTRITION FACTS
One serving (1 sandwich) equals:
247 calories
7 g fat
2 g saturated fat
45 mg cholesterol
553 mg sodium
32 g carbohydrate
2 g fiber
14 g protein

DIABETIC EXCHANGES
2 starch
1-1/2 lean meat

SLOPPY JOES IN MINUTES

The slow cooker is great for fix-and-forget-it meals. You can run errands or even have fun while the slow cooker does the work. But, if you want the great taste of Turkey Sloppy Joes and don't have 4 hours to wait, you can make it on the stovetop. Follow all the directions in step 1. Then, bring the mixture to a boil. Reduce heat; cover and simmer for 20 minutes to heat through and allow the flavors to blend. You'll have a tasty dinner in about 35 minutes.

PREP/TOTAL TIME
20 min.
YIELD 6 servings

NUTRITION FACTS
One serving
(1-1/3 cups) equals:
342 calories
5 g fat
2 g saturated fat
78 mg cholesterol
526 mg sodium
36 g carbohydrate
4 g fiber
35 g protein

DIABETIC EXCHANGES
4 very lean meat
2 starch
1 vegetable

Chicken Pasta Primavera

Canned soup, frozen vegetables and other kitchen staples bring this popular family meal together in no time. Add a green salad, and dinner is ready.

Margaret Wilson, Hemet, California

6 ounces uncooked spaghetti

1 can (10-3/4 ounces) reduced-fat reduced-sodium condensed cream of chicken soup, undiluted

3/4 cup water

1 tablespoon lemon juice

1-1/2 teaspoons dried basil

3/4 teaspoon garlic powder

1/2 teaspoon salt

1/4 teaspoon pepper

1 package (16 ounces) frozen California-blend vegetables, thawed

4 cups cubed cooked chicken breast

3 tablespoons grated Parmesan cheese

1. Cook spaghetti according to package directions. Meanwhile, in a large saucepan, combine the soup, water, lemon juice, basil, garlic powder, salt and pepper. Stir

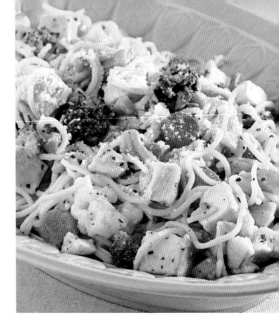

in vegetables; bring to a boil. Reduce heat; cover and simmer for 3-5 minutes or until vegetables are tender.

2. Stir in the chicken; heat through. Drain spaghetti; add to chicken mixture and toss to coat. Sprinkle with Parmesan cheese.

PREP/TOTAL TIME
20 min.
YIELD 1 dozen

NUTRITION FACTS
One serving
(1 taco) equals:
146 calories
2 g fat
0 g saturated fat
22 mg cholesterol
228 mg sodium
20 g carbohydrate
0 g fiber
13 g protein

DIABETIC EXCHANGES
1 starch
1 lean meat
1 vegetable

Chicken 'n' Bean Tacos

These mouthwatering tacos are a wonderful change of pace. We love the combination of black beans, chicken and tomatoes.

Wendy Hines, Chesnee, South Carolina

1 pound boneless skinless chicken breasts, cut into bite-size pieces

1/2 cup chopped onion

2 garlic cloves, minced

1 can (15 ounces) black beans, undrained

1/4 cup minced fresh parsley

1 to 2 teaspoons ground cumin

1/4 teaspoon pepper

12 corn tortillas (6 inches), warmed

1/2 cup shredded reduced-fat cheddar cheese

1 cup chopped fresh tomatoes

1. In a nonstick skillet, saute the chicken, onion and garlic until juices run clear. Stir in the beans, parsley, cumin and pepper; heat through.

2. Spoon 1/3 cup down the center of each tortilla; sprinkle with cheese and tomatoes. Fold in half; serve immediately.

CHANGE OUT THE BEANS

Out of canned black beans? You can use pinto beans, kidney beans, cannellini beans or even chickpeas for these tacos. All these beans will provide your diet with a good source of fiber.

Italian Turkey and Noodles

A jar of meatless spaghetti sauce makes this easy dish a perfect supper during the week. Just add a green salad, and dinner is set. Best of all, my whole family loves it.

Cindi Roshia, Racine, Wisconsin

1-1/4	pounds lean ground turkey
1-1/2	cups sliced fresh mushrooms
1/2	cup chopped onion
1/2	cup chopped green pepper
1	jar (26 ounces) meatless spaghetti sauce
1/2	teaspoon onion salt
3	cups cooked yolk-free wide noodles
1	cup (4 ounces) shredded part-skim mozzarella cheese

1. In a large nonstick skillet, cook turkey, mushrooms, onion and green pepper until turkey is no longer pink. Add spaghetti sauce and onion salt; bring to a boil. Reduce heat; simmer, uncovered, for 15 minutes.

2. Place cooked noodles in the bottom of a 2-1/2-qt. baking dish coated with cooking spray. Pour the meat mixture over the noodles. Sprinkle with cheese. Cover and bake at 350° for 20 minutes. Uncover; bake 10-15 minutes longer or until heated through.

PREP/TOTAL TIME
Prep: 35 min.
Bake: 30 min.
YIELD 6 servings

NUTRITION FACTS
One serving equals:
392 calories
12 g fat
5 g saturated fat
86 mg cholesterol
798 mg sodium
39 g carbohydrate
5 g fiber
28 g protein

DIABETIC EXCHANGES
3 lean meat
3 vegetable
1-1/2 starch
1/2 fat

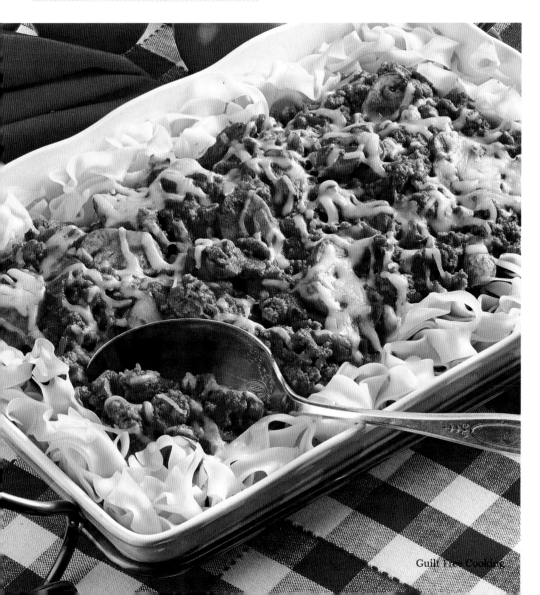

Chicken Cacciatore

For a special Italian entree, try this chicken simmered in a well-seasoned sauce.

Taste of Home Test Kitchen

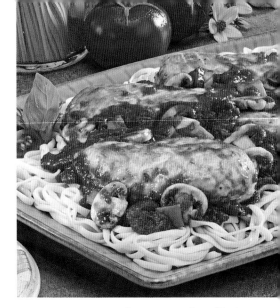

NUTRITION FACTS
One serving
(1 chicken breast
half with 1/2 cup
sauce, calculated
without spaghetti)
equals:
  248 calories
    8 g fat
    1 g saturated fat
  67 mg cholesterol
857 mg sodium
  18 g carbohydrate
    3 g fiber
  29 g protein

DIABETIC EXCHANGES
  3 lean meat
  3 vegetable

- 6 boneless skinless chicken breast halves (4 ounces *each*)
- 1 teaspoon salt, *divided*
- 1/8 teaspoon pepper
- 2 tablespoons olive oil, *divided*
- 1 medium green pepper, chopped
- 1/2 pound fresh mushrooms, sliced
- 4 garlic cloves, minced
- 1 can (15 ounces) tomato puree
- 1 can (14-1/2 ounces) stewed tomatoes, cut up
- 1 tablespoon balsamic vinegar
- 2 teaspoons sugar
- 1-1/2 teaspoons dried basil
- 1-1/2 teaspoons dried oregano
- 1/4 teaspoon crushed red pepper flakes
- 1/4 cup minced fresh parsley

Hot cooked spaghetti, optional

1. Sprinkle chicken with 1/4 teaspoon salt and pepper. In a large nonstick skillet, brown chicken in 1 tablespoon oil. Remove and set aside. In the same skillet, saute the green pepper, mushrooms and garlic in remaining oil until vegetables are tender.

2. Add the tomato puree, stewed tomatoes, vinegar, sugar, basil, oregano, red pepper flakes, remaining salt and reserved chicken. Bring to a boil. Reduce heat; cover and simmer for 30 minutes.

3. Stir in parsley. Simmer, uncovered, 15 minutes longer or until sauce is thickened. Serve over spaghetti if desired.

Chicken in Creamy Gravy

You only need a few ingredients and a few minutes to put this pleasing main dish on the table. A burst of lemon in every bite makes it a popular standby in my home.

Jean Little, Charlotte, North Carolina

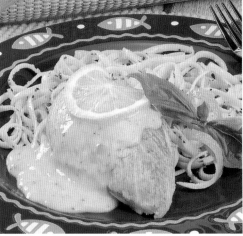

NUTRITION FACTS
One serving equals:
  232 calories
    7 g fat
    1 g saturated fat
  72 mg cholesterol
644 mg sodium
  18 g carbohydrate
    5 g fiber
  30 g protein

DIABETIC EXCHANGES
  3 lean meat
  1 starch

- 4 boneless skinless chicken breast halves (1 pound)
- 1 tablespoon canola oil
- 1 can (10-3/4 ounces) reduced-fat reduced-sodium condensed cream of chicken and broccoli soup, undiluted
- 1/4 cup fat-free milk
- 2 teaspoons lemon juice
- 1/8 teaspoon pepper
- 4 lemon slices

1. In a large nonstick skillet, cook chicken in oil until browned on both sides, about 10 minutes; drain. In a large bowl, combine soup, milk, juice and pepper. Pour over chicken. Top each chicken breast with a lemon slice. Reduce heat; cover and simmer until chicken juices run clear, about 5 minutes.

Turkey Tetrazzini

Your family will flip over this tasty turkey and mushroom casserole. It's so good!

Irene Banegas, Las Cruces, New Mexico

1/2 pound uncooked spaghetti

1/4 cup finely chopped onion

1 garlic clove, minced

1 tablespoon butter

3 tablespoons cornstarch

1 can (14-1/2 ounces) reduced-sodium chicken broth

1 can (12 ounces) fat-free evaporated milk

2-1/2 cups cubed cooked turkey breast

1 can (4 ounces) mushroom stems and pieces, drained

1/2 teaspoon seasoned salt

Dash pepper

2 tablespoons grated Parmesan cheese

1/4 teaspoon paprika

1. Cook spaghetti according to package directions; drain. In a large saucepan, saute onion and garlic in butter until tender. Combine cornstarch and broth until smooth; stir into the onion mixture. Bring to a boil; cook and stir for 2 minutes or until thickened. Reduce heat to low. Add the milk; cook and stir for 2-3 minutes. Stir in the spaghetti, turkey, mushrooms, seasoned salt and pepper.

2. Transfer to an 8-in. square baking dish coated with cooking spray. Cover and bake at 350° for 20 minutes. Uncover; sprinkle with cheese and paprika. Bake 5-10 minutes longer or until heated through.

LOW FAT

PREP/TOTAL TIME
Prep: 25 min.
Bake: 25 min.

YIELD 6 servings

NUTRITION FACTS
One serving
(1-1/4 cups) equals:
331 calories
5 g fat
2 g saturated fat
51 mg cholesterol
544 mg sodium
41 g carbohydrate
1 g fiber
28 g protein

DIABETIC EXCHANGES
3 very lean meat
2 starch
1 vegetable
1/2 fat-free milk

Mushroom Cheese Chicken

There's a delightful surprise tucked inside these rolled chicken breasts. The mushroom and mozzarella filling is perked up with chives and pimientos. A crumb topping adds a bit of crunch to the moist, tender bundles.

Anna Free, Plymouth, Ohio

4 boneless skinless chicken breast halves (5 ounces *each*)

1/2 teaspoon salt

Dash pepper

2 tablespoons all-purpose flour

1/2 cup reduced-fat plain yogurt

1/2 cup shredded part-skim mozzarella cheese

1/2 cup canned mushroom stems and pieces

1 tablespoon diced pimientos

1 tablespoon minced fresh parsley

1 tablespoon minced chives

TOPPING:

1 tablespoon reduced-fat plain yogurt

1 tablespoon dry bread crumbs

1/8 teaspoon paprika

1. Flatten chicken to 1/8-in. thickness; sprinkle with salt and pepper. In a small bowl, combine the flour and yogurt until smooth. Stir in the cheese, mushrooms, pimientos, parsley and chives. Spread down the center of each piece of chicken. Roll up and tuck in ends; secure with toothpicks. Place seam side down in an 11-in. x 7-in. x 2-in. baking dish coated with cooking spray.

2. Brush yogurt over chicken. Combine bread crumbs and paprika; sprinkle over the top. Bake, uncovered, at 350° for 20-25 minutes or until chicken juices run clear. Discard toothpicks before serving.

LOW FAT

PREP/TOTAL TIME
Prep: 15 min.
Bake: 20 min.

YIELD 4 servings

NUTRITION FACTS
One serving equals:
222 calories
5 g fat
2 g saturated fat
92 mg cholesterol
544 mg sodium
4 g carbohydrate
Trace fiber
39 g protein

DIABETIC EXCHANGE
4 lean meat

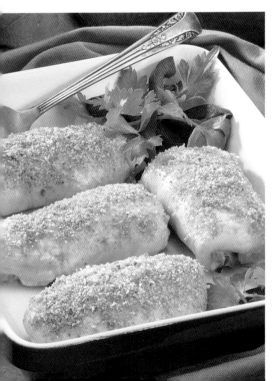

Penne Sausage Bake

This hearty pasta dish was inspired by the sausage rolls served at our favorite Italian restaurant. I serve it often because it's easy to fix and my husband loves it.

Vicky Benscoter, Birmingham, Alabama

1. Cook pasta according to package directions; drain. In a large skillet, saute green pepper and onion in oil for 6-7 minutes. Add sausage; cook and stir until sausage is no longer pink. Drain. Stir in spaghetti sauce and pasta.

2. Transfer to a 3-qt. baking dish coated with cooking spray. Cover and bake at 350° for 15-20 minutes. Uncover; sprinkle with the cheeses. Bake 5-10 minutes longer or until cheese is melted.

1 package (16 ounces) uncooked penne pasta
1 medium green pepper, chopped
1 small onion, chopped
1 tablespoon olive oil
1 pound Italian turkey sausage links, casings removed
3 cups fat-free meatless spaghetti sauce
1-1/2 cups (6 ounces) shredded part-skim mozzarella cheese
1/4 cup grated Parmesan cheese

NUTRITION FACTS
One serving
(1 cup) equals:
276 calories
11 g fat
4 g saturated fat
40 mg cholesterol
948 mg sodium
25 g carbohydrate
1 g fiber
18 g protein

DIABETIC EXCHANGES
2 lean meat
1-1/2 starch
1 fat

Tender Chicken Nuggets

With just four ingredients, you can prepare these moist, golden bites that are healthier than fast food. I serve them with light ranch dressing and barbecue sauce for dipping.

Lynne Hahn, Winchester, California

- 1/2 cup seasoned bread crumbs
- 2 tablespoons grated Parmesan cheese
- 1 egg white
- 1 pound boneless skinless chicken breasts, cut into 1-inch cubes

1. In a large resealable plastic bag, combine the bread crumbs and Parmesan cheese. In a shallow bowl, beat the egg white. Dip chicken pieces in egg white, then place in bag and shake to coat.

2. Place in a 15-in. x 10-in. x 1-in. baking pan coated with cooking spray. Bake, uncovered, at 400° for 12-15 minutes or until chicken is no longer pink, turning once.

CUTTING CHICKEN BREASTS

Chicken breasts are easier to cube if they are partially frozen. Place the breasts flat on a cutting board. With a sharp knife, cut lengthwise into 1-inch strips, then cut crosswise, making 1-inch cubes.

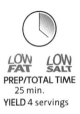

LOW FAT LOW SALT

PREP/TOTAL TIME
25 min.
YIELD 4 servings

NUTRITION FACTS
One serving
(6 nuggets) equals:
194 calories
3 g fat
1 g saturated fat
68 mg cholesterol
250 mg sodium
10 g carbohydrate
Trace fiber
30 g protein

DIABETIC EXCHANGES
3 lean meat
1/2 starch

Mushroom Chicken Pizza

Who doesn't like pizza? This is a terrific alternative to the greasy, high-fat variety.

Vickie Madrigal, Shreveport, Louisiana

- 1 tube (13.8 ounces) refrigerated pizza crust
- 1 can (6 ounces) Italian tomato paste
- 1-1/2 cups cubed cooked chicken breast
- 2 cups grape tomatoes, halved
- 1/2 cup sliced fresh mushrooms
- 1/4 cup sliced ripe olives
- 1/8 teaspoon garlic salt
- 1/8 teaspoon salt
- 1/8 teaspoon pepper
- 1 tablespoon olive oil
- 1-1/2 cups (6 ounces) shredded part-skim mozzarella cheese

1. Press dough onto the bottom of a 15-in. x 10-in. x 1-in. baking pan coated with cooking spray. Prick crust with a fork. Bake at 400° for 5 minutes.

2. Spread tomato paste over crust to within 1/2 in. of edges. Top with the chicken, tomatoes, mushrooms, olives, garlic salt, salt and pepper. Drizzle with oil. Sprinkle with cheese. Bake 13-16 minutes longer or until cheese is melted.

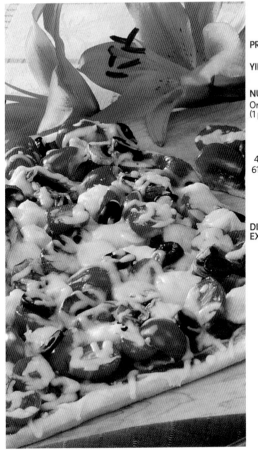

PREP/TOTAL TIME
30 min.
YIELD 6 servings

NUTRITION FACTS
One serving
(1 piece) equals:
319 calories
10 g fat
4 g saturated fat
46 mg cholesterol
618 mg sodium
32 g carbohydrate
3 g fiber
23 g protein

DIABETIC EXCHANGES
2 lean meat
1-1/2 starch
1 vegetable
1/2 fat

Chicken Pepper Fajitas

This spicy entree is fun to serve sizzling at the table, just like they do in restaurants. I fill the fajitas with peppers, onions and chicken that's quickly marinated for a flavor boost.

Lucinda Price, Tracy, California

PREP/TOTAL TIME
Prep: 10 min. + marinating
Cook: 15 min.
YIELD 6 servings

NUTRITION FACTS
One serving
(1 fajita) equals:
199 calories
2 g fat
Trace saturated fat
44 mg cholesterol
96 mg sodium
23 g carbohydrate
3 g fiber
22 g protein

DIABETIC EXCHANGES
3 meat
1 starch
1 vegetable

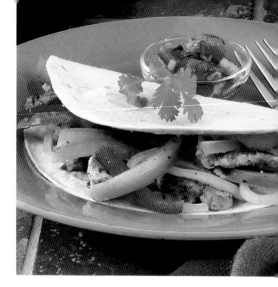

2/3 cup lime juice
1 tablespoon salt-free seasoning blend
1 tablespoon ground cumin
1 teaspoon chili powder
1 teaspoon pepper
1/2 teaspoon garlic powder
1 pound boneless skinless chicken breasts, cut into 1/4-inch strips
1 large onion, halved and thinly sliced
1 medium green pepper, julienned
1 medium sweet red pepper, julienned
6 flour tortillas (6 inches), warmed

1. In a bowl, combine the first six ingredients; set aside 2 tablespoons marinade. Pour remaining marinade into a large resealable plastic bag; add chicken. Seal bag and turn to coat; refrigerate for 30 minutes, turning occasionally.

2. In a large skillet coated with cooking spray, saute onion and peppers until crisp-tender; remove and set aside. Add chicken and reserved marinade to skillet; cook for 3-5 minutes or until no longer pink. Return vegetables to the pan; heat through. Serve on tortillas.

Hot Swiss Chicken Sandwiches

I've been fixing these tasty open-faced sandwiches for years. I like the filling on slices of sourdough and inside pitas, too.

Edith Tabor, Vancouver, Washington

PREP/TOTAL TIME
20 min.
YIELD 6 servings

NUTRITION FACTS
One serving
(1 sandwich) equals:
218 calories
9 g fat
3 g saturated fat
44 mg cholesterol
438 mg sodium
17 g carbohydrate
1 g fiber
17 g protein

DIABETIC EXCHANGES
2 lean meat
1 starch
1/2 fat

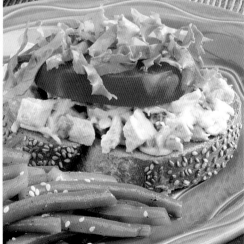

1/4 cup reduced-fat mayonnaise
1/4 teaspoon salt
1/4 teaspoon lemon juice
1-1/2 cups diced cooked chicken breast
2/3 cup chopped celery
1/2 cup shredded reduced-fat Swiss cheese
4 teaspoons butter, softened
6 slices Italian bread (about 3/4 inch thick)
6 slices tomato
3/4 cup shredded lettuce

1. In a bowl, combine mayonnaise, salt and lemon juice. Stir in the chicken, celery and cheese. Spread butter on each slice of bread; top each with 1/3 cup chicken mixture.

2. Place in a 15-in. x 10-in. x 1-in. baking pan. Broil 4-6 in. from the heat for 3-4 minutes or until heated through. Top with tomato and lettuce. Serve immediately.

Marinated Barbecued Chicken

Whenever I make this tender, grilled chicken, people rave about the flavor and ask for the recipe. A friend of mine received it from her sister-in-law, who's from the Philippines.

Deborah DiLaura English, Casper, Wyoming

- 2/3 cup sugar
- 2/3 cup reduced-sodium soy sauce
- 1/2 cup lemon-lime soda
- 1/2 cup lemon juice
- 2 tablespoons garlic powder
- 1 teaspoon pepper
- 1/2 teaspoon salt
- 8 bone-in skinless chicken breast halves (7 ounces *each*)
- 2 tablespoons barbecue sauce

1. In a bowl, combine the first seven ingredients. Pour 1-1/2 cups marinade into a large resealable plastic bag; add the chicken. Seal bag and turn to coat; refrigerate overnight. Cover and refrigerate remaining marinade.

2. Coat grill rack with cooking spray before starting the grill. Drain and discard marinade from chicken. Add barbecue sauce to reserved marinade.

3. Grill chicken, covered, over indirect medium heat for 35-50 minutes or until a meat thermometer reads 170°, turning and basting occasionally with marinade. Before serving, brush with remaining marinade.

LOW FAT

PREP/TOTAL TIME
Prep: 15 min. + marinating
Grill: 35 min.
YIELD 8 servings

NUTRITION FACTS
One serving
(1 chicken breast half) equals:
- 205 calories
- 3 g fat
- 1 g saturated fat
- 79 mg cholesterol
- 590 mg sodium
- 12 g carbohydrate
- Trace fiber
- 30 g protein

DIABETIC EXCHANGES
- 4 lean meat
- 1/2 starch

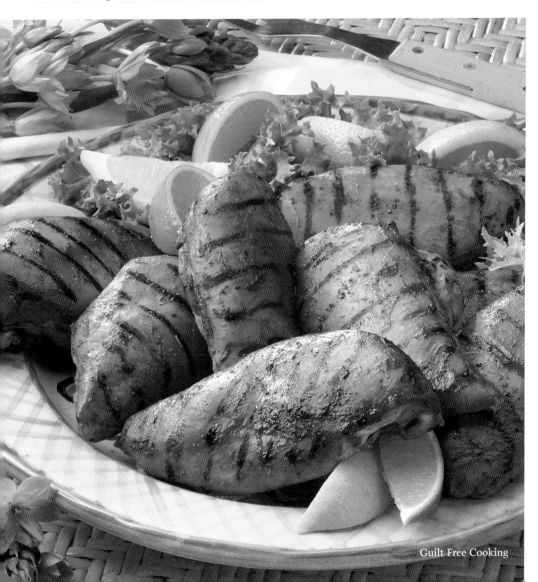

Chicken Dressing Casserole

PREP/TOTAL TIME
Prep: 10 min.
Bake: 50 min.
YIELD 6 servings

NUTRITION FACTS
One serving
(1-1/2 cups) equals:
303 calories
6 g fat
2 g saturated fat
49 mg cholesterol
930 mg sodium
39 g carbohydrate
3 g fiber
21 g protein

**DIABETIC
EXCHANGES**
2-1/2 starch
2 very lean
meat
1/2 fat

This hearty bake is perfect after a day in the crisp autumn air. Topped with bread crumbs, the combination of chicken, mixed veggies and stuffing makes it a one-dish wonder.

Angela Oelschlaeger, Tonganoxie, Kansas

- 1 can (14-1/2 ounces) reduced-sodium chicken broth
- 1 can (10-3/4 ounces) reduced-fat reduced-sodium condensed cream of chicken soup, undiluted
- 1 can (10-3/4 ounces) reduced-fat reduced-sodium condensed cream of mushroom soup, undiluted
- 1 package (6 ounces) reduced-sodium stuffing mix
- 2 cups cubed cooked chicken breast
- 1-1/2 cups frozen mixed vegetables, thawed
- 1/2 cup soft whole wheat bread crumbs
- 1 tablespoon butter, melted

1. In a bowl, combine the broth and soups; set aside. In a 2-qt. baking dish coated with cooking spray, layer half of the stuffing mix, 1 cup chicken, 3/4 cup mixed vegetables and half of the soup mixture. Repeat layers (dish will be full).

2. Cover and bake at 350° for 30 minutes. Uncover; bake for 15 minutes. In a small bowl, combine the bread crumbs and butter. Sprinkle over casserole. Bake 5-10 minutes longer or until heated through and topping is golden brown. Let stand for 5 minutes before serving.

Turkey 'n' Beef Loaf

PREP/TOTAL TIME
Prep: 20 min.
Bake: 40 min. +
standing
YIELD 8 servings

NUTRITION FACTS
One serving
(1 slice) equals:
249 calories
12 g fat
4 g saturated fat
92 mg cholesterol
539 mg sodium
9 g carbohydrate
1 g fiber
25 g protein

**DIABETIC
EXCHANGES**
3 lean meat
1-1/2 vegetable
1/2 starch

This moist, tender meat loaf tastes so good. I like the combination of beef and turkey.

C. White, Nashotah, Wisconsin

- 1 large onion, chopped
- 3/4 cup chopped sweet red or green pepper
- 2 garlic cloves, minced
- 2 teaspoons canola oil
- 1 egg, lightly beaten
- 1/4 cup egg substitute
- 1 cup soft whole wheat bread crumbs (2 slices)
- 1/4 cup minced fresh parsley
- 1 tablespoon minced fresh marjoram or 1 teaspoon dried marjoram
- 1 tablespoon minced fresh thyme or 1 teaspoon dried thyme
- 1 teaspoon salt
- 1/4 teaspoon pepper
- 1 pound lean ground beef
- 1 pound lean ground turkey
- 1/4 cup ketchup

Additional parsley, optional

1. In a nonstick skillet, saute the onion, red pepper and garlic in oil for 3 minutes. Place in a bowl; cool slightly. Add egg, egg substitute, bread crumbs, parsley, marjoram, thyme, salt and pepper. Crumble beef and turkey over mixture and mix well.

2. Shape into a 9-in. x 5-in. loaf; place in a 13-in. x 9-in. x 2-in. baking dish. Bake, uncovered, at 350° for 40 minutes. Top with ketchup. Bake 35-40 minutes longer or until no pink remains and a meat thermometer reads 160°. Let stand for 15 minutes before slicing. Sprinkle with parsley if desired.

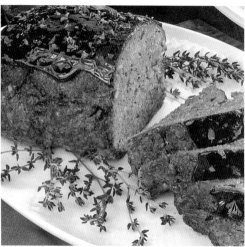

Chicken 'n' Biscuits

This comforting dish features homemade biscuits over chunks of chicken and veggies.

Marilyn Minnick, Hillsboro, Indiana

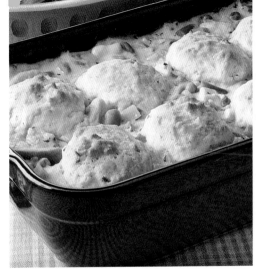

1 medium onion, chopped
2 teaspoons canola oil
1/4 cup all-purpose flour
1/2 teaspoon dried basil
1/2 teaspoon dried thyme
1/4 teaspoon pepper
2-1/2 cups fat-free milk
1 tablespoon Worcestershire sauce
1 package (16 ounces) frozen mixed vegetables
2 cups cubed cooked chicken
2 tablespoons grated Parmesan cheese

BISCUITS:

1 cup all-purpose flour
1 tablespoon sugar
1-1/2 teaspoons baking powder
1/4 teaspoon salt
1/3 cup fat-free milk
3 tablespoons canola oil
1 tablespoon minced fresh parsley

1. In a large saucepan, saute onion in oil until tender. Stir in flour, basil, thyme and pepper until blended. Gradually stir in milk and Worcestershire sauce until smooth. Bring to a boil; cook and stir for 2 minutes or until thickened. Reduce heat to low; stir in vegetables, chicken and Parmesan cheese.

2. Meanwhile, in a large bowl, combine flour, sugar, baking powder and salt. Combine milk, oil and parsley; stir into dry ingredients just until combined.

3. Transfer the hot chicken mixture to a greased 2-1/2-qt. baking dish. Drop the batter by rounded tablespoonfuls onto the chicken mixture. Bake, uncovered, at 375° for 30-40 minutes or until biscuits are lightly browned.

LOW SALT

PREP/TOTAL TIME
Prep: 25 min.
Bake: 30 min.
YIELD 8 servings

NUTRITION FACTS
One serving equals:
246 calories
8 g fat
0 g saturated fat
24 mg cholesterol
284 mg sodium
31 g carbohydrate
0 g fiber
13 g protein

DIABETIC EXCHANGES
2 starch
1 meat
1/2 fat

Grilled Breaded Chicken

When I got married, my husband's aunt gave us all of her favorite recipes. This chicken dish is one we especially enjoy.

Kristy McClellan, Morgan, Utah

1 cup (8 ounces) reduced-fat sour cream
1/4 cup lemon juice
4 teaspoons Worcestershire sauce
2 teaspoons paprika
1 teaspoon celery salt
1/8 teaspoon garlic powder
8 boneless skinless chicken breast halves (4 ounces *each*)
2 cups crushed herb-seasoned stuffing
Refrigerated butter-flavored spray

1. In a large resealable plastic bag, combine the sour cream, lemon juice, Worcestershire sauce, paprika, celery salt and garlic powder; add chicken. Seal bag and turn to coat; refrigerate for at least 8 hours or overnight.

2. Coat grill rack with cooking spray before starting the grill. Drain and discard marinade from chicken. Coat both sides of chicken with the stuffing crumbs; spritz with butter-flavored spray.

3. Grill, covered, over medium heat for 4 minutes on each side or until the juices run clear.

LOW FAT

PREP/TOTAL TIME
Prep: 15 min. + marinating
Grill: 10 min.
YIELD 8 servings

NUTRITION FACTS
One serving
(1 chicken breast half) equals:
224 calories
5 g fat
2 g saturated fat
75 mg cholesterol
419 mg sodium
12 g carbohydrate
1 g fiber
30 g protein

DIABETIC EXCHANGES
3 lean meat
1 starch

Wild Rice Chicken Bake

PREP/TOTAL TIME
Prep: 10 min.
Bake: 35 min.
YIELD 6 servings

NUTRITION FACTS
One serving equals:
314 calories
5 g fat
1 g saturated fat
68 mg cholesterol
762 mg sodium
34 g carbohydrate
4 g fiber
31 g protein

DIABETIC EXCHANGES
3 lean meat
2 starch
1 vegetable

This home-style combination is one of my most-requested chicken recipes. It's a snap to assemble using a boxed rice mix.

Joyce Unruh, Shipshewana, Indiana

1 package (6 ounces) long grain and wild rice mix

2 medium carrots, shredded

3/4 cup frozen peas

1 can (8 ounces) sliced water chestnuts, drained

1-1/4 cups water

1 can (10-3/4 ounces) reduced-fat reduced-sodium condensed cream of mushroom soup, undiluted

6 boneless skinless chicken breast halves (4 ounces *each*)

1/8 teaspoon paprika

1/8 teaspoon pepper

1 garlic clove, minced

1 tablespoon olive oil

1. In a bowl, combine rice mix with contents of seasoning packet, carrots, peas and water chestnuts. Combine water and soup; pour over rice mixture and mix well. Transfer to a shallow 3-qt. baking dish coated with cooking spray. Cover and bake at 350° for 25 minutes.

2. Meanwhile, sprinkle chicken with paprika and pepper. In a large nonstick skillet, cook chicken and garlic in oil for 5-6 minutes on each side or until lightly browned. Arrange chicken over rice mixture. Cover and bake 10-15 minutes longer or until chicken juices run clear and rice is tender.

Pork
Pleasers

If spicy sausages, home-style ham, crisp bacon, tender roasts and other pork mainstays always draw your family to the table, you'll love the rave-winning recipes in this chapter.

154
Mediterranean Pork and Orzo

147
Pepper-Crusted Pork Tenderloin

162
Cranberry-Mustard Pork Medallions

chapter *8*

Tangy Pork Barbecue

A dear neighbor shared this zesty recipe with me many years ago. This barbecue has always been a hit with my family. I usually serve it with French fries and coleslaw.

Carmine Walters, San Jose, California

LOW FAT   LOW SALT

PREP/TOTAL TIME
Prep: 20 min.
Cook: 3 hours
YIELD 12 servings

NUTRITION FACTS
One serving
(3/4 cup prepared
without salt,
calculated without
bun) equals:
245 calories
5 g fat
0 g saturated fat
80 mg cholesterol
141 mg sodium
5 g carbohydrate
0 g fiber
29 g protein

DIABETIC EXCHANGES
4 lean meat
1 vegetable

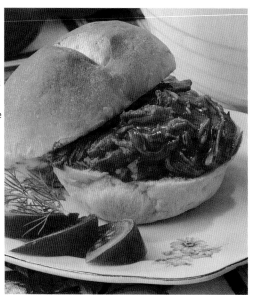

2	tablespoons margarine
3	tablespoons all-purpose flour
1	bottle (28 ounces) no-salt-added ketchup
2	cups boiling water
1/4	cup white vinegar
1/4	cup Worcestershire sauce
1	medium onion, chopped
1	garlic clove, minced
2	teaspoons chili powder
1	teaspoon salt, optional
1	teaspoon ground mustard
1/8	teaspoon cayenne pepper
1	boneless pork loin roast (3-1/2 to 4 pounds), cut in half
12	sandwich buns, split

1. In a Dutch oven over medium heat, melt margarine. Stir in flour until smooth. Add the ketchup, water, vinegar, Worcestershire sauce, onion, garlic and seasonings; bring to a boil. Add roast. Reduce the heat; cover and simmer for 3 hours or until the meat is very tender.

2. Remove meat; shred with two forks. Skim fat from cooking juices; return meat to pan and heat through. Serve with a slotted spoon on buns.

SHREDDING EASE

To shred the pork roast for Tangy Pork Barbecue, remove the meat from the Dutch oven and place it in a shallow baking pan. Holding an ordinary dinner fork in each hand, pull the meat into fine shreds.

Pork Picante

Lots of outdoor activity on our farm whets the appetites of my husband and three teenage kids. This supper always satisfies them.

Susan Miller, Marion, Illinois

LOW SALT

PREP/TOTAL TIME
25 min.
YIELD 6 servings

NUTRITION FACTS
One serving
(2/3 cup calculated
without rice) equals:
237 calories
6 g fat
2 g saturated fat
63 mg cholesterol
236 mg sodium
19 g carbohydrate
2 g fiber
23 g protein

DIABETIC EXCHANGES
3 lean meat
1 vegetable
1/2 starch
1/2 fruit

1/3	cup all-purpose flour
1	teaspoon chili powder
1/2	teaspoon ground cumin
1/4	teaspoon garlic powder
1/4	teaspoon cayenne pepper
1-1/2	pounds pork tenderloin, cut into 3/4-inch cubes
1	tablespoon canola oil
1	cup salsa
1/3	cup peach preserves

Hot cooked rice, optional

1. In a large resealable plastic bag, combine the flour, chili powder, cumin, garlic powder and cayenne. Add the pork a few pieces at a time and shake to coat.

2. In a large nonstick skillet or wok, brown pork in oil. Add salsa and peach preserves; cover and simmer for 10-15 minutes or until meat is no longer pink. Serve over rice if desired.

SPICE IT UP

To give Pork Picante even more zip and heat, use hot salsa rather than mild and add a diced jalapeno pepper. You can also add some dried chipotle chili pepper to the seasoning mix.

Pork Lo Mein

This full-flavored stir-fry is sure to bring rave reviews. Snappy snow peas, sweet pepper and pork are spiced up with ginger, sesame oil, red pepper flakes and soy sauce. If you like, try rice as an alternative to the pasta.

Linda Trainer, Phoenix, Arizona

- 1 pork tenderloin (1 pound)
- 1/4 cup reduced-sodium soy sauce
- 3 garlic cloves, minced
- 1 teaspoon minced fresh gingerroot
- 1/4 teaspoon crushed red pepper flakes
- 2 cups fresh snow peas
- 1 medium sweet red pepper, julienned
- 3 cups cooked thin spaghetti
- 1/3 cup reduced-sodium chicken broth
- 2 teaspoons sesame oil

1. Cut tenderloin in half lengthwise. Cut each half widthwise into 1/4-in. slices; set aside. In a large resealable plastic bag, combine the soy sauce, garlic, ginger and pepper flakes; add pork. Seal bag and turn to coat; refrigerate for 20 minutes.

2. In a large nonstick skillet or wok coated with cooking spray, stir-fry pork and marinade for 4-5 minutes or until meat is no longer pink. Add peas and red pepper; stir-fry for 1 minute. Stir in spaghetti and broth; cook 1 minute longer. Remove from the heat; stir in sesame oil.

PREP/TOTAL TIME
Prep: 10 min. + marinating
Cook: 10 min.
YIELD 4 servings

NUTRITION FACTS
One serving
(1-1/2 cups) equals:
343 calories
7 g fat
2 g saturated fat
74 mg cholesterol
716 mg sodium
37 g carbohydrate
3 g fiber
31 g protein

DIABETIC EXCHANGES
3 lean meat
2 starch
1 vegetable

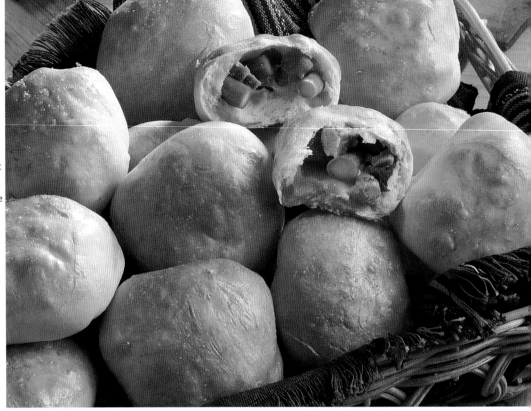

PREP/TOTAL TIME
Prep: 20 min. + rising
Bake: 20 min.
YIELD 2 dozen

NUTRITION FACTS
One serving
(1 roll) equals:

129 calories
3 g fat
1 g saturated fat
17 mg cholesterol
237 mg sodium
18 g carbohydrate
1 g fiber
7 g protein

DIABETIC EXCHANGES
1 starch
1/2 lean meat

Asparagus Ham Rolls

Chock-full of fresh flavor, these scrumptious rolls are perfect to pack for a picnic, ball game or even lunch at the office. When I'm pressed for time, I prepare the dough in my bread machine.

Amy Davis, Folsom, New Mexico

- 3 to 4 cups all-purpose flour
- 2 tablespoons sugar
- 1 package (1/4 ounce) active dry yeast
- 1 teaspoon salt
- 1/2 cup milk
- 1/2 cup water
- 2 tablespoons canola oil
- 2 egg whites, *divided*
- 1 egg
- 1 pound fresh asparagus, trimmed and cut into 1/2-inch pieces
- 1 block (4 ounces) cheddar cheese, cubed
- 2 cups diced fully cooked lean ham

1. In a large mixing bowl, combine 2-1/2 cups flour, sugar, yeast and salt. In a saucepan, heat milk, water and oil to 120°-130°. Add to dry ingredients; beat just until moistened. Add one egg white and the egg, beating until smooth. Stir in enough remaining flour to form a soft dough.

2. Turn onto a floured surface; knead until smooth and elastic, about 6-8 minutes. Place in a greased bowl, turning once to grease top. Cover and let rise in a warm place until doubled, about 1 hour.

3. Punch dough down. Turn onto a lightly floured surface. Cover and let stand for 15 minutes. Meanwhile, place 1/2 in. of water and asparagus in a saucepan; bring to a boil. Reduce heat; cover and simmer for 3-5 minutes. Drain.

4. Divide dough into 24 pieces; roll each piece into a 5-in. circle. Place a few pieces of asparagus, a cheese cube and a tablespoon of ham in the center of each circle. Wrap dough around filling, pinching seams to seal. Place rolls seam side down 2 in. apart on baking sheets coated with cooking spray. Cover and let rise in a warm place until doubled, about 30 minutes.

5. Beat remaining egg white; brush over rolls. Bake at 350° for 18-20 minutes or until golden brown. Remove to wire racks. Refrigerate leftovers.

Italian-Sausage Pepper Sandwiches

I don't remember where I got this recipe, but I sure am glad I did! The popular sandwiches are great on a busy weeknight because they are easy to prepare yet very tasty.

Molly Gee, Plainwell, Michigan

- 2 uncooked Italian sausage links
- 1 small red onion, thinly sliced
- 1/2 medium green pepper, julienned
- 1/2 medium sweet red pepper, julienned
- 1 garlic clove, chopped
- 1 tablespoon canola oil
- 1 large tomato, seeded and chopped
- 1/2 teaspoon dried oregano

Salt and pepper to taste, optional

- 2 French *or* submarine rolls, split and toasted

1. In a skillet, cook sausage over medium heat until browned. Let stand until cool enough to handle. Cut into 1/2-in. slices. Return to pan and cook until no longer pink; drain and set aside.

2. In same skillet, saute the onion, green pepper, red pepper and garlic in oil until crisp-tender. Add the sausage, tomato, oregano and salt and pepper if desired. Cook until tomatoes are heated through. Spoon sausage mixture into rolls.

EXTRA LINKS

Generally, Italian Sausage is purchased in packages of 5 to 6 links. Since only two links are used for these delicious sandwiches, you'll have a few left over. For long-term storage, wrap each link individually in plastic wrap and place them in a freeze bag. They can be frozen for up to 2 months.

PREP/TOTAL TIME
25 min.
YIELD 2 sandwiches

NUTRITION FACTS
One serving
(1 sandwich) equals:
- 291 calories
- 12 g fat
- 2 g saturated fat
- 15 mg cholesterol
- 466 mg sodium
- 38 g carbohydrate
- 4 g fiber
- 11 g protein

DIABETIC EXCHANGES
- 2 starch
- 2 lean meat
- 1 vegetable

Breaded Pork Chops

A bread crumb coating gives a nice golden look to these tender pork chops. Parmesan and hot pepper sauce add just the right spark of flavor.

Taste of Home Test Kitchen

- 2 tablespoons all-purpose flour
- 4 egg whites
- 1/2 teaspoon Worcestershire sauce
- 1/2 teaspoon balsamic vinegar
- 1/8 teaspoon hot pepper sauce
- 3/4 cup dry bread crumbs
- 3 tablespoons grated Parmesan cheese
- 1/2 teaspoon dried thyme
- 1/4 teaspoon salt
- 1/4 teaspoon paprika
- 6 boneless pork loin chops (1/2 inch thick and 4 ounces *each*)

Refrigerated butter-flavored spray

1. Place flour in a shallow dish. In another shallow dish, beat the egg whites, Worcestershire sauce, vinegar and hot pepper sauce. In a third dish, combine the bread crumbs, cheese, thyme, salt and paprika. Coat pork chops with flour. Dip into egg mixture, then coat with crumb mixture. Place on a plate; cover and refrigerate for 1 hour.

2. Place chops in a 13-in. x 9-in. x 2-in. baking dish coated with cooking spray; spritz chops with butter-flavored spray. Bake, uncovered, at 350° for 25-28 minutes or until juices run clear.

PREP/TOTAL TIME
Prep: 10 min. + chilling
Bake: 25 min.
YIELD 6 servings

NUTRITION FACTS
One serving
(1 pork chop) equals:
- 250 calories
- 8 g fat
- 3 g saturated fat
- 74 mg cholesterol
- 372 mg sodium
- 12 g carbohydrate
- 1 g fiber
- 29 g protein

DIABETIC EXCHANGES
- 3 lean meat
- 1 starch

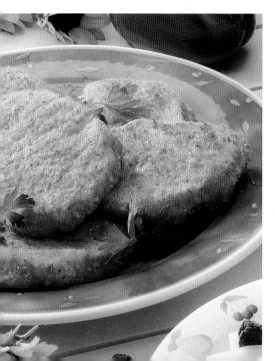

Ham with Orange Sauce

With a light and citrusy glaze and sauce, this ham is wonderful for special occasions.

Gloria Warczak, Cedarburg, Wisconsin

PREP/TOTAL TIME
Prep: 25 min.
Bake: 1 hour
20 min.
YIELD 20 servings
(about 3 cups
sauce)

NUTRITION FACTS
One serving equals:
211 calories
5 g fat
0 g saturated fat
43 mg cholesterol
907 mg sodium
22 g carbohydrate
0 g fiber
20 g protein

DIABETIC EXCHANGES
2 lean meat
1-1/2 fruit

1 reduced-sodium semi-boneless fully cooked ham (6 pounds)
1 cup orange juice
1 cup reduced-sodium chicken broth
1/4 teaspoon ground cloves

GLAZE:

1 cup reduced-sugar orange marmalade
1 tablespoon lemon juice
1 tablespoon Worcestershire sauce
1 teaspoon horseradish mustard
1/8 teaspoon garlic powder

SAUCE:

1/4 cup orange juice
1/4 cup packed brown sugar
1/2 teaspoon ground ginger
1 can (11 ounces) mandarin oranges, drained
1/2 cup golden raisins

1. Remove skin from ham. Place on a rack in a shallow roasting pan. Combine orange juice and broth; pour over ham. Sprinkle with cloves. Cover and bake at 325° for 1 to 1-1/2 hours.

2. Combine glaze ingredients; spoon over ham. Bake, uncovered, 20-30 minutes longer or until a meat thermometer reads 140° and ham is heated through.

3. Remove ham to a serving platter and keep warm. Strain pan drippings; skim fat. In a saucepan, combine orange juice, brown sugar and ginger. Stir in pan drippings, oranges and raisins. Bring to a boil. Reduce heat; simmer, uncovered, for 15-20 minutes. Thicken if desired. Serve with the ham.

SEMI-BONELESS HAM

Not familiar with a semi-boneless ham also known as partially boned ham? This is a whole or half ham that has just the leg bone. The hip or shank bones have been removed. A semi-boneless ham is easier to carve than a bone-in ham. Some feel that the bone adds to the flavor of the ham.

BLT Tortillas

I first sampled these at a bridal luncheon years ago. Now I frequently make them for our weekly neighborhood dinners.

Darla Wester, Meriden, Iowa

PREP/TOTAL TIME
15 min.
YIELD 8 servings

NUTRITION FACTS
One serving
(1 tortilla prepared
with three strips
of green pepper)
equals:
232 calories
9 g fat
0 g saturated fat
12 mg cholesterol
511 mg sodium
28 g carbohydrate
0 g fiber
9 g protein

DIABETIC EXCHANGES
1-1/2 starch
1 vegetable
1 fat
1/2 meat

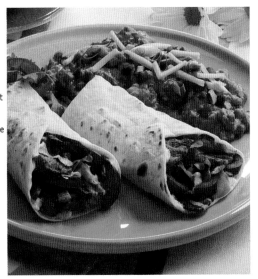

1/2 cup fat-free mayonnaise
1/2 cup fat-free sour cream
2 tablespoons ranch salad dressing mix
1/4 teaspoon crushed red pepper flakes
8 flour tortillas (8 inches), room temperature
16 bacon strips, cooked and drained
2 to 3 cups shredded lettuce
2 cups chopped tomato

Green and sweet red pepper strips, optional

1. In a large bowl, combine mayonnaise, sour cream, salad dressing mix and red pepper flakes; spread on tortillas. Layer with bacon, lettuce and tomato. Top with peppers if desired. Roll up tortillas.

Pepper-Crusted Pork Tenderloin

Guests are sure to be impressed by this elegant, crumb-coated entree. The meat slices up so moist and tender, you can serve it without sauce and still have a taste-tempting main course.

Taste of Home Test Kitchen

- 2 pork tenderloins (3/4 pound *each*)
- 3 tablespoons Dijon mustard
- 1 tablespoon buttermilk
- 2 teaspoons minced fresh thyme
- 1 to 2 teaspoons coarsely ground pepper
- 1/4 teaspoon salt
- 2/3 cup soft bread crumbs

1. Place tenderloins side by side and tie together with kitchen string. In a small bowl, combine the mustard, buttermilk, thyme, pepper and salt; spread over surface of meat. Press crumbs onto meat.

2. Place on a rack in a shallow roasting pan. Cover and bake at 425° for 15 minutes.

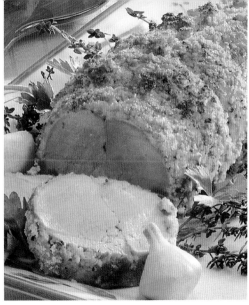

LOW FAT

PREP/TOTAL TIME
Prep: 5 min.
Bake: 50 min. + standing
YIELD 6 servings

NUTRITION FACTS
One serving
(3 ounces cooked pork) equals:
178 calories
5 g fat
1 g saturated fat
67 mg cholesterol
383 mg sodium
6 g carbohydrate
Trace fiber
25 g protein

DIABETIC EXCHANGES
3 lean meat
1/2 starch

Uncover; bake 35-40 minutes longer or until a meat thermometer reads 160°. Let stand for 5 minutes. Remove string before slicing.

Pork Chops with Red Cabbage

I add shredded sweet-and-sour cabbage and pineapple to these tender pork chops. It's a complete meal in one pan.

Steve Rose, Mesa, Arizona

- 5 boneless pork loin chops (4 ounces *each*)
- 1 tablespoon olive oil
- 1 jar (16 ounces) shredded sweet-and-sour red cabbage, undrained
- 1 can (8 ounces) unsweetened pineapple chunks, drained
- 1 tablespoon minced fresh parsley
- 1 teaspoon dried minced onion
- 1 teaspoon dried oregano
- 1/4 teaspoon coarsely ground pepper
- Dash celery seed
- 1 small onion, peeled and halved

1. In a large nonstick skillet, brown pork chops on both sides in oil. In a bowl, combine the cabbage, pineapple, parsley, dried onion, oregano, pepper and celery seed. Cut each onion half into eight wedges; place over pork chops. Top with cabbage mixture.

2. Bring to a boil. Reduce heat; cover and simmer for 15-20 minutes or until meat juices run clear and onions are tender.

LOW SALT

PREP/TOTAL TIME
30 min.
YIELD 5 servings

NUTRITION FACTS
One serving
(1 pork chop with 1/2 cup cabbage mixture) equals:
336 calories
8 g fat
2 g saturated fat
57 mg cholesterol
67 mg sodium
43 g carbohydrate
1 g fiber
23 g protein

DIABETIC EXCHANGES
3 lean meat
2 vegetable
1-1/2 starch
1/2 fruit

Ham Mushroom Fettuccine

I like the fact that I can make this creamy pasta toss in about half an hour, yet it tastes like I spent hours in the kitchen. It's also a great way to use up leftover ham.

Michelle Armistead, Keyport, New Jersey

NUTRITION FACTS
One serving
(1–1/3 cups) equals:
334 calories
8 g fat
1 g saturated fat
29 mg cholesterol
876 mg sodium
46 g carbohydrate
3 g fiber
21 g protein

DIABETIC EXCHANGES
2 starch
2 lean meat
1 fat
1/2 vegetable

12 ounces uncooked fettuccine

3/4 pound fully cooked lean ham, cubed

2 tablespoons olive oil

1 medium onion, finely chopped

1/2 pound fresh mushrooms, sliced

1 tablespoon all-purpose flour

1/2 teaspoon dried rosemary, crushed

1/4 teaspoon pepper

1-1/4 cups fat-free evaporated milk

1/2 cup frozen peas, thawed

2 tablespoons reduced-fat sour cream

1. Cook fettuccine according to package directions. Meanwhile, in a large skillet, saute ham in oil until lightly browned. Remove with a slotted spoon and set aside. Add onion to skillet; saute for 4 minutes. Add mushrooms; saute 3 minutes longer.

2. Stir in the flour, rosemary and pepper until blended. Gradually add milk. Bring to a boil; cook and stir for 2 minutes or until thickened. Reduce heat; add peas and sour cream. Cook 2 minutes longer. Drain fettuccine; stir into the mushroom mixture. Add ham; heat through.

Pork 'n' Veggie Packets

I love the flavor of grilled food, especially these all-in-one pork packets with their delicious sesame and ginger sauce.

Andrea Bolden, Unionville, Tennessee

1   pound pork tenderloin, sliced

2   cups fresh broccoli florets

2   cups sliced fresh carrots

1   can (8 ounces) sliced water chestnuts, drained

1   medium green pepper, julienned

2   green onions, sliced

1/4   cup reduced-sodium soy sauce

4   teaspoons sesame oil

1   teaspoon ground ginger

Hot cooked rice, optional

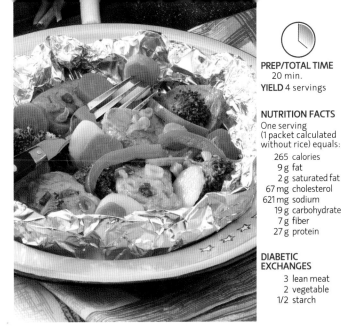

1. Divide pork, broccoli, carrots, water chestnuts, green pepper and onions evenly among four pieces of double-layered heavy-duty foil (about 18 in. x 12 in.). Combine the soy sauce, sesame oil and ginger; drizzle over pork and vegetables. Fold foil around filling and seal tightly.

2. Grill, covered, over medium heat for 10-12 minutes or until vegetables are tender and pork is no longer pink. Serve with rice if desired.

PREP/TOTAL TIME
20 min.
YIELD 4 servings

NUTRITION FACTS
One serving
(1 packet calculated without rice) equals:

265 calories
9 g fat
2 g saturated fat
67 mg cholesterol
621 mg sodium
19 g carbohydrate
7 g fiber
27 g protein

DIABETIC EXCHANGES
3 lean meat
2 vegetable
1/2 starch

Caramelized Pork Slices

This easy treatment for pork caught my eye when I was paging through a cookbook and saw the word "caramelized." The glaze is slightly sweet and so yummy. I serve the meat over noodles or alongside potatoes.

Elisa Lochridge, Aloha, Oregon

1   pork tenderloin (1 pound), cut into 1-inch slices

2   teaspoons canola oil

2   garlic cloves, minced

2   tablespoons brown sugar

1   tablespoon orange juice

1   tablespoon molasses

1/2   teaspoon salt

1/4   teaspoon pepper

1. Flatten the pork slices to 1/2-in. thickness. In a nonstick skillet, brown the pork in oil over medium-high heat. Remove the pork and keep warm.

2. In the same skillet, saute the garlic for 1 minute; stir in the brown sugar, orange juice, molasses, salt and pepper. Return pork to pan; cook, uncovered, for 3-4 minutes or until meat is no longer pink.

PREP/TOTAL TIME
15 min.
YIELD 4 servings

NUTRITION FACTS
One serving
(3 ounces cooked pork) equals:

200 calories
6 g fat
2 g saturated fat
74 mg cholesterol
355 mg sodium
11 g carbohydrate
1 g fiber
24 g protein

DIABETIC EXCHANGES
3 lean meat
1/2 starch

Sweet and Sour Ham

PREP/TOTAL TIME
15 min.
YIELD 4 servings

NUTRITION FACTS
One serving
(1 cup calculated
without rice) equals:
288 calories
7 g fat
2 g saturated fat
39 mg cholesterol
946 mg sodium
36 g carbohydrate
2 g fiber
18 g protein

DIABETIC
EXCHANGES
2 lean meat
1-1/2 fruit
1 starch

This quick-to-fix dinner is a great way to use up leftover ham. The recipe also works well with cooked chicken or beef.

Joyce Peugh, Woodstock, Maryland

1 can (20 ounces) pineapple chunks
3 tablespoons brown sugar
2 tablespoons cornstarch
1/2 teaspoon ground ginger
1/2 cup water
3 tablespoons white vinegar
2 cups cubed fully cooked ham
1 small green pepper, cut into julienne strips
1/4 cup thinly sliced halved onion
1 tablespoon canola oil
Hot cooked rice

1. Drain the pineapple, reserving juice and pineapple chunks. In a bowl, combine the brown sugar, cornstarch and ginger. Stir in the water, vinegar and reserved juice until smooth; set aside.

2. In a large nonstick skillet, saute the ham, green pepper and onion in hot oil over medium-high heat for 3 minutes or until ham is lightly browned and vegetables are crisp-tender. Stir reserved pineapple chunks into skillet; heat through. Stir juice mixture. Gradually stir into skillet. Bring to a boil; cook and stir for 1-2 minutes or until thickened. Serve over rice.

Teriyaki Pork

PREP/TOTAL TIME
Prep: 10 min. +
marinating
Cook: 20 min.
YIELD 4 servings

NUTRITION FACTS
One serving
(1-1/2 cups
calculated without
rice) equals:
302 calories
11 g fat
3 g saturated fat
63 mg cholesterol
802 mg sodium
20 g carbohydrate
5 g fiber
30 g protein

DIABETIC
EXCHANGES
3 lean meat
3 vegetable
1/2 starch
1/2 fat

I season tender pork loin and an assortment of crisp-tender vegetables with soy sauce and a garlic marinade for this savory stir-fry.

Molly Gee, Plainwell, Michigan

3/4 cup reduced-sodium chicken broth, *divided*
1/3 cup reduced-sodium soy sauce
2 tablespoons red wine vinegar
2 teaspoons honey
2 teaspoons garlic powder
1 pound boneless pork loin chops, cut into thin strips
1 tablespoon canola oil
2 cups broccoli florets
3 medium carrots, sliced
3 celery ribs, sliced
4 cups shredded cabbage
6 green onions, sliced
1 tablespoon cornstarch
Hot cooked rice, optional

1. In a bowl, combine 1/4 cup broth, soy sauce, vinegar, honey and garlic powder; mix well. Pour 1/3 cup marinade into a large resealable plastic bag; add the pork. Seal bag and turn to coat; refrigerate for 1 hour. Cover and refrigerate remaining marinade.

2. Drain and discard marinade from pork. In a large nonstick skillet or wok, stir-fry pork in oil for 2-3 minutes or until no longer pink. Remove and keep warm.

3. In the same pan, stir-fry broccoli and carrots in reserved marinade for 2 minutes. Add celery; stir-fry for 2 minutes. Add cabbage and green onions; stir-fry 2-3 minutes longer or until vegetables are crisp-tender.

4. Combine cornstarch and remaining broth until smooth; stir into vegetable mixture. Bring to a boil; cook and stir for 2 minutes or until thickened. Return pork to the pan; heat through. Serve over rice if desired.

Sausage Bow Tie Salad

I made this flavorful main-dish salad for a first date. He liked it so much, he took the leftovers home...and his roommates raved about it, too! If you prefer, substitute turkey sausage for the kielbasa.

Christina Campeau, Simi Valley, California

1 pound fully cooked reduced-fat kielbasa *or* Polish sausage, cut into 1/4-inch slices

1 large onion, finely chopped

1 tablespoon water

1-1/2 teaspoons minced garlic, *divided*

1/2 cup balsamic vinegar

1 to 3 teaspoons fennel seed, crushed

5 cups cooked bow tie pasta

7 plum tomatoes, diced

1/4 cup minced fresh basil *or* 4 teaspoons dried basil

1 cup (4 ounces) crumbled feta cheese

1. In a large nonstick skillet, cook the sausage, onion, water and 3/4 teaspoon garlic over medium heat for 10 minutes. Add vinegar and fennel seed. Reduce heat; cover and simmer for 5 minutes. Remove from the heat.

2. Stir in the pasta until coated. Add the tomatoes, basil and remaining garlic; stir gently. Cover and refrigerate until serving. Sprinkle with feta cheese.

LOW FAT

PREP/TOTAL TIME
25 min.
YIELD 9 servings

NUTRITION FACTS
One serving (1 cup) equals:
235 calories
5 g fat
2 g saturated fat
29 mg cholesterol
582 mg sodium
35 g carbohydrate
2 g fiber
13 g protein

DIABETIC EXCHANGES
2 starch
1 lean meat
1 vegetable

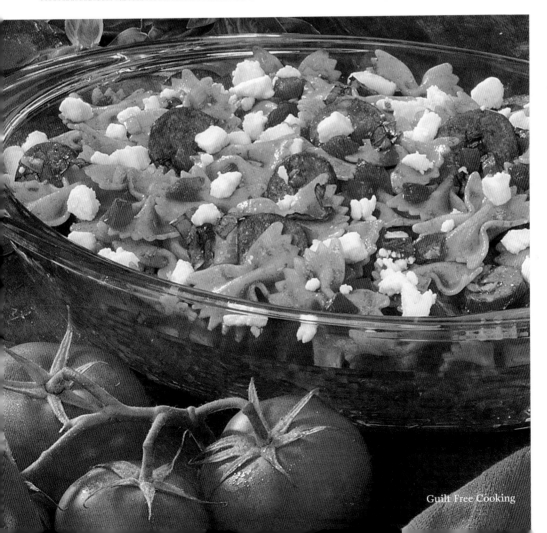

Polynesian Kabobs

PREP/TOTAL TIME
30 min.
YIELD 6 servings

NUTRITION FACTS
One serving
(2 kabobs) equals:
147 calories
6 g fat
0 g saturated fat
43 mg cholesterol
531 mg sodium
14 g carbohydrate
0 g fiber
11 g protein

**DIABETIC
EXCHANGES**
1 meat
1 vegetable
1/2 fruit

With their explosion of tastes and textures, these kabobs make a quick, filling entree. I've also served them as a fun appetizer.

Chris Anderson, Morton, Illinois

1 can (8 ounces) unsweetened pineapple chunks

1 package (12 ounces) light pork breakfast sausage links

1 can (8 ounces) whole water chestnuts, drained

1 large sweet red pepper, cut into 1-inch chunks

2 tablespoons honey

2 teaspoons reduced-sodium soy sauce

1/8 teaspoon ground nutmeg

Dash pepper

1. Drain pineapple, reserving 1 tablespoon juice. Thread sausages, water chestnuts, pineapple and the red pepper alternately onto 12 metal or soaked wooden skewers.

2. Grill kabobs, uncovered, over medium-hot heat for 7 minutes. Meanwhile, in a small bowl, combine honey, soy sauce, nutmeg, pepper and reserved pineapple juice. Turn kabobs; brush with the honey mixture. Grill 5-6 minutes longer or until the sausages are browned.

Black Beans 'n' Rice

**LOW
FAT**

PREP/TOTAL TIME
Prep: 20 min. +
standing
Cook: 1-1/2
hours
YIELD 12 servings

NUTRITION FACTS
One serving (1 cup
bean mixture with
1/2 cup rice) equals:
324 calories
5 g fat
2 g saturated fat
12 mg cholesterol
843 mg sodium
53 g carbohydrate
7 g fiber
17 g protein

**DIABETIC
EXCHANGES**
3 starch
1 meat
1 vegetable

A co-worker who was born in Cuba helped me perfect the recipe for this hearty dish. Now it's one of our family's favorites.

Helen Simms, Lyons, Michigan

1 pound dried black beans, rinsed

7 cups water

1 cup diced fully cooked lean ham

5 garlic cloves, minced

1-1/4 teaspoons pepper

1-1/4 teaspoons ground cumin

1 teaspoon salt

1 bay leaf

1/2 teaspoon Liquid Smoke, optional

4 cups chicken broth

2 cups uncooked long grain rice

1 tablespoon red wine vinegar

2 teaspoons olive oil

3/4 cup shredded reduced-fat cheddar cheese

3/4 cup chopped sweet red pepper

2 tablespoons chopped jalapeno peppers

1. Place beans in a Dutch oven or soup kettle; add water to cover by 2 in. Bring to a boil; boil for 2 minutes. Remove from the heat; cover and let stand for 1 to 4 hours or until softened. Drain and rinse beans, discarding liquid.

2. Return beans to the pan. Add 7 cups water, ham, garlic, pepper, cumin, salt, bay leaf and Liquid Smoke if desired. Bring to a boil. Reduce heat; cover and simmer for 1-1/2 hours or until beans are tender.

3. Meanwhile, in a saucepan, bring broth and rice to a boil. Reduce heat; cover and simmer for 20 minutes or until rice is tender. Just before serving, discard bay leaf from bean mixture; add vinegar and oil. Serve over rice. Sprinkle each serving with 1 tablespoon cheese, 1 tablespoon red pepper and 1 teaspoon jalapenos.

Editor's Note: When cutting hot peppers, disposable gloves are recommended. Avoid touching your face.

Mustard-Glazed Pork Chops

When I was a child, one of my friends would invite me to dinner, and her mother made the most delicious barbecue sauce with mustard. I finally asked for the recipe!

Jeri-Lynn Sandusky, Georgetown, Texas

- 1/2 cup packed brown sugar
- 1/3 cup Dijon mustard
- 5 tablespoons cider vinegar
- 2 tablespoons molasses
- 1 tablespoon ground mustard
- 6 bone-in pork loin chops
  (6 ounces *each*)

1. In a small saucepan, whisk the brown sugar, Dijon mustard, vinegar, molasses and ground mustard until blended. Bring to a boil over medium heat, stirring frequently. Reduce heat; cover and simmer for 2-3 minutes or until thickened.

2. Place pork chops in a 13-in. x 9-in. x 2-in. baking dish coated with cooking spray. Top with sauce; turn to coat. Bake, uncovered, at 350° for 18-22 minutes or until juices run clear, basting occasionally.

PREP/TOTAL TIME
30 min.
YIELD 6 servings

NUTRITION FACTS
One serving
(1 pork chop) equals:
  258 calories
  9 g fat
  3 g saturated fat
  58 mg cholesterol
397 mg sodium
  25 g carbohydrate
Trace fiber
  21 g protein

DIABETIC EXCHANGES
  3 lean meat
1-1/2 fruit

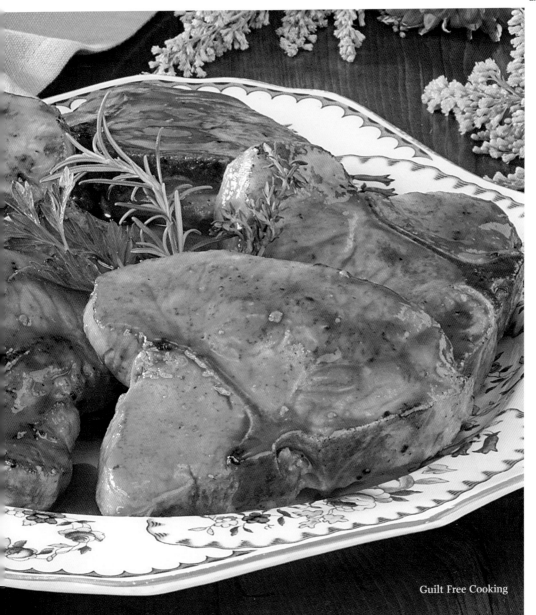

Mediterranean Pork And Orzo

PREP/TOTAL TIME
30 min.
YIELD 6 servings

Is there a food group NOT represented in this flavorful and fabulous meal-in-a-bowl? It's one of my family's wholesome favorites.

Mary Relyea, Canastota, New York

NUTRITION FACTS
One serving (2/3 cup pork mixture with 2/3 cup orzo) equals:
372 calories
11 g fat
4 g saturated fat
71 mg cholesterol
306 mg sodium
34 g carbohydrate
3 g fiber
31 g protein

DIABETIC EXCHANGES
3 lean meat
2 starch
1 fat

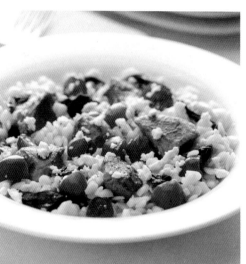

2 pork tenderloins (3/4 pound *each*)
1 teaspoon coarsely ground pepper
2 tablespoons olive oil
3 quarts water
1-1/4 cups uncooked orzo pasta
1/4 teaspoon salt
1 package (6 ounces) fresh baby spinach
1 cup grape tomatoes, halved
3/4 cup crumbled feta cheese

1. Rub pork with pepper; cut into 1-in. cubes. In a large nonstick skillet, cook pork in oil over medium heat for 8-10 minutes or until no longer pink.

2. Meanwhile, in a large saucepan, bring water to a boil. Stir in orzo and salt; cook, uncovered, for 8 minutes. Stir in spinach; cook 45-60 seconds longer or until orzo is tender and spinach is wilted.

3. Add tomatoes to the pork; cook and stir for 1 minute or until heated through. Drain orzo mixture; toss with pork mixture and feta cheese.

Slow-Cooked Pork Roast

PREP/TOTAL TIME
Prep: 20 min.
Cook: 4 hours +
standing
YIELD 12 servings

This roast makes a wonderful summer meal because you don't need to heat the oven. The pork is fall-apart tender.

Marion Lowery, Medford, Oregon

NUTRITION FACTS
One serving (3 ounces cooked pork with 1/4 cup sauce) equals:
202 calories
7 g fat
2 g saturated fat
6 mg cholesterol
306 mg sodium
8 g carbohydrate
1 g fiber
26 g protein

DIABETIC EXCHANGES
3 lean meat
1/2 starch

2 cans (8 ounces *each*) unsweetened crushed pineapple, undrained
1 cup barbecue sauce
2 tablespoons unsweetened apple juice
1 tablespoon minced fresh rosemary *or* 1 teaspoon dried rosemary, crushed
2 teaspoons grated lemon peel
1 teaspoon minced garlic
1 teaspoon Liquid Smoke, optional
1/2 teaspoon salt
1/4 teaspoon pepper
1 boneless pork top loin roast (3 pounds), cut in half

1. In a saucepan, combine the pineapple, barbecue sauce, apple juice, rosemary, lemon peel, garlic, Liquid Smoke if desired, salt and pepper. Bring to a boil. Reduce heat; simmer, uncovered, for 3 minutes. Meanwhile, in a nonstick skillet coated with cooking spray, brown the pork roast.

2. Place the roast in a 5-qt. slow cooker. Pour sauce over roast and turn to coat. Cook on high for 4 hours or on low for 6-7 hours. Let stand for 15 minutes before carving.

SMOKY FLAVOR

Liquid Smoke is made from smoke created during a control burn of wood that is typically used for barbecuing or smoking, such as hickory, mesquite, pecan or apple. Once the smoke is collected, it is processed into a liquid. Then it's aged, filtered and bottled. Since it is a concentrated flavor, a little goes a long way.

Pork Soft-Shell Tacos

It's hard to find recipes that have enough spicy flavor to satisfy my husband but don't overwhelm our kids. This Southwestern fare earned a thumbs-up from them all!

Margaret Steele, North Vancouver, British Columbia

- 1 pork tenderloin (1 pound), cut into 1-inch strips
- 1 small onion, chopped
- 1 teaspoon canola oil
- 2/3 cup enchilada sauce
- 1 tablespoon dry roasted peanuts
- 1 tablespoon semisweet chocolate chips
- 1 tablespoon raisins
- 1 garlic clove, minced
- 1 teaspoon ground cumin
- 1/4 teaspoon crushed red pepper flakes
- 1/2 cup frozen corn, thawed
- 8 corn tortillas (6 inches), warmed
- 1 cup shredded lettuce
- 1/4 cup reduced-fat sour cream
- 1/4 cup sliced green onions

1. In a large nonstick skillet or wok, stir-fry the pork strips and onion in oil for 3-4 minutes or until the pork is no longer pink; drain and keep warm.

2. In the same skillet, combine the enchilada sauce, peanuts, chocolate chips, raisins, garlic, cumin and red pepper flakes. Cook and stir over medium heat for 2-3 minutes or until chocolate is melted. Pour into a blender; cover and process until smooth. Return to skillet. Stir in corn and pork mixture; cook until heated through.

3. Spoon pork mixture down one half of each tortilla; fold the remaining side over the filling. Serve with lettuce, sour cream and green onions.

LOW SALT

PREP/TOTAL TIME
20 min.
YIELD 4 servings

NUTRITION FACTS
One serving
(2 tacos) equals:
370 calories
10 g fat
3 g saturated fat
67 mg cholesterol
263 mg sodium
41 g carbohydrate
5 g fiber
30 g protein

DIABETIC EXCHANGES
3 lean meat
2-1/2 starch

Baked Pork Chimichangas

Plenty of shredded pork and pinto beans combine with Southwestern ingredients like green chilies, chili powder and picante sauce in these from-scratch chimichangas. Because the recipe makes a lot, I can freeze some for when I don't feel like cooking.

LaDonna Reed, Ponca City, Oklahoma

PREP/TOTAL TIME
Prep: 15 min. +
standing
Bake: 2 hours
25 min.
YIELD 2-1/2 dozen

NUTRITION FACTS
One serving
(1 chimichanga)
equals:

276 calories
8 g fat
4 g saturated fat
36 mg cholesterol
475 mg sodium
30 g carbohydrate
6 g fiber
20 g protein

DIABETIC EXCHANGES
2 starch
2 lean meat

1 pound dried pinto beans
1 boneless pork loin roast (3 pounds), trimmed
3 cans (4 ounces *each*) chopped green chilies
1 large onion, chopped
1/3 cup chili powder
1/2 cup reduced-sodium chicken broth
30 flour tortillas (6 inches)
4 cups (16 ounces) shredded reduced-fat cheddar cheese
2 cups picante sauce
1 egg white
2 teaspoons water

1. Place beans in a soup kettle; add water to cover by 2 in. Bring to a boil; boil for 2 minutes. Remove from the heat; cover and let stand for 1 to 4 hours or until softened. Drain and rinse beans, discarding liquid.

2. Place roast in a Dutch oven. In a bowl, combine chilies, onion, chili powder and beans. Spoon over roast. Cover and bake at 325° for 1-1/2 hours. Stir in broth; cover and bake 30-45 minutes longer or until a meat thermometer reads 160°. Increase oven temperature to 350°.

3. Remove meat and shred with two forks; set aside. Mash bean mixture; stir in shredded pork. Spoon 1/3 cup mixture down the center of each tortilla; top with picante sauce. Fold sides and ends over filling and roll up. Place seam side down on two 15-in. x 10-in. x 1-in. baking pans coated with cooking spray.

4. In a bowl, whisk egg white and water; brush over top. Bake, uncovered, at 350° for 25-30 minutes or until heated through. Serve immediately or cool, wrap and freeze for up to 3 months.

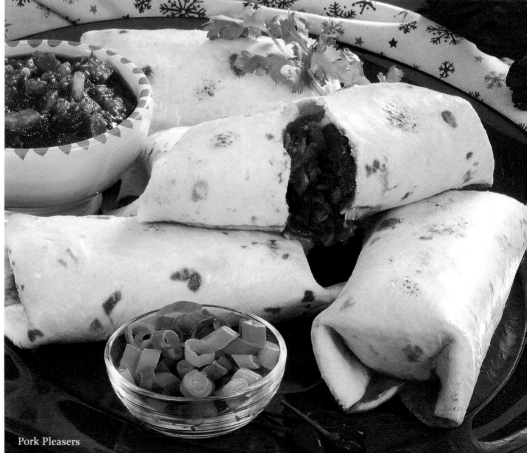

One-Pot Pork and Rice

No one will guess that this filling entree is low on fat and calories. Green pepper and onion enhance the rice and chops, which are covered with diced tomatoes and gravy.

Duna Stephens, Palisade, Colorado

- 6 boneless pork loin chops (5 ounces *each*)
- 2 teaspoons canola oil
- 1 cup uncooked long grain rice
- 1 large onion, sliced
- 1 large green pepper, sliced
- 1 envelope pork gravy mix
- 1 can (28 ounces) diced tomatoes, undrained
- 1-1/2 cups water

1. In a Dutch oven, brown pork chops in oil on both sides; drain. Remove chops.

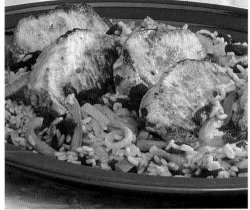

2. Layer rice, onion and green pepper in Dutch oven; top with pork chops. Combine the gravy mix, tomatoes and water; pour over chops. Cover and bake at 350° for 1 hour or until meat juices run clear and rice is tender.

PREP/TOTAL TIME
Prep: 20 min.
Bake: 1 hour
YIELD 6 servings

NUTRITION FACTS
One serving
(1 pork chop with
1/2 cup rice) equals:
391 calories
10 g fat
3 g saturated fat
83 mg cholesterol
545 mg sodium
40 g carbohydrate
3 g fiber
33 g protein

DIABETIC EXCHANGES
3-1/2 lean meat
2 starch
2 vegetable

Ham and Red Beans

I've cut some of the fat and calories from this traditional Southern dish. But after one bite, people agree it still has plenty of flavor.

June Robinson, Bastrop, Louisiana

- 3 cans (15-1/2 ounces *each*) kidney beans, rinsed and drained
- 1 can (14-1/2 ounces) Cajun *or* Mexican stewed tomatoes
- 2 cups diced fully cooked lean ham
- 1/2 cup water
- 1/2 teaspoon garlic powder
- 1/2 teaspoon ground cumin
- 1/2 teaspoon dried thyme
- 1/2 teaspoon dried oregano
- 1/4 teaspoon pepper
- 3 dashes hot pepper sauce

1. In a large saucepan or Dutch oven, bring all ingredients to a boil. Reduce heat; cover and simmer for 30 minutes.

TOMATO TYPES

Stewed tomatoes are available not only in Cajun and Mexican flavors, but also in a no-sodium-added variety. When making Ham and Red Beans, choose whichever stewed tomatoes appeal to you most. Feel free to experiment with the seasonings in the recipe and adjust them to suit your taste.

PREP/TOTAL TIME
Prep: 10 min.
Cook: 30 min.
YIELD 10 servings

NUTRITION FACTS
One serving
(3/4 cup) equals:
207 calories
2 g fat
0 g saturated fat
13 mg cholesterol
474 mg sodium
32 g carbohydrate
0 g fiber
15 g protein

DIABETIC EXCHANGES
2 starch
1 lean meat

Creamy Ham Turnovers

Refrigerated pizza crust makes these tasty turnovers a time-saver. The golden-brown bundles look like you fussed, but they're actually very simple to prepare.

Earnestine Jackson, Beaumont, Texas

PREP/TOTAL TIME
30 min.
YIELD 4 servings

NUTRITION FACTS
One serving equals:
308 calories
9 g fat
4 g saturated fat
27 mg cholesterol
967 mg sodium
37 g carbohydrate
1 g fiber
17 g protein

DIABETIC EXCHANGES
2-1/2 starch
2 lean meat

4 ounces reduced-fat cream cheese, softened
2 tablespoons fat-free milk
1 teaspoon dill weed
1 cup cubed fully cooked lean ham
2 tablespoons diced onion
1 celery rib, diced
2 tablespoons diced pimientos
1 tube (13.8 ounces) refrigerated pizza crust
1 egg white, beaten

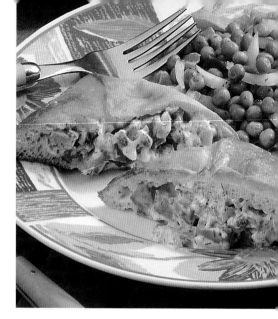

1. In a large mixing bowl, beat cream cheese, milk and dill until blended. Stir in the ham, onion, celery and pimientos. Roll out pizza dough into a 12-in. x 10-in. rectangle; cut in half lengthwise and widthwise. Place the rectangles on a baking sheet coated with cooking spray.

2. Divide ham mixture evenly between the four rectangles. Fold opposite corners over ham mixture; pinch to seal. Brush with egg white. Bake at 400° for 20-25 minutes or until golden brown.

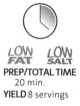

Tomato Ham Pasta

I got this recipe from a cooking show years ago and have been making it frequently ever since. I like to use my garden tomatoes.

Colleen Harvel, Big Bear City, California

PREP/TOTAL TIME
20 min.
YIELD 8 servings

NUTRITION FACTS
One serving
(1 cup) equals:
157 calories
3 g fat
0 g saturated fat
13 mg cholesterol
254 mg sodium
24 g carbohydrate
0 g fiber
10 g protein

DIABETIC EXCHANGES
2 starch
1 lean meat

3 cups uncooked penne pasta
2 garlic cloves, minced
2 tablespoons canola oil
4 medium tomatoes, peeled, seeded and chopped
1 cup diced fully cooked low-sodium ham
1/2 teaspoon salt-free seasoning blend
1/4 teaspoon pepper
1/8 teaspoon crushed red pepper flakes

1. Cook pasta according to the package directions. Meanwhile, in a skillet, saute garlic in oil until tender. Add tomatoes; simmer for 5 minutes.

2. Stir in ham and seasonings. Cook 8 minutes longer or until heated through. Drain pasta; add to ham mixture.

GREAT GARLIC

Garlic brings fabulous flavor to many different kinds of dishes. When a recipe calls for minced garlic, you may use either minced garlic from the grocery store or fresh garlic that's been finely chopped by hand or put through a press. Choose whichever variety is convenient for you.

Moist Ham Loaf

Not only is this main dish special enough for company, but I can assemble it early in the day and simply pop it in the oven before dinner. Plus, the cherry sauce really dresses it up, so my guests think I fussed.

Nancy Brown, Dahinda, Illinois

- 1/2 cup fat-free milk
- 1/3 cup dry bread crumbs
- 1/4 cup egg substitute
- 1/2 teaspoon onion powder
- 1/4 teaspoon pepper
- 1 pound ground fully cooked lean ham
- 1/2 pound ground turkey

CHERRY SAUCE:

- 1/2 cup cherry preserves
- 1 tablespoon cider vinegar
- 1/8 teaspoon ground cloves

1. In a bowl, combine the milk, bread crumbs, egg substitute, onion powder and pepper. Crumble ham and turkey over mixture and mix well. Press into a 9-in. x 5-in. x 3-in. loaf pan coated with cooking spray. Bake, uncovered, at 375° for 50-55 minutes or until a meat thermometer reads 160°.

2. In a saucepan, combine the preserves, vinegar and cloves. Cook and stir over medium heat for 5 minutes or until heated through. Serve with ham loaf.

PREP/TOTAL TIME
Prep: 15 min.
Bake: 50 min.
YIELD 6 servings

NUTRITION FACTS
One serving (1 slice with 1 tablespoon sauce) equals:

- 269 calories
- 7 g fat
- 2 g saturated fat
- 53 mg cholesterol
- 980 mg sodium
- 25 g carbohydrate
- Trace fiber
- 25 g protein

DIABETIC EXCHANGES
- 3 lean meat
- 1 starch
- 1/2 fruit

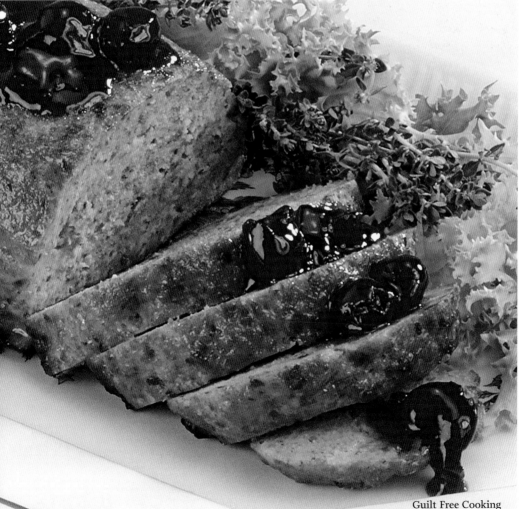

LOW FAT

PREP/TOTAL TIME
30 min.
YIELD 5 servings

NUTRITION FACTS
One serving
(1-1/2 cups
(calculated without
rice) equals:
   227 calories
   5 g fat
   1 g saturated fat
   32 mg cholesterol
952 mg sodium
   31 g carbohydrate
   7 g fiber
   16 g protein

DIABETIC EXCHANGES
   4 vegetable
   2 lean meat
   1/2 starch

Creole Sausage and Vegetables

If you're a fan of okra, you'll get a kick out of this zippy smoked sausage and vegetable medley. Served over rice, this dish makes a hearty meal with generous portions.

Jill Holland, Florence, Alabama

- 1 pound reduced-fat fully cooked sausage, cut into 1/2-inch slices
- 1 large onion, chopped
- 1/2 cup chopped green pepper
- 1/2 cup chopped sweet red pepper
- 2 garlic cloves, minced
- 2 teaspoons canola oil
- 4 cups chopped fresh tomatoes
- 1 tablespoon Worcestershire sauce
- 1/2 teaspoon sugar
- 1/2 teaspoon lemon juice
- 1/4 teaspoon salt
- 1/4 teaspoon crushed red pepper flakes
- 1/4 teaspoon pepper
- 1/4 teaspoon seafood seasoning
- 4 cups frozen cut okra

Hot cooked rice, optional

1. In a large skillet, cook the sausage, onion, green pepper, sweet red pepper and garlic in oil over medium heat until vegetables are tender. Stir in the tomatoes, Worcestershire sauce, sugar, lemon juice and seasonings. Bring to a boil. Reduce the heat; simmer, uncovered, for 15 minutes.

2. Add the okra; return to a boil. Reduce the heat; simmer, uncovered, for 7 minutes or just until the okra is tender. Serve with rice if desired.

NICE RICE

For fluffier rice to serve with your Creole Sausage and Vegetables, remove the saucepan from the heat after the cooking time is complete and let it stand for 5 to 10 minutes. Then fluff the rice with a fork.

Herb-Stuffed Pork Loin

I serve this impressive pork roast often when I'm entertaining. It's especially good with fresh herbs, but dried work nicely as well.

Michele Montgomery, Lethbridge, Alberta

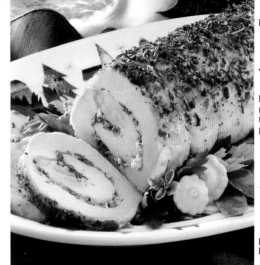

1	boneless pork loin roast (3 pounds)
1/4	cup Dijon mustard
4	garlic cloves, minced
1/3	cup minced chives
1/4	cup minced fresh sage *or* 4 teaspoons rubbed sage
2	tablespoons minced fresh thyme *or* 2 teaspoons dried thyme
1	tablespoon minced fresh rosemary *or* 1 teaspoon dried rosemary, crushed
2-3/4	teaspoons pepper, *divided*
1	teaspoon salt, *divided*
1	tablespoon olive oil

1. Starting about a third in from one side, make a lengthwise slit down the roast to within 1/2 in. of the bottom. Turn roast over and make another lengthwise slit, starting about a third in from the opposite side. Open roast so it lies flat; cover with plastic wrap. Flatten to 3/4-in. thickness; remove plastic wrap.

2. Combine mustard and garlic; rub two-thirds of the mixture over roast. Combine the chives, sage, thyme, rosemary, 3/4 teaspoon pepper and 1/2 teaspoon salt.

Sprinkle two-thirds of the herb mixture over roast. Roll up jelly-roll style, starting with a long side; tie several times with kitchen string. Rub oil over roast; sprinkle with remaining salt and pepper.

3. If grilling the roast, coat the grill rack with cooking spray before starting the grill. Grill the roast, covered, over indirect medium heat or bake, uncovered, at 350° for 1 hour.

4. Brush remaining mustard mixture over roast; sprinkle with remaining herb mixture. Grill or bake 20-25 minutes longer or until a meat thermometer reads 160°. Let stand for 10 minutes before slicing.

PREP/TOTAL TIME
Prep: 20 min.
Bake: 1 hour
20 min. +
standing
YIELD 12 servings

NUTRITION FACTS
One serving
(3 ounces cooked
pork) equals:
199 calories
10 g fat
3 g saturated fat
69 mg cholesterol
372 mg sodium
2 g carbohydrate
1 g fiber
25 g protein

DIABETIC EXCHANGE
3 lean meat

Ham Noodle Casserole

My mom used to make the original version of this mild curry casserole, which I loved. It didn't fit my healthier eating habits until I made a few changes. Now our whole family can enjoy it without the guilt.

Sheri Switzer, Crawfordsville, Indiana

6	cups uncooked no-yolk medium noodles
1	can (10-3/4 ounces) reduced-fat reduced-sodium condensed cream of celery soup, undiluted
1	cup cubed fully cooked lean ham
2/3	cup cubed reduced-fat process cheese (Velveeta)
1/2	cup fat-free milk
1/4	cup thinly sliced green onions
1/2	teaspoon curry powder

1. Cook noodles according to package directions; drain and place in a large bowl. Stir in the remaining ingredients.

2. Transfer to a 2-1/2-qt. baking dish coated with cooking spray. Cover and bake at 375° for 20-30 minutes or until heated through.

PROCESS POINTER

Process cheese is made from natural cheeses with added emulsifiers, and is pasteurized to increase storage life. Generally, it is stable at room temperature and stays smooth and creamy when heated. The most common brand name of process American cheese is Velveeta.

LOW FAT
PREP/TOTAL TIME
Prep: 15 min.
Bake: 20 min.
YIELD 6 servings

NUTRITION FACTS
One serving
(1 cup) equals:
241 calories
4 g fat
2 g saturated fat
20 mg cholesterol
725 mg sodium
35 g carbohydrate
3 g fiber
15 g protein

DIABETIC EXCHANGES
2-1/2 starch
1 lean meat

NUTRITION FACTS

One serving
(3 ounces cooked
pork with 1/4 cup
sauce) equals:

332 calories
11 g fat
4 g saturated fat
71 mg cholesterol
419 mg sodium
34 g carbohydrate
1 g fiber
23 g protein

DIABETIC EXCHANGES

3 lean meat
1 starch
1 fruit
1 fat

Cranberry-Mustard Pork Medallions

This pretty pork entree makes a great holiday dish. Topped with cranberry sauce, the pork medallions are light and filling, but they're so delicious, guests always want more.

Tami Morrison, Kent, Washington

2/3 cup water

1/3 cup unsweetened apple juice concentrate

1/3 cup cranberry juice concentrate

1/3 cup port wine *or* 1 tablespoon additional cranberry juice concentrate plus 1/4 cup water

1 pork tenderloin (1 pound)

1/4 teaspoon garlic salt

1/8 teaspoon pepper

1 tablespoon olive oil

1 tablespoon butter

2 to 3 tablespoons Dijon mustard

1/3 cup dried cranberries

1. In a bowl, combine the first four ingredients; set aside. Cut pork into 1-in. slices; flatten to 1/4-in. thickness. Sprinkle with garlic salt and pepper.

2. In a large nonstick skillet, saute the pork in oil and butter in batches for 2-3 minutes on each side or until juices run clear. Remove and keep warm.

3. Add reserved juice mixture to the skillet; bring to a boil. Reduce heat; simmer for 3 minutes.

4. Stir in mustard; cook and stir for 6-8 minutes or until slightly thickened. Add cranberries. Return the pork to the pan; cover and simmer for 5 minutes or until heated through.

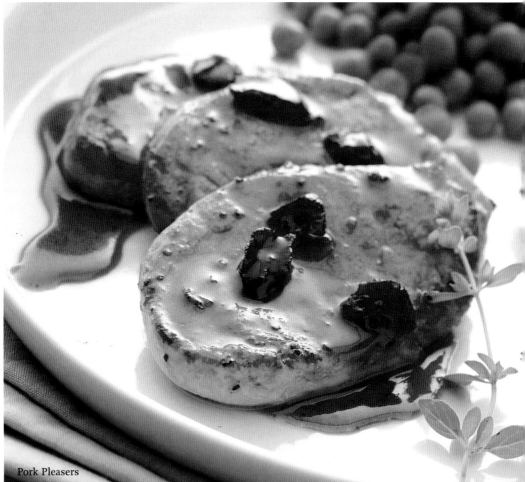

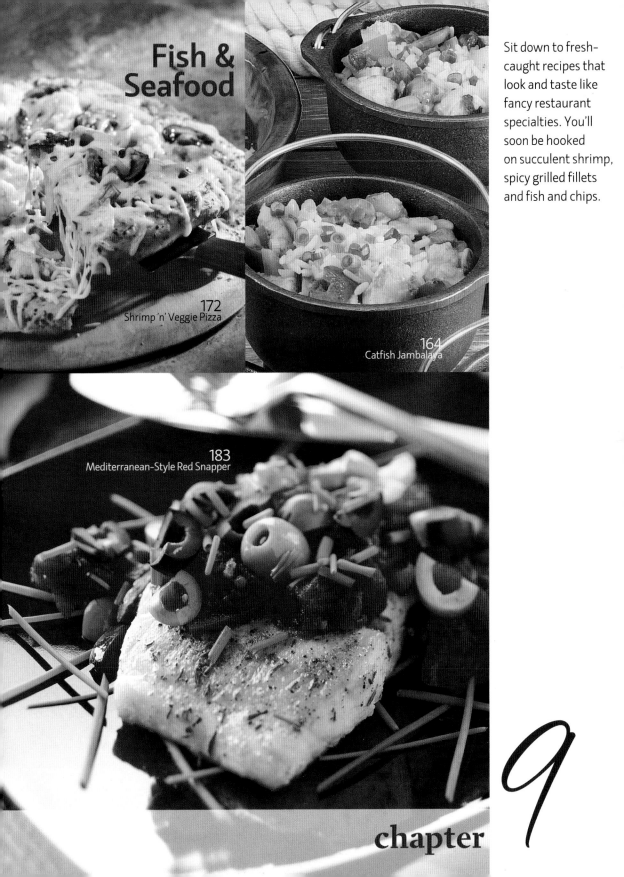

Fish & Seafood

Sit down to fresh-caught recipes that look and taste like fancy restaurant specialties. You'll soon be hooked on succulent shrimp, spicy grilled fillets and fish and chips.

172
Shrimp 'n' Veggie Pizza

164
Catfish Jambalaya

183
Mediterranean-Style Red Snapper

chapter *9*

LOW FAT

PREP/TOTAL TIME
15 min.
YIELD 4 servings

NUTRITION FACTS
One serving
(prepared with
reduced-sodium
broth) equals:
162 calories
4 g fat
0 g saturated fat
38 mg cholesterol
321 mg sodium
10 g carbohydrate
1 g fiber
21 g protein

DIABETIC EXCHANGES
3 very lean
meat
1/2 starch

Crumb-Topped Scallops

A pretty crumb topping blankets this tasty seafood entree. The recipe is so good, I won't make scallops any other way.

Kathy Brodin, Wauwatosa, Wisconsin

1/4 cup dry bread crumbs
1 tablespoon margarine, melted
1 to 2 teaspoons dried parsley flakes
1 pound sea scallops
6 fresh mushrooms, quartered
1 tablespoon white wine *or*
   reduced-sodium chicken broth
1-1/2 teaspoons lemon juice
1/4 teaspoon dried thyme
1/8 teaspoon garlic powder
1/8 teaspoon seasoned salt
1/8 teaspoon pepper
Lemon wedges, optional

1. In a small bowl, combine bread crumbs, margarine and parsley; set aside. Place scallops and mushrooms in a 9-in. microwave-safe pie plate. Combine wine or broth, lemon juice and seasonings; pour over the scallop mixture.

2. Cover and microwave at 50% power for 1-1/2 minutes; drain. Sprinkle with crumb mixture. Cover and microwave at 50% power 3-1/2 minutes longer or until scallops are opaque, stirring once. Serve with lemon if desired.

Editor's Note: This recipe was tested in a 1,100-watt microwave.

SIZING UP SCALLOPS

Scallops are typically referred to as sea and bay scallops. Sea scallops are the large ones and bay the small ones, about 1/2 inch in diameter. Sea scallops vary in size and you may find some markets refer to them as jumbo, large and medium.

LOW FAT

PREP/TOTAL TIME
30 min.
YIELD 4 servings

NUTRITION FACTS
One serving
(calculated without
salt, rice and green
onions) equals:
161 calories
4 g fat
0 g saturated fat
66 mg cholesterol
395 mg sodium
12 g carbohydrate
0 g fiber
21 g protein

DIABETIC EXCHANGES
3 very lean
meat
2 vegetable

Catfish Jambalaya

My family owns a catfish processing plant. This colorful, zippy main dish featuring that fish is an all-time favorite of ours.

Mrs. Bill Saul, Macon, Mississippi

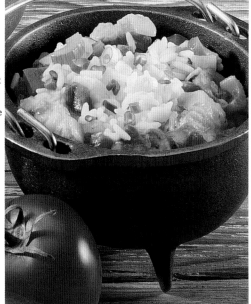

2 cups chopped onion
1/2 cup chopped celery
1/2 cup chopped green pepper
2 garlic cloves, minced
1/4 cup butter
1 can (10 ounces) diced tomatoes and
   green chilies, undrained
1 cup sliced fresh mushrooms
1/4 teaspoon cayenne pepper
1/2 teaspoon salt, optional
1 pound catfish fillets, cubed
Hot cooked rice, optional
Sliced green onions, optional

1. In a saucepan coated with cooking spray over medium-high heat, saute onion, celery, green pepper and garlic in butter until tender, about 10 minutes. Add the tomatoes, mushrooms, cayenne and salt if desired; bring to a boil. Add catfish.

2. Reduce heat; cover and simmer until fish flakes easily with a fork, about 10 minutes. If desired, serve with hot rice and top with sliced green onions.

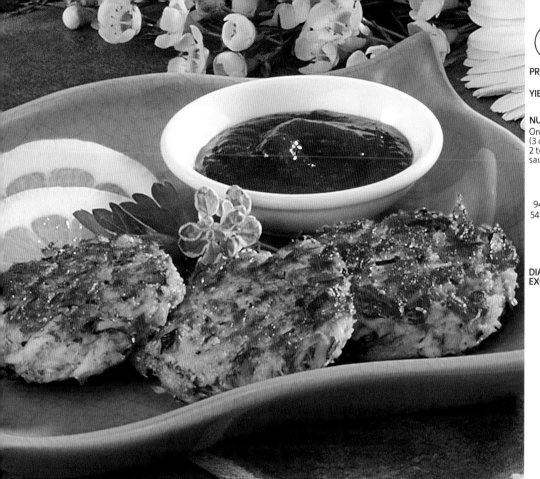

LOW FAT

PREP/TOTAL TIME
20 min.
YIELD 9 servings

NUTRITION FACTS
One serving
(3 crab cakes with
2 teaspoons seafood
sauce) equals:
139 calories
5 g fat
1 g saturated fat
94 mg cholesterol
547 mg sodium
7 g carbohydrate
1 g fiber
17 g protein

DIABETIC EXCHANGES
2 very lean
meat
1/2 starch
1/2 fat

Crab Cakes

My family really likes crab cakes, but some recipes have too much breading and not enough crab. So I experimented until I finally hit on the right light combination.

Kathy Buchanan, Hartsville, South Carolina

1 egg, lightly beaten
1/4 cup fat-free mayonnaise
1/2 cup soft bread crumbs
2 green onions, finely chopped
1 tablespoon minced fresh parsley
1 teaspoon ground mustard
1/4 teaspoon salt
1/4 teaspoon pepper
4 cans (6 ounces *each*) crabmeat, drained, flaked and cartilage removed
1 tablespoon butter
1 tablespoon canola oil
6 tablespoons seafood sauce

1. In a bowl, combine the egg, mayonnaise, bread crumbs, green onions, parsley, mustard, salt and pepper. Add the crab; mix gently. Shape rounded tablespoonfuls into 2-in. patties.

2. In a large nonstick skillet, cook patties in butter and oil over medium heat for 3-4 minutes on each side or until golden brown. Serve with seafood sauce.

FLAVOR TWIST

If you want to add a special flavor to crab cakes, try adding some Old Bay seasoning along with the other herbs and spices. A little will go a long way, so add a 1/4 to 1/2 teaspoon.

LOW SALT

PREP/TOTAL TIME
25 min.
YIELD 4 servings

NUTRITION FACTS
One serving (1 fillet
with 3 tablespoons
relish) equals:

   222 calories
     9 g fat
     4 g saturated fat
 168 mg cholesterol
 241 mg sodium
     1 g carbohydrate
Trace fiber
   33 g protein

**DIABETIC
EXCHANGES**
   4 very lean
     meat
   2 fat

Perch with Cucumber Relish

I give fish a flavor lift with homemade relish. Tangy vinegar and tarragon lend zest to the condiment, while chopped cucumber and radishes add from-the-garden color.

Mildred Sherrer, Fort Worth, Texas

2/3	cup chopped seeded cucumber
1/2	cup chopped radishes
2	tablespoons white vinegar
1	teaspoon canola oil
1/4	teaspoon sugar
1/4	teaspoon dried tarragon
1/8	teaspoon salt
2	tablespoons butter
4	perch *or* tilapia fillets (6 ounces *each*)

1. For relish, in a bowl, combine cucumber, radishes, vinegar, oil, sugar, tarragon and salt; set aside.

2. In a large skillet, melt butter over medium-high heat. Cook fillets for 3-4 minutes on each side or until fish flakes easily with a fork. Serve with relish.

Tuna Noodle Casserole

Your family will love the creamy texture and comforting taste of this traditional tuna casserole that goes together in a jiffy. I serve it with a green salad and warm rolls.

Ruby Wells, Cynthiana, Kentucky

- 1 can (10-3/4 ounces) reduced-fat reduced-sodium condensed cream of celery soup, undiluted
- 1/2 cup fat-free milk
- 2 cups cooked yolk-free wide noodles
- 1 cup frozen peas, thawed
- 1 can (6 ounces) light water-packed tuna, drained and flaked
- 1 jar (2 ounces) diced pimientos, drained
- 2 tablespoons dry bread crumbs
- 1 tablespoon butter, melted

1. In a large bowl, combine soup and milk until smooth. Add the noodles, peas, tuna and pimientos; mix well.

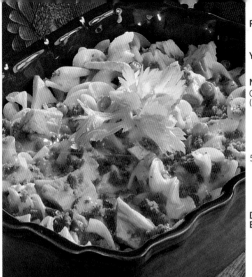

2. Pour into a 1-1/2-qt. baking dish coated with cooking spray. Bake, uncovered, at 400° for 25 minutes. Toss crumbs and butter; sprinkle over the top. Bake 5 minutes longer or until golden brown.

PREP/TOTAL TIME
Prep: 10 min.
Bake: 30 min.
YIELD 4 servings

NUTRITION FACTS
One serving
(1 cup) equals:
255 calories
6 g fat
3 g saturated fat
29 mg cholesterol
582 mg sodium
31 g carbohydrate
4 g fiber
18 g protein

DIABETIC EXCHANGES
2 starch
2 lean meat

Creole Catfish Fillets

I rub catfish fillets with a pleasant mixture of seasonings before cooking them quickly on the grill. The moist fish gets added flavor from a spicy sauce and lemon wedges.

Dave Bremstone, Plantation, Florida

- 3 tablespoons reduced-fat plain yogurt
- 2 tablespoons finely chopped onion
- 1 tablespoon fat-free mayonnaise
- 1 tablespoon Dijon mustard
- 1 tablespoon ketchup
- 1/2 teaspoon dried thyme
- 1/4 teaspoon grated lemon peel
- 1 teaspoon paprika
- 1/2 teaspoon onion powder
- 1/4 teaspoon salt
- 1/8 teaspoon cayenne pepper
- 4 catfish fillets (4 ounces *each*)
- 4 lemon wedges

1. In a small bowl, combine the yogurt, onion, mayonnaise, mustard, ketchup, thyme and lemon peel. Cover and refrigerate until serving. In another bowl, combine the paprika, onion powder, salt and cayenne; rub over both sides of fillets.

2. Grill, covered, in a grill basket coated with cooking spray over medium-hot heat for 5-6 minutes on each side or until fish flakes easily with a fork. Serve with lemon wedges and yogurt sauce.

WHEN IT'S DONE

When cooking catfish fillets, check for doneness by inserting a fork at an angle into the thickest portion of the fish and gently parting the meat. When it flakes into sections, it's cooked completely.

PREP/TOTAL TIME
15 min.
YIELD 4 servings

NUTRITION FACTS
One serving
(1 fillet with about
1 tablespoon sauce)
equals:
182 calories
9 g fat
2 g saturated fat
54 mg cholesterol
382 mg sodium
5 g carbohydrate
1 g fiber
19 g protein

DIABETIC EXCHANGES
3 lean meat
1/2 fat

Tuna Patties with Dill Sauce

These tender, golden tuna patties have a great blend of flavors. Parsnips are the "secret ingredient." They replace part of the traditional bread crumbs and add moisture, fiber and extra nutrition.

Taste of Home Test Kitchen

  2 large parsnips, peeled and cut into 1/2-inch slices
  2 egg whites, lightly beaten
  1/2 cup soft bread crumbs
  1/4 cup finely chopped green onions
  1 tablespoon dried parsley flakes
  2 teaspoons lemon juice
  1/2 teaspoon grated lemon peel
  1/2 teaspoon dill weed
  1/4 teaspoon pepper
  2 cans (6 ounces *each*) light water-packed tuna, drained and flaked
  2 teaspoons olive oil

DILL SAUCE:
  1/2 cup fat-free mayonnaise
  1 teaspoon lemon juice
  1 teaspoon grated lemon peel
  1/2 teaspoon dill weed

1. Place parsnips in a saucepan and cover with water; bring to a boil. Reduce heat; cover and simmer for 30-35 minutes or

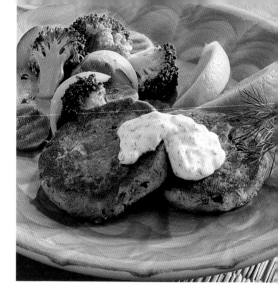

until tender. Drain well and cool slightly; place the parsnips in a food processor or blender; cover and process until smooth.

2. In a bowl, combine 1 cup pureed parsnips, egg whites, bread crumbs, onions, parsley, lemon juice and peel, dill and pepper. Add tuna and mix well. Shape into eight 1/2-in.-thick patties (patties will be soft).

3. In a large nonstick skillet, heat oil over medium heat. Cook patties for 5-6 minutes on each side or until lightly browned. Combine the sauce ingredients in a small bowl; serve with tuna patties.

Cilantro Lime Cod

My daughter loves to cook and especially likes dishes with Mexican flair. She bakes these wonderfully seasoned fillets in foil to keep them moist and cut down on cleanup.

Donna Hackman, Huddleston, Virginia

  4 cod *or* flounder fillets (2 pounds)
  1/4 teaspoon pepper
  1 tablespoon dried minced onion
  1 garlic clove, minced
  1 tablespoon olive oil
  1-1/2 teaspoons ground cumin
  1/4 cup minced fresh cilantro
  2 limes, thinly sliced
  2 tablespoons reduced-fat margarine, melted

1. Place each fillet on a 15-in. x 12-in. piece of heavy-duty foil. Sprinkle with pepper. In a small saucepan, saute onion and garlic in oil; stir in cumin. Spoon over fillets; sprinkle with cilantro. Place lime slices over each; drizzle with margarine. Fold foil around fish and seal tightly.

2. Place on a baking sheet. Bake at 375° for 35-40 minutes or until fish flakes easily with a fork.

SAVOR CILANTRO

Also known as coriander and Chinese parsley, zesty-flavored cilantro adds a distinctive flavor not only to fish, but also to chili, Mexican dishes, sauces and more.

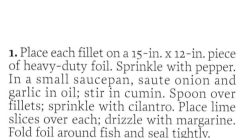

Zippy Shrimp Linguine

I won a community recipe contest several years ago with this spicy dish. Red pepper flakes put a little zing in the shrimp, and the veggies are crisp-tender and colorful.

Jackie Selover, Sidney, Ohio

1	package (16 ounces) linguine
1	pound uncooked large shrimp, peeled and deveined
2	garlic cloves, minced
1/2	to 1 teaspoon crushed red pepper flakes
2	tablespoons olive oil
1	teaspoon butter
1-1/2	cups sliced zucchini
1	cup sliced yellow summer squash
1	cup julienned carrots
1	cup fresh broccoli florets
1	tablespoon minced fresh parsley
1	tablespoon minced fresh basil
3/4	teaspoon salt
1/2	cup shredded Parmesan cheese

1. Cook pasta according to package directions. Meanwhile, in a large nonstick skillet, stir-fry the shrimp, garlic and pepper flakes in oil and butter for 3-5 minutes or until the shrimp turn pink. Remove shrimp; keep warm.

2. Add the zucchini, summer squash, carrots and broccoli to same skillet; stir-fry for 8-10 minutes or until crisp-tender.

3. Return shrimp to skillet. Drain the pasta; add to skillet along with the parsley, basil and salt. Heat through. Sprinkle with shredded Parmesan cheese.

PREP/TOTAL TIME
20 min.
YIELD 8 servings

NUTRITION FACTS
One serving
(1-1/2 cups) equals:
312 calories
7 g fat
2 g saturated fat
73 mg cholesterol
407 mg sodium
45 g carbohydrate
3 g fiber
18 g protein

DIABETIC EXCHANGES
2-1/2 starch
1 lean meat
1 vegetable
1 fat

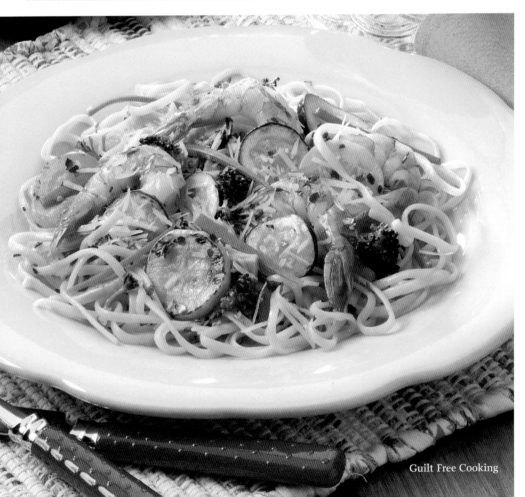

PREP/TOTAL TIME
10 min.
YIELD 4 servings

NUTRITION FACTS
One serving equals:
201 calories
3 g fat
0 g saturated fat
80 mg cholesterol
465 mg sodium
19 g carbohydrate
0 g fiber
23 g protein

DIABETIC EXCHANGES
2 very lean meat
1-1/2 starch

Shrimp Salad Bagels

Dill adds fresh taste to the shrimp and cream cheese topping I spread on bagels. I usually prepare these open-faced sandwiches for a fast lunch. You can heat them quickly in the microwave or pop them under the broiler if you'd like a crispier version.

Angie Hansen, Gildford, Montana

> 1 package (3 ounces) fat-free cream cheese
> 3 tablespoons fat-free mayonnaise
> 1 tablespoon lemon juice
> 1/2 teaspoon dill weed
> 1 can (6 ounces) small shrimp, rinsed and drained
> 2 bagels, split and toasted
> 1/4 cup shredded reduced-fat Swiss cheese

1. In a bowl, combine the cream cheese, mayonnaise, lemon juice and dill. Stir in the shrimp; spread over bagels.

2. Microwave, uncovered, on high for 1 minute or broil 4 in. from the heat until hot and bubbly. Sprinkle with the Swiss cheese.

Editor's Note: This recipe was tested in a 1,100-watt microwave.

CUT BACK THE SODIUM

To reduce the sodium in Shrimp Salad Bagels, substitute frozen cooked small shrimp. There is only about 64 mg of sodium per ounce of the frozen shrimp. To use the frozen shrimp, thaw 6 ounces and shell if necessary. Since these will be slight larger than the canned shrimp, you will need to chop them.

PREP/TOTAL TIME
Prep: 15 min. + chilling
Bake: 15 min.
YIELD 4 servings

NUTRITION FACTS
One serving equals:
217 calories
3 g fat
1 g saturated fat
52 mg cholesterol
382 mg sodium
21 g carbohydrate
1 g fiber
25 g protein

DIABETIC EXCHANGES
3 very lean meat
1-1/2 reduced-fat milk

Homemade Fish Fingers

Once you've tried these mouthwatering morsels, you'll never buy fish sticks again! We coated pieces of cod in a tasty Parmesan, herb and bread crumb mixture that's sure to get raves.

Taste of Home Test Kitchen

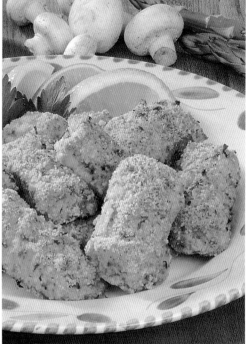

> 1 pound frozen cod fillets, partially thawed
> 1/2 cup seasoned bread crumbs
> 2 tablespoons grated Parmesan cheese
> 1 tablespoon minced fresh parsley
> 1 teaspoon grated lemon peel
> 1/2 teaspoon paprika
> 1/2 teaspoon dried thyme
> 1/4 teaspoon garlic salt
> 1/2 cup buttermilk
> 1/4 cup plus 2 tablespoons all-purpose flour

1. Cut fillets into 3/4-in. strips; set aside. In a shallow bowl, combine the bread crumbs, Parmesan cheese, parsley, lemon peel, paprika, thyme and garlic salt. Place buttermilk in another shallow bowl and flour in a third bowl. Coat fish strips with flour; dip into buttermilk, then coat with crumb mixture. Place on a baking sheet coated with cooking spray. Refrigerate for 20 minutes.

2. Bake at 425° for 15-20 minutes or until the fish flakes easily with a fork. Let stand for 2 minutes before removing from baking sheets.

Scallops and Asparagus Stir-Fry

Savory scallops, crisp-tender asparagus and cherry tomatoes blend together beautifully in this fresh-tasting stir-fry. Sesame oil and soy sauce delicately accent the colorful combo that's special enough for company.

Lisa Lancaster, Tracy, California

- 3/4 pound fresh asparagus, trimmed and cut into 2-inch pieces
- 1 tablespoon cornstarch
- 3/4 cup chicken broth
- 1 teaspoon reduced-sodium soy sauce
- 3/4 pound sea scallops, halved
- 1 cup sliced fresh mushrooms
- 1 garlic clove, minced
- 2 teaspoons canola oil
- 1 cup halved cherry tomatoes
- 2 green onions, sliced
- 1 teaspoon sesame oil
- 1/8 teaspoon pepper
- 2 cups hot cooked rice

1. Place asparagus in a saucepan and cover with water; bring to a boil. Cook, uncovered, for 3-5 minutes or until crisp-tender; drain and set aside. In a small

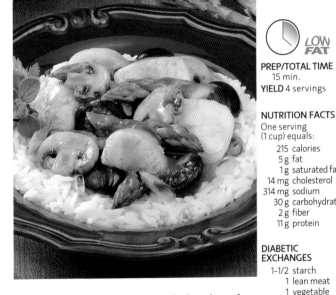

bowl, combine the cornstarch, broth and soy sauce until smooth; set aside.

2. In a large nonstick skillet or wok, stir-fry scallops, mushrooms and garlic in canola oil until scallops are opaque and mushrooms are tender. Stir cornstarch mixture; add to skillet. Bring to a boil; cook and stir until sauce is thickened.

3. Add the asparagus, tomatoes, onions, sesame oil and pepper; heat through. Serve over rice.

LOW FAT

PREP/TOTAL TIME
15 min.
YIELD 4 servings

NUTRITION FACTS
One serving
(1 cup) equals:
215 calories
5 g fat
1 g saturated fat
14 mg cholesterol
314 mg sodium
30 g carbohydrate
2 g fiber
11 g protein

DIABETIC EXCHANGES
1-1/2 starch
1 lean meat
1 vegetable
1/2 fat

Open-Face Tuna Melts

I created this recipe when I got married over 20 years ago and have served it countless times since then. Sometimes I add a little chili powder, heap the tuna mixture over tortilla chips instead of English muffins and microwave it for hearty nachos. It's a no-fuss snack.

Marilyn Smelser, Albany, Oregon

- 2 cans (6 ounces *each*) light water-packed tuna, drained and flaked
- 3/4 cup chopped sweet red pepper
- 1/2 cup chopped fresh mushrooms
- 1/2 cup shredded reduced-fat cheddar cheese
- 1/4 cup sliced pimiento-stuffed olives
- 4-1/2 teaspoons reduced-fat mayonnaise
- 4 English muffins, split and toasted
- 8 thin slices tomato

1. In a bowl, combine the tuna, red pepper, mushrooms, cheese and olives. Fold in mayonnaise. Spread over English muffin halves. Top each with a tomato slice. Broil 6 in. from the heat for 7-9 minutes or until lightly browned. Serve immediately.

MORE MUFFINS

Want another tempting idea for English muffins? Top them with a little pizza sauce, add your favorite chopped vegetables and sprinkle on some part-skim mozzarella cheese. Then just pop the muffins under the broiler, and you'll have great mini pizzas.

LOW FAT

PREP/TOTAL TIME
20 min.
YIELD 8 servings

NUTRITION FACTS
One serving equals:
165 calories
5 g fat
2 g saturated fat
24 mg cholesterol
413 mg sodium
16 g carbohydrate
2 g fiber
14 g protein

DIABETIC EXCHANGES
2 lean meat
1 starch

Shrimp 'n' Veggie Pizza

Just 30 minutes are all you'll need to put together this simple, colorful pizza. It's a great way to use up leftover veggies.

Terri Webber, Miami, Florida

PREP/TOTAL TIME
30 min.
YIELD 6 servings

NUTRITION FACTS
One serving
(1 slice) equals:
215 calories
7 g fat
2 g saturated fat
38 mg cholesterol
426 mg sodium
24 g carbohydrate
1 g fiber
13 g protein

DIABETIC EXCHANGES
1-1/2 starch
1 lean meat
1 fat

1/2 cup sliced onion

1/2 cup sliced fresh mushrooms

3 asparagus spears, trimmed and cut into 1-inch pieces

1 garlic clove, minced

2 teaspoons olive oil

4 ounces uncooked medium shrimp, peeled, deveined and halved lengthwise

1 prebaked thin Italian bread shell crust (10 ounces)

1/2 cup pizza sauce

1 cup (4 ounces) shredded part-skim mozzarella cheese

1. In a nonstick skillet, saute onion, mushrooms, asparagus and garlic in oil until almost tender. Add shrimp; cook until shrimp turn pink. Remove from the heat.

2. Place the crust on a pizza pan or baking sheet. Spread with pizza sauce. Top with shrimp mixture. Sprinkle with cheese. Bake at 450° for 8-10 minutes or until cheese is melted.

Lemon Dill Walleye

In our region, walleye is popular and abundant. This tasty version is moist and nicely enhanced with lemon and dill.

Dawn Piasta, Dauphin, Manitoba

- 1 large onion, halved and thinly sliced
- 1 tablespoon butter
- 4 cups water
- 1 tablespoon snipped fresh dill *or 1 teaspoon dill weed*
- 3/4 cup fat-free milk
- 2 medium lemons, thinly sliced
- 1/8 teaspoon pepper
- 2 pounds walleye, cod, halibut *or* orange roughy fillets

1. In a large skillet, saute onion in butter until tender. Add water and dill; bring to a boil. Reduce heat; simmer, uncovered, for 4-5 minutes. Add milk; stir in lemon slices and pepper. Top with fillets. Cover and simmer for 12-15 minutes or until fish flakes easily with a fork.

2. Transfer fish to a serving platter and keep warm. Strain the cooking liquid, reserving lemons, onion and dill; serve with fish.

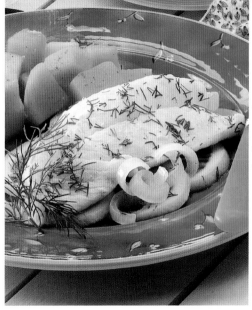

LOW FAT **LOW SALT**

PREP/TOTAL TIME
30 min.
YIELD 8 servings

NUTRITION FACTS
One serving (calculated with walleye) equals:
- 116 calories
- 2 g fat
- Trace saturated fat
- 70 mg cholesterol
- 113 mg sodium
- 5 g carbohydrate
- 1 g fiber
- 18 g protein

DIABETIC EXCHANGES
- 2-1/2 very lean meat
- 1 vegetable

Tomato-Topped Cod

Fresh tomato slices and a buttery topping jazz up plain fish fillets in this easy oven entree. Preparing it this way helps keep the cod moist and delicious.

Kathleen Taugher, East Troy, Wisconsin

- 1-1/2 cups water
- 2 tablespoons lemon juice
- 1-1/2 pounds cod fillets

Pepper to taste

- 1 small onion, finely chopped
- 2 large tomatoes, sliced
- 1/2 cup chopped green pepper
- 1/2 cup seasoned bread crumbs
- 1/4 cup grated Parmesan cheese
- 1/2 teaspoon dried basil
- 1 tablespoon canola oil

1. In a bowl, combine the water and lemon juice. Add fish; soak for 5 minutes. Drain and place fish in an 11-in. x 7-in. x 2-in. baking dish coated with cooking spray.

2. Sprinkle with pepper. Layer with onion, tomatoes and green pepper. Combine the remaining ingredients; sprinkle over top. Bake, uncovered, at 375° for 20-30 minutes or until fish flakes easily with a fork.

LOW FAT

PREP/TOTAL TIME
Prep: 15 min.
Bake: 20 min.
YIELD 6 servings

NUTRITION FACTS
One serving equals:
- 158 calories
- 4 g fat
- 0 g saturated fat
- 33 mg cholesterol
- 391 mg sodium
- 13 g carbohydrate
- Trace fiber
- 16 g protein

DIABETIC EXCHANGES
- 2 lean meat
- 1 starch

LOW FAT

PREP/TOTAL TIME
15 min.
YIELD 3 servings

NUTRITION FACTS
One serving
(4 ounces cooked
scallops with
4 mushrooms)
equals:
170 calories
4 g fat
2 g saturated fat
57 mg cholesterol
407 mg sodium
6 g carbohydrate
1 g fiber
27 g protein

DIABETIC EXCHANGES
3 lean meat
1 vegetable

Sea Scallops and Mushrooms

This is a foolproof yet elegant way to make sea scallops. The no-fuss dish couldn't be simpler because it uses the microwave.

Lynnae Neuberger, Marshfield, Wisconsin

1	pound fresh *or* frozen sea scallops, thawed and rinsed
12	small fresh mushrooms, halved
1	tablespoon white wine *or* chicken broth
1-1/2	teaspoons lemon juice
1/2	teaspoon lemon-pepper seasoning
1/4	teaspoon dried thyme
1/8	teaspoon garlic powder
1/8	teaspoon seasoned salt
2	teaspoons butter, melted

1. Place the scallops and mushrooms in a 9-in. glass pie plate or dish. Combine the wine or broth, lemon juice and seasonings; pour over scallop mixture.

2. Cover and microwave at 50% power for 2 minutes; stir. Cover and microwave at 50% power 4 to 4-1/2 minutes longer or until scallops turn opaque. Stir in melted butter.

Editor's Note: This recipe was tested in a 1,100-watt microwave.

PREP/TOTAL TIME
Prep: 15 min.
Bake: 25 min.
YIELD 4 servings

NUTRITION FACTS
One serving equals:
280 calories
11 g fat
4 g saturated fat
91 mg cholesterol
442 mg sodium
15 g carbohydrate
1 g fiber
30 g protein

DIABETIC EXCHANGES
4 lean meat
1 starch

Stuffed Mountain Trout

You can substitute any whole fish in this recipe, but I like to make it with fresh-caught trout from our local mountain stream. The moist stuffing makes this nice for company.

Loretta Walters, Ogden, Utah

2	trout (10 to 11 ounces *each*)
4	tablespoons plus 1-1/2 teaspoons lemon juice, *divided*
3	teaspoons dill weed, *divided*
2	teaspoons lemon-pepper seasoning, *divided*
1	small onion, chopped
1	tablespoon butter
1/2	cup minced fresh parsley
2	cups soft bread crumbs

1. Place trout in a 13-in. x 9-in. x 2-in. baking dish coated with cooking spray. Sprinkle 3 tablespoons lemon juice, 1-1/2 teaspoons dill and 1-1/2 teaspoons lemon-pepper in the fish cavities and over outside of fish; set aside.

2. In a nonstick skillet, saute onion in butter until tender. Add the parsley and remaining dill and lemon-pepper. Stir in bread crumbs; heat through. Sprinkle with remaining lemon juice; stir gently until moistened. Stuff into fish cavities. Bake, uncovered, at 400° for 25-30 minutes or until fish flakes easily with a fork.

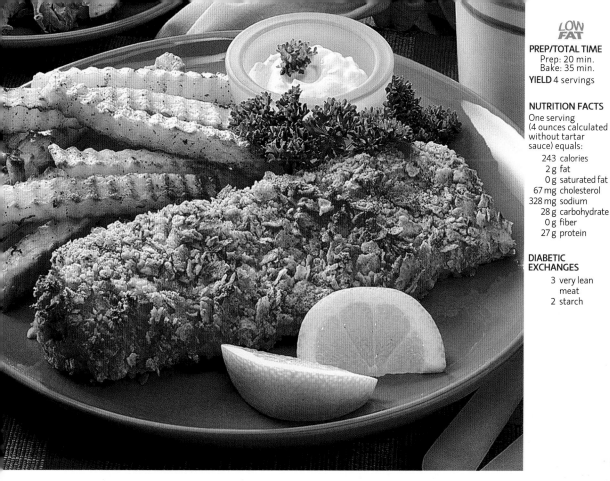

LOW FAT

PREP/TOTAL TIME
Prep: 20 min.
Bake: 35 min.
YIELD 4 servings

NUTRITION FACTS
One serving
(4 ounces calculated
without tartar
sauce) equals:

243 calories
2 g fat
0 g saturated fat
67 mg cholesterol
328 mg sodium
28 g carbohydrate
0 g fiber
27 g protein

DIABETIC EXCHANGES
3 very lean
   meat
2 starch

Oven Fish 'n' Chips

This great fish coating is as crunchy and golden as the deep-fried variety. Your family is sure to love the crisp "fries," too!

Janice Mitchell, Aurora, Colorado

2	tablespoons olive oil
1/4	teaspoon pepper
4	medium baking potatoes (1 pound), peeled

FISH:

1/3	cup all-purpose flour
1/4	teaspoon pepper
1/4	cup egg substitute
2	tablespoons water
2/3	cup crushed cornflakes
1	tablespoon grated Parmesan cheese
1/8	teaspoon cayenne pepper
1	pound frozen haddock fillets, thawed

Tartar sauce, optional

1. In a large bowl, combine oil and pepper. Cut potatoes lengthwise into 1/2-in. strips. Add to oil mixture; toss to coat. Place on a 15-in. x 10-in. x 1-in. baking pan coated with cooking spray. Bake, uncovered, at 425° for 25-30 minutes or until golden brown and crisp.

2. Meanwhile, combine flour and pepper in a shallow dish. In a second dish, beat egg substitute and water. In a third dish, combine cornflakes, cheese and cayenne. Dredge fish in flour, then dip in egg mixture and roll in crumb mixture.

3. Place on a baking sheet coated with cooking spray. Bake at 425° for 10-15 minutes or until fish flakes easily with a fork. Serve with chips and tartar sauce if desired.

LOW SALT

PREP/TOTAL TIME
10 min.
YIELD 2 servings

NUTRITION FACTS
One serving
(1 steak prepared
without salt) equals:

192 calories
9 g fat
0 g saturated fat
68 mg cholesterol
185 mg sodium
5 g carbohydrate
0 g fiber
22 g protein

DIABETIC EXCHANGES
3 lean meat
1 vegetable

Confetti Salmon Steaks

I rely on my microwave to cook this tasty salmon in a jiffy. With its sprinkling of bright peppers, the mildly seasoned dish makes a pretty and satisfying entree for two.

Mary Kay Dixson, Decatur, Alabama

2 salmon steaks (6 ounces *each*)
1/2 teaspoon Worcestershire sauce
1/2 teaspoon lemon juice
1/2 teaspoon Cajun *or* Creole seasoning
1/4 teaspoon salt, optional
1/2 cup diced green pepper
1/2 cup diced sweet red pepper

1. Place the salmon in an ungreased 8-in. square microwave-safe dish. Rub with Worcestershire sauce and lemon juice; sprinkle with Cajun seasoning and salt if desired. Sprinkle peppers over top.

2. Cover and microwave on high for 5-1/2 to 6 minutes, turning once, or until fish flakes easily with a fork. Let stand, covered, for 2 minutes.

Editor's Note: The following spices may be substituted for the Creole seasoning: 1/2 teaspoon *each* paprika and garlic powder, and a pinch *each* cayenne pepper, dried thyme and ground cumin. This recipe was tested in a 1,100-watt microwave.

Skinny Crab Quiche

Crabmeat, zucchini, cheddar cheese and green onions star in this savory, crustless quiche. I like to take this to potlucks and cut it into appetizer-size slices.

Nancy Romero, Clarkston, Washington

- 1 can (6 ounces) crabmeat, drained, flaked and cartilage removed
- 1-1/2 cups (6 ounces) shredded reduced-fat cheddar cheese
- 1/2 cup shredded zucchini
- 1/3 cup chopped green onions
- 1-1/2 cups egg substitute
- 1 can (12 ounces) fat-free evaporated milk
- 3/4 teaspoon ground mustard
- 1/2 teaspoon salt
- 1/4 teaspoon salt-free lemon-pepper seasoning

Dash paprika

1. In a bowl, combine the crab, cheese, zucchini and onions. Press onto the bottom and up the sides of a 9-in. deep-dish pie plate coated with cooking spray.

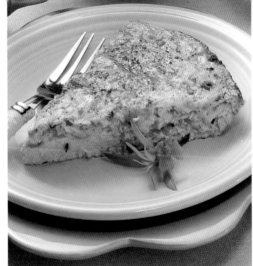

In another bowl, combine egg substitute, milk, mustard, salt and lemon-pepper; mix well. Pour into crust and sprinkle with paprika.

2. Bake, uncovered, at 400° for 25-30 minutes or until a knife inserted near the center comes out clean. Let stand for 10 minutes before cutting.

PREP/TOTAL TIME
Prep: 15 min.
Bake: 25 min. +
standing
YIELD 6 servings

NUTRITION FACTS
One serving
(1 slice) equals:
223 calories
9 g fat
5 g saturated fat
50 mg cholesterol
736 mg sodium
10 g carbohydrate
1 g fiber
26 g protein

DIABETIC EXCHANGES
3 lean meat
1/2 fat-free milk

Tomato Baked Haddock

This is one of my husband's favorite fish dishes, so I usually prepare this simple main course at least once a month.

Diana MacDonald, Westville, Nova Scotia

- 1 medium green pepper, chopped
- 1 small onion, chopped
- 1 tablespoon butter
- 1 tablespoon all-purpose flour
- 1 can (14-1/2 ounces) diced tomatoes, undrained
- 1 pound fresh or frozen haddock fillets, thawed
- 1/2 teaspoon salt

Pepper to taste

- 1/2 cup shredded part-skim mozzarella cheese

1. In a nonstick skillet, saute the green pepper and onion in butter until tender. Stir in flour until blended. Add tomatoes; cook and stir until thickened, about 3 minutes.

2. Place the fillets skin side down in an 11-in. x 7-in. x 2-in. baking dish coated with cooking spray. Sprinkle with salt and pepper; top with tomato mixture. Bake, uncovered, at 350° for 20-25 minutes or until fish flakes easily with a fork. Sprinkle with cheese. Bake 2 minutes longer or until cheese is melted.

PREP/TOTAL TIME
Prep: 25 min.
Bake: 30 min.
YIELD 4 servings

NUTRITION FACTS
One serving equals:
204 calories
6 g fat
4 g saturated fat
80 mg cholesterol
625 mg sodium
10 g carbohydrate
2 g fiber
27 g protein

DIABETIC EXCHANGES
3 very lean meat
2 vegetable
1 fat

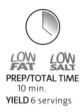

LOW FAT LOW SALT

PREP/TOTAL TIME
10 min.
YIELD 6 servings

NUTRITION FACTS
One serving
(1/2 cup) equals:
122 calories
1 g fat
0 g saturated fat
11 mg cholesterol
153 mg sodium
10 g carbohydrate
0 g fiber
19 g protein

DIABETIC EXCHANGES
2 very lean meat
1/2 starch
1/2 vegetable

Salsa Tuna Salad

I like to perk up my tuna salad with flavorful salsa. Bright corn and green pepper give pretty color to the mixture. Served on a bed of lettuce, it makes a great light lunch.

Jennifer Harris, Skellytown, Texas

- 1/2 cup plain fat-free yogurt
- 1/4 cup salsa
- 1/4 teaspoon pepper
- 2 cans (6 ounces *each*) tuna, drained and flaked
- 1 cup frozen corn, thawed
- 1 cup chopped green pepper

Lettuce leaves, optional

1. In a bowl, combine yogurt, salsa and pepper; mix well. Add tuna, corn and green pepper; toss to coat. Serve in a lettuce-lined bowl if desired.

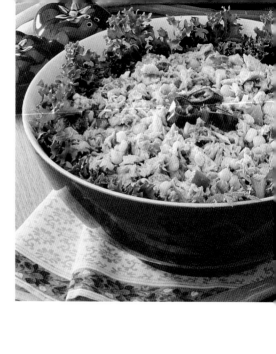

LOW SALT

PREP/TOTAL TIME
Prep: 5 min. + marinating
Grill: 10 min.
YIELD 8 servings

NUTRITION FACTS
One serving
(4 ounces salmon) equals:
254 calories
12 g fat
2 g saturated fat
67 mg cholesterol
179 mg sodium
12 g carbohydrate
Trace fiber
23 g protein

DIABETIC EXCHANGES
3 lean meat
1 starch

Maple-Glazed Grilled Salmon

When I made up my mind to serve my family more nutritious fare, I decided to use more fish. Everyone likes this marinated salmon.

Kate Selner, St. Paul, Minnesota

- 3/4 cup maple syrup
- 2 tablespoons ketchup
- 1 tablespoon brown sugar
- 1 tablespoon cider vinegar
- 1 tablespoon Worcestershire sauce
- 1/2 teaspoon salt
- 1/2 teaspoon ground mustard
- 1/8 teaspoon hot pepper sauce
- 1 salmon fillet (2 pounds)

1. In a bowl, combine the first eight ingredients; mix well. Pour 1/2 cup into a large resealable plastic bag; add the salmon. Seal bag and turn to coat; refrigerate for up to 2 hours. Cover and refrigerate remaining marinade.

2. Before starting the grill, coat grill rack with cooking spray. Drain and discard marinade from salmon. Grill salmon skin side up over medium-hot heat for 2-4 minutes. Transfer to a double thickness of heavy-duty foil (about 17 in. x 21 in.).

3. Spoon some of the reserved marinade over salmon. Fold foil around fillet and seal tightly. Grill 5-6 minutes longer or until fish flakes easily with a fork. Brush with remaining marinade.

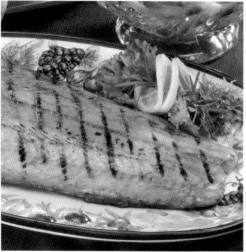

Spicy Shrimp Wraps

Here's a quick and easy recipe that's big on seafood flavor and the sunny sweetness of mango. Coated with taco seasoning, the shrimp are tucked inside a tortilla wrap along with coleslaw and dressed-up salsa.

Frankie Allen Mann, Warrior, Alabama

- 1 cup salsa
- 1 medium ripe mango, peeled, pitted and diced
- 1 tablespoon ketchup
- 1 envelope reduced-sodium taco seasoning
- 1 tablespoon olive oil
- 1 pound uncooked medium shrimp, peeled and deveined
- 6 flour tortillas (10 inches), warmed
- 1-1/2 cups coleslaw mix
- 6 tablespoons reduced-fat sour cream

1. In a small bowl, combine the salsa, mango and ketchup; set aside. In a large resealable plastic bag, combine the taco seasoning and oil; add shrimp. Seal bag and shake to coat.

2. In a nonstick skillet or wok, cook shrimp over medium-high heat for 2-3 minutes or until shrimp turn pink. Top tortillas with coleslaw mix, salsa mixture and shrimp. Fold bottom third of tortilla up over filling; fold sides over. Serve with sour cream.

PREP/TOTAL TIME
20 min.
YIELD 6 servings

NUTRITION FACTS
One serving (1 wrap with 1 tablespoon sour cream) equals:

- 367 calories
- 8 g fat
- 2 g saturated fat
- 117 mg cholesterol
- 1,074 mg sodium
- 45 g carbohydrate
- 8 g fiber
- 19 g protein

DIABETIC EXCHANGES

- 2 starch
- 2 very lean meat
- 1 fat
- 1/2 fruit

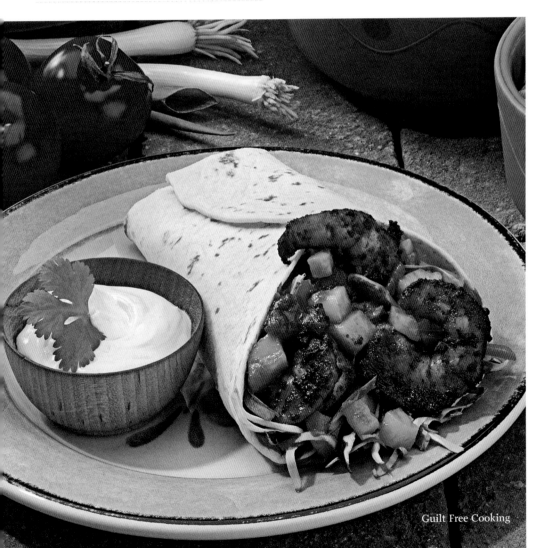

NUTRITION FACTS
One serving
(1 roll-up) equals:

321 calories
10 g fat
3 g saturated fat
26 mg cholesterol
696 mg sodium
34 g carbohydrate
4 g fiber
25 g protein

**DIABETIC
EXCHANGES**
3 lean meat
2 starch

Broccoli Tuna Roll-Ups

For a family-pleasing main dish that's on the lighter side, consider these cheesy tortilla wraps. They're a fun, delicious alternative to the usual tuna-noodle casserole.

Mary Wilhelm, Sparta, Wisconsin

1 can (10-3/4 ounces) reduced-fat reduced-sodium condensed cream of mushroom soup, undiluted

1 cup fat-free milk

2 cans (6 ounces *each*) light water-packed tuna, drained and flaked

1 package (10 ounces) frozen chopped broccoli, thawed and drained

2/3 cup shredded reduced-fat cheddar cheese, *divided*

1/3 cup sliced almonds, *divided*

6 flour tortillas (7 inches)

1 large tomato, seeded and chopped

1. In a small bowl, combine soup and milk; set aside. Combine the tuna, broccoli, 1/3 cup cheese and 3 tablespoons almonds. Stir in half of the soup mixture.

2. Spoon filling down the center of each tortilla; roll up. Place seam side down in an 11-in. x 7-in. x 2-in. baking dish coated with cooking spray. Pour remaining soup mixture over top; sprinkle with tomato.

3. Cover and bake at 350° for 35 minutes. Uncover; sprinkle with remaining cheese and almonds. Bake 5 minutes longer or until cheese is melted.

Lime Fish Tacos

The secret to getting my family to eat fish is tucked inside these tempting tacos. The flavors and textures in this unusual entree blend in a surprisingly pleasing way. Lime adds a zippy twist to the fillets and sauce.

Tammy Hayden, Carmichael, California

- 1 pound red snapper *or* orange roughy fillets
- 1 garlic clove, minced
- 2 tablespoons butter
- 7 teaspoons lime juice, *divided*
- 1/4 teaspoon white pepper
- 2 tablespoons reduced-fat sour cream
- 2 tablespoons fat-free mayonnaise

Dash hot pepper sauce

- 7 flour tortillas (8 inches), warmed
- 1 cup shredded lettuce
- 1 cup chopped fresh tomato

1. Remove skin from fish and cut fish into 1-in. cubes. In a nonstick skillet, saute garlic in butter and 5 teaspoons lime juice for 30 seconds. Add the fish and pepper. Cook for 6-8 minutes over medium heat until the fish flakes easily with a fork, gently stirring occasionally.

2. Meanwhile, combine the sour cream, mayonnaise, hot pepper sauce and remaining lime juice. Place a spoonful of fish on each tortilla. Top each with lettuce, tomato and sour cream sauce; fold over.

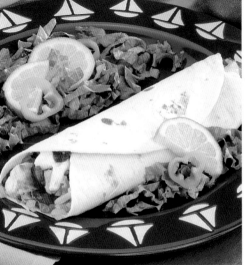

PREP/TOTAL TIME
20 min.
YIELD 7 servings

NUTRITION FACTS
One serving
(1 taco) equals:
238 calories
7 g fat
3 g saturated fat
24 mg cholesterol
366 mg sodium
28 g carbohydrate
1 g fiber
15 g protein

DIABETIC EXCHANGES
2 starch
1-1/2 lean meat

Spicy Haddock

I'm originally from Louisiana, where much of the food is spicy. So I like the spark that the chili powder and green chilies give these better-for-you baked fillets.

Kathleen Plake, Fort Wayne, Indiana

- 2 pounds fresh *or* frozen haddock fillets, thawed
- 1 can (4 ounces) chopped green chilies
- 2 tablespoons canola oil
- 2 tablespoons soy sauce
- 2 tablespoons Worcestershire sauce
- 1 teaspoon paprika
- 1/2 teaspoon garlic powder
- 1/2 teaspoon chili powder

Dash hot pepper sauce

1. Place fillets in a 13-in. x 9-in. x 2-in. baking dish coated with cooking spray. Combine remaining ingredients; spoon over fish. Bake, uncovered, at 350° for 20-25 minutes or until fish flakes easily with a fork.

GO FISH

When buying fresh fish fillets or steaks, look for firm flesh that appears moist. Don't purchase fish that looks dried out. When buying frozen fish, look for packages that are solidly frozen, tightly sealed and free of freezer burn and odor.

PREP/TOTAL TIME
30 min.
YIELD 8 servings

NUTRITION FACTS
One serving
(4 ounces) equals:
139 calories
4 g fat
0 g saturated fat
65 mg cholesterol
501 mg sodium
2 g carbohydrate
0 g fiber
22 g protein

DIABETIC EXCHANGES
3 very lean meat
1/2 vegetable

PREP/TOTAL TIME
20 min.
YIELD 4 servings

NUTRITION FACTS
One serving
(6 ounces halibut
with 2 tablespoons
sauce) equals:
   224 calories
     7 g fat
     1 g saturated fat
  57 mg cholesterol
447 mg sodium
     3 g carbohydrate
Trace fiber
   36 g protein

DIABETIC EXCHANGES
   5 lean meat
   1 fat

Grilled Halibut with Mustard Dill Sauce

Halibut steaks are draped with a thick and creamy sauce in this sensational recipe. The topping makes a wonderful alternative to store-bought tartar sauce.

Laura Perry, Exton, Pennsylvania

1/3 cup fat-free plain yogurt

2 tablespoons reduced-fat mayonnaise

2 tablespoons snipped fresh dill *or* 2 teaspoons dill weed

2 teaspoons Dijon mustard

4 halibut steaks (6 ounces *each*)

1/4 teaspoon salt

1/8 teaspoon pepper

1. For sauce, in a small bowl, combine the yogurt, mayonnaise, dill and mustard; cover and refrigerate.

2. Sprinkle halibut with salt and pepper. Coat grill rack with cooking spray before starting the grill. Grill halibut, covered, over medium heat for 4-6 minutes on each side or until fish flakes easily with a fork. Serve sauce with halibut.

Mediterranean-Style Red Snapper

This entree is both time-saving and nutritious. Seasoned with spices and served with a zesty sauce, it's a favorite at our house.

Josephine Piro, Easton, Pennsylvania

- 1 teaspoon lemon-pepper seasoning
- 1/2 teaspoon garlic powder
- 1/2 teaspoon dried thyme
- 1/8 teaspoon cayenne pepper
- 4 red snapper fillets (6 ounces *each*)
- 2 teaspoons olive oil, *divided*
- 1/2 medium sweet red pepper, julienned
- 3 green onions, chopped
- 1 garlic clove, minced
- 1 can (14-1/2 ounces) diced tomatoes, undrained
- 1/2 cup chopped pimiento-stuffed olives
- 1/4 cup chopped ripe olives
- 1/4 cup minced fresh chives

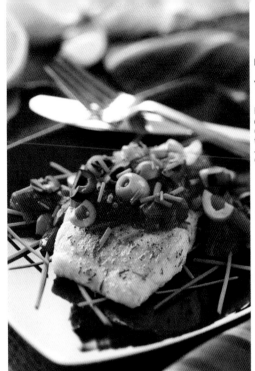

1. Combine the lemon-pepper, garlic powder, thyme and cayenne; rub over fillets. In a large nonstick skillet coated with cooking spray, cook fillets in 1 teaspoon oil over medium heat for 4-5 minutes on each side or until fish flakes easily with a fork. Remove and keep warm.

2. In the same pan, saute the red pepper, onions and garlic in remaining oil until crisp-tender. Stir in tomatoes. Bring to a boil. Reduce heat; simmer, uncovered, for 3 minutes or until liquid has evaporated. Serve over snapper. Sprinkle with olives and chives.

PREP/TOTAL TIME
30 min.
YIELD 4 servings

NUTRITION FACTS
One serving
(1 fillet with 1/3 cup tomato mixture and 3 tablespoons olives) equals:

258 calories
9 g fat
1 g saturated fat
60 mg cholesterol
754 mg sodium
10 g carbohydrate
3 g fiber
35 g protein

DIABETIC EXCHANGES
5 very lean meat
1-1/2 fat
1 vegetable

Crab Rice Primavera

I try to take a lunch along to work as often as possible. This delicious and colorful entree reheats so well, its leftovers have become one of my brown-bag favorites.

Michelle Armistead, Keyport, New Jersey

- 1-1/2 cups frozen vegetable blend (broccoli, red pepper, onions and mushrooms)
- 1/4 cup water
- 1-1/2 cups fat-free milk
- 1/2 cup grated Parmesan cheese
- 2 tablespoons butter
- 1 teaspoon dried basil
- 1/2 teaspoon garlic powder
- 3/4 pound flaked imitation crabmeat
- 1-1/2 cups uncooked instant rice

1. In a large saucepan, bring vegetables and water to a boil. Reduce heat; cover and simmer for 3 minutes.

2. Stir in milk, Parmesan cheese, butter, basil, garlic powder and crab. Bring to a boil. Stir in rice. Remove from the heat; cover and let stand for 5 minutes. Fluff with a fork. Serve immediately.

FABULOUS CRAB

Imitation crabmeat is most often made with Alaskan pollock. It can be substituted for real crab in equal proportions in recipes if you keep in mind that the flavor and texture will be a bit different than the real thing. Also, the cooking time in your recipe may need to be adjusted because imitation crabmeat is already cooked.

PREP/TOTAL TIME
30 min.
YIELD 5 servings

NUTRITION FACTS
One serving
(1 cup) equals:

325 calories
9 g fat
5 g saturated fat
55 mg cholesterol
483 mg sodium
41 g carbohydrate
1 g fiber
19 g protein

DIABETIC EXCHANGES
2 starch
2 lean meat
1 vegetable
1/2 fat

PREP/TOTAL TIME
30 min.
YIELD 4 servings

NUTRITION FACTS
One serving
(1 fillet) equals:
199 calories
5 g fat
2 g saturated fat
41 mg cholesterol
684 mg sodium
9 g carbohydrate
Trace fiber
28 g protein

DIABETIC EXCHANGES
4 very lean
meat
1/2 starch
1/2 fat

Taco Fish

I live near a lake and have a husband who's an avid angler, so fish always tops my list of mealtime ingredients. Here, I use delicate fillets as the base for a tempting bake that has mild taco taste and a crunchy topping.

Evelyn Eyermann, Cuba, Missouri

4   orange roughy *or* bass fillets
    (6 ounces *each*)

1/2 teaspoon salt

1/4 teaspoon chili powder

1/2 cup taco sauce

1/3 cup tortilla chips, crushed

1/3 cup shredded reduced-fat cheddar
    cheese

1. Place the fish in a 13-in. x 9-in. x 2-in. baking dish coated with cooking spray; sprinkle with salt and chili powder. Cover and bake at 350° for 20 minutes.

2. Uncover; pour the taco sauce over the fish. Bake 5-8 minutes longer or until heated through. Immediately sprinkle with tortilla chips and cheese.

SUBSTITUTE FISH
Orange roughy is a mild flavored, lean fish (which means it has a low-fat content). Other fish that can be used in place of orange roughy are cod, flounder, haddock, ocean perch, pollock and tilapia.

PREP/TOTAL TIME
20 min.
YIELD 6 servings

NUTRITION FACTS
One serving
(1 fillet) equals:
158 calories
1 g fat
1 g saturated fat
23 mg cholesterol
400 mg sodium
16 g carbohydrate
1 g fiber
20 g protein

DIABETIC EXCHANGES
3 very lean
meat
1 starch

Breaded Orange Roughy

My whole family loves fish, so I serve it often. Seasoned pepper really adds to the flavor of these tasty orange roughy fillets.

Joann Frazier Hensley, McGaheysville, Virginia

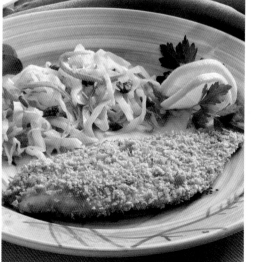

1   cup crushed cornflakes

2   teaspoons seasoned pepper

1/4 teaspoon salt

4   egg whites

1/4 cup water

6   fresh *or* frozen orange roughy
    fillets (4 ounces *each*)

1/4 cup all-purpose flour

1. In a shallow dish, combine the cornflakes, seasoned pepper and salt. In another shallow dish, beat egg whites and water. Sprinkle fish with flour; dip in egg white mixture, then roll in the cornflake mixture.

2. Place on a baking sheet coated with cooking spray. Bake at 425° for 9-11 minutes or until fish flakes easily with a fork.

Salmon with Dill Sauce

This moist, tender salmon is a savory treat draped with a smooth, creamy dill sauce. When my daughter served this tempting main course for dinner one evening, I was surprised to learn how simple the recipe is.

Janet Painter, Three Springs, Pennsylvania

1	salmon fillet (1 pound)
1-1/2	teaspoons dill weed, *divided*
1/2	cup reduced-fat plain yogurt
1/2	teaspoon sugar
1/2	teaspoon salt-free seasoning blend

1. Place salmon in a 13-in. x 9-in. x 2-in. baking dish coated with cooking spray; sprinkle with 1/2 teaspoon dill. Cover and bake at 375° for 20-25 minutes or until fish flakes easily with a fork.

2. Meanwhile, in a small saucepan, combine the yogurt, sugar, seasoning blend and remaining dill. Cook and stir over low heat until warmed. Serve with the salmon.

LOW SALT

PREP/TOTAL TIME
30 min.
YIELD 4 servings

NUTRITION FACTS
One serving
(4 ounces) equals:
227 calories
12 g fat
3 g saturated fat
77 mg cholesterol
76 mg sodium
3 g carbohydrate
0 g fiber
24 g protein

DIABETIC EXCHANGES
2-1/2 lean meat
2 fat

PREP/TOTAL TIME
30 min.
YIELD 4 servings

NUTRITION FACTS
One serving
(1 fillet) equals:

304 calories
6 g fat
1 g saturated fat
63 mg cholesterol
552 mg sodium
27 g carbohydrate
Trace fiber
35 g protein

DIABETIC EXCHANGES
5 very lean
  meat
2 fruit

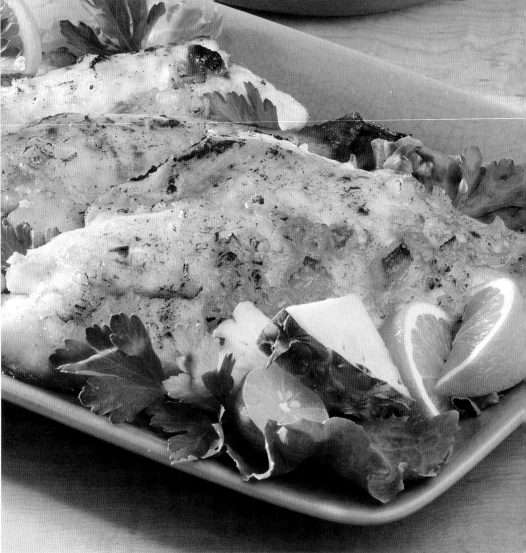

Snapper with Spicy Pineapple Glaze

Ginger and cayenne give some spice to this tangy treatment for red snapper fillets. Sweet pineapple preserves round out the delicious combination of flavors.

Taste of Home Test Kitchen

1/2 cup pineapple preserves

2 tablespoons rice wine vinegar

2 teaspoons minced fresh gingerroot

2 garlic cloves, minced

3/4 teaspoon salt, *divided*

1/4 teaspoon cayenne pepper

4 fresh *or* frozen red snapper fillets
   (6 ounces *each*), thawed

3 teaspoons olive oil

1. In a small bowl, combine the preserves, vinegar, ginger, garlic, 1/2 teaspoon salt and cayenne; set aside. Place fillets on a broiler pan coated with cooking spray. Spoon oil over both sides of fillets; sprinkle with remaining salt.

2. Broil 4-6 in. from the heat for 5 minutes. Baste with half of the glaze. Broil 5-7 minutes longer or until fish flakes easily with a fork. Baste with remaining glaze.

Meatless Main Dishes

Don't eat meatless because you have to...eat it because you want to! You will after sampling these mouth-watering entrees. You'll be amazed at the wide range of dinners your whole family will enjoy.

189
Asparagus Tofu Stir-Fry

202
Mexican Bean 'n' Barley Chili

196
Southwest Lasagna Rolls

chapter *10*

Black Bean Fajitas

PREP/TOTAL TIME
10 min.
YIELD 4 servings

NUTRITION FACTS
One serving
(1 fajita) equals:
257 calories
6 g fat
2 g saturated fat
13 mg cholesterol
671 mg sodium
36 g carbohydrate
6 g fiber
13 g protein

DIABETIC EXCHANGES
2 starch
1 lean meat
1 vegetable

For lunch one day, I came up with these fajitas using leftover beans and vegetables from my visit to the local farmers market. They made a fast and satisfying light meal.

Linda Rock, Stratford, Wisconsin

1/2 cup *each* julienned sweet yellow and red pepper

1 can (15 ounces) black beans, rinsed and drained

4 flour tortillas (6 inches), warmed

1 medium tomato, seeded and chopped

1/2 cup salsa

1/2 cup shredded reduced-fat cheddar cheese

1/4 cup fat-free sour cream

1. Place the yellow and red pepper in a microwave-safe bowl. Cover and microwave on high for 2 minutes or until crisp-tender. Add beans; cover and cook 1 minute longer or until heated through.

2. Spoon 1/2 cupful down the center of each tortilla; top with tomato, salsa, cheese and sour cream. Fold in half.

Editor's Note: This recipe was tested in a 1,100-watt microwave.

PEPPER POWER

Sweet red and yellow peppers are nutrient-dense vegetables. They are high in vitamin C, vitamin A, vitamin B6, potassium and beta-carotene.

Spinach Cheese Enchiladas

PREP/TOTAL TIME
Prep: 20 min.
Bake: 35 min.
YIELD 10 servings

NUTRITION FACTS
One serving
(1 enchilada) equals:
334 calories
12 g fat
6 g saturated fat
26 mg cholesterol
754 mg sodium
40 g carbohydrate
2 g fiber
19 g protein

DIABETIC EXCHANGES
2 starch
2 lean meat
1 vegetable
1 fat

This scrumptious dish is great because it's easy to prepare and low in fat. Plus, it travels well to potlucks and often prompts recipe requests.

Carol Jackson, Eden Prairie, Minnesota

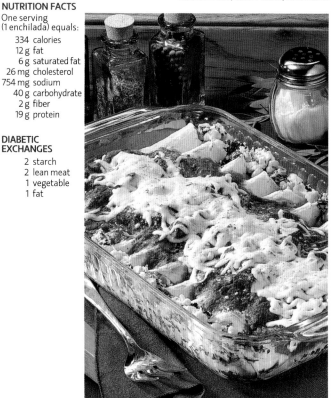

1 carton (15 ounces) reduced-fat ricotta cheese

1 package (10 ounces) frozen chopped spinach, thawed and drained

2 cups frozen corn, thawed and drained

2 cups (8 ounces) shredded part-skim mozzarella cheese, *divided*

1/4 cup egg substitute

10 fat-free flour tortillas (8 inches)

1 can (14-1/2 ounces) Italian diced tomatoes, undrained

1 can (8 ounces) tomato sauce

1 teaspoon dried basil

1/4 cup grated Parmesan cheese

1. In a bowl, combine ricotta, spinach, corn, 1 cup mozzarella and egg substitute. Spoon about 1/2 cup on each tortilla; roll up tightly. Place the seam side down in a 13-in. x 9-in. x 2-in. baking dish coated with cooking spray.

2. Combine tomatoes, tomato sauce and basil; spoon over tortillas. Sprinkle with Parmesan and the remaining mozzarella. Bake, uncovered, at 375° for 35 minutes or until heated through.

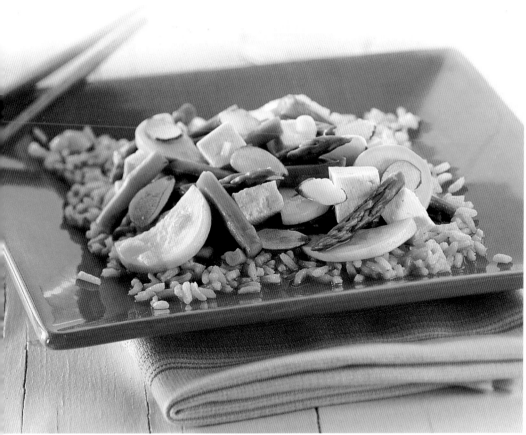

PREP/TOTAL TIME
Prep: 15 min.
Cook: 20 min.
YIELD 4 servings

NUTRITION FACTS
One serving
(1 cup stir-fry with
1/2 cup rice) equals:

278	calories
11 g	fat
1 g	saturated fat
0	cholesterol
682 mg	sodium
34 g	carbohydrate
4 g	fiber
14 g	protein

DIABETIC EXCHANGES

2	starch
1	lean meat
1	vegetable
1	fat

Asparagus Tofu Stir-Fry

With its flavorful ginger sauce and fresh vegetables, this tasty dish is a favorite. My family is always happy to see this on the table, and it doesn't bother my husband's food allergies.

Phyllis L. Smith, Chimacum, Washington

- 1 tablespoon cornstarch
- 1/2 teaspoon sugar
- 1-1/4 cups vegetable broth
- 4 teaspoons reduced-sodium soy sauce
- 2 teaspoons minced fresh gingerroot, *divided*
- 3 teaspoons canola oil, *divided*
- 1 pound fresh asparagus, trimmed and cut into 1-inch pieces
- 1 medium yellow summer squash, halved and sliced
- 2 green onions, thinly sliced
- 1 package (14 ounces) extra-firm tofu, drained and cut into 1/2-inch cubes
- 1/4 teaspoon salt
- 1/4 teaspoon pepper
- 2 cups hot cooked brown rice
- 2 tablespoons sliced almonds, toasted

1. In a small bowl, combine the cornstarch, sugar, broth and soy sauce until smooth; set aside.

2. In a large nonstick skillet or wok, stir-fry 1 teaspoon ginger in 1 teaspoon oil for 1 minute. Add asparagus; stir-fry for 2 minutes. Add squash; stir-fry 2 minutes longer. Add onions; stir-fry 1 minute longer or until vegetables are crisp-tender. Remove and keep warm.

3. In the same pan, stir-fry tofu, salt, pepper and remaining ginger in remaining oil for 7-9 minutes or until tofu is lightly browned. Remove and keep warm.

4. Stir cornstarch mixture and add to the pan. Bring to a boil; cook and stir for 2 minutes or until thickened. Add reserved asparagus mixture and tofu; heat through. Serve with rice; sprinkle with almonds.

PREP/TOTAL TIME
Prep: 10 min.
Cook: 35 min.
YIELD 6 servings

NUTRITION FACTS
One serving
(2 tacos) equals:
361 calories
12 g fat
5 g saturated fat
25 mg cholesterol
874 mg sodium
44 g carbohydrate
12 g fiber
19 g protein

DIABETIC EXCHANGES
2-1/2 starch
2 lean meat
1 vegetable
1 fat

Tasty Lentil Tacos

When my husband's cholesterol numbers rose, I quickly lowered the fat in our diet. This fun taco recipe was a huge hit with him as well as all our children.

Michelle Thomas, Bangor, Maine

1 cup finely chopped onion
1 garlic clove, minced
1 teaspoon canola oil
1 cup dried lentils, rinsed
1 tablespoon chili powder
2 teaspoons ground cumin
1 teaspoon dried oregano
2-1/2 cups vegetable broth
1 cup salsa
12 taco shells
1-1/2 cups shredded lettuce
1 cup chopped fresh tomato
1-1/2 cups (6 ounces) shredded reduced-fat cheddar cheese
6 tablespoons fat-free sour cream

1. In a large nonstick skillet, saute the onion and garlic in oil until tender. Add the lentils, chili powder, cumin and the oregano; cook and stir for 1 minute. Add broth; bring to a boil. Reduce heat; cover and simmer for 25-30 minutes or until the lentils are tender.

2. Uncover; cook for 6-8 minutes or until mixture is thickened. Mash lentils slightly. Stir in the salsa. Spoon about 1/4 cup lentil mixture into each taco shell. Top with the lettuce, tomato, cheese and sour cream.

Tortellini Primavera

This decadent tortellini with spinach, mushrooms and tomatoes always brings compliments. Dressed up with fresh Parmesan cheese, no one even notices it's meatless!

Susie Pietrowski, Belton, Texas

- 1 package (19 ounces) frozen cheese tortellini
- 1/2 pound sliced fresh mushrooms
- 1 small onion, chopped
- 2 garlic cloves, minced
- 2 teaspoons butter
- 2/3 cup fat-free milk
- 1 package (8 ounces) fat-free cream cheese, cubed
- 1 package (10 ounces) frozen chopped spinach, thawed and squeezed dry
- 1 teaspoon Italian seasoning
- 1 large tomato, chopped
- 1/4 cup shredded Parmesan cheese

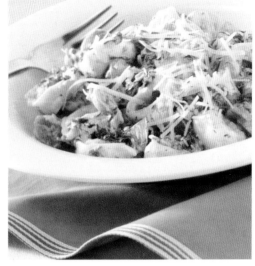

1. Cook tortellini according to package directions. Meanwhile, in a large nonstick skillet coated with cooking spray, saute mushrooms, onion and garlic in butter until tender. Reduce heat. Stir in milk; heat through (do not boil). Stir in cream cheese until blended. Add spinach and Italian seasoning; heat through (do not boil).

2. Drain the tortellini; toss with sauce and tomato. Sprinkle with Parmesan cheese.

PREP/TOTAL TIME
Prep: 30 min.
YIELD 5 servings

NUTRITION FACTS
One serving
(1-1/4 cups) equals:
341 calories
10 g fat
5 g saturated fat
28 mg cholesterol
671 mg sodium
41 g carbohydrate
4 g fiber
23 g protein

DIABETIC EXCHANGES
2-1/2 starch
2 lean meat
1 vegetable

Veggie Pockets

Even our five children enjoy the crunchy vegetable filling in these handy meatless sandwiches. It's a terrific way to use up your homegrown garden produce.

June Ballard, Weston, Idaho

- 3 medium onions, thinly sliced
- 2 tablespoons canola oil
- 2 tablespoons barbecue sauce
- 4 cups broccoli florets, cooked and drained
- 2 cups cauliflowerets, cooked and drained
- 1/4 cup reduced-fat mayonnaise
- 1/2 cup *each* grated carrot, red cabbage and yellow summer squash
- 6 pita breads (6 inches), halved and warmed
- 2 cups shredded lettuce

1. In a saucepan, cook onions in oil until tender. Add barbecue sauce; cook and stir for 2 minutes. Add the broccoli and cauliflower; heat through.

2. Stir in the mayonnaise, carrot, cabbage and squash; heat through. Fill each pita half with about 2 tablespoons lettuce and 1/2 cup vegetable mixture.

MORE ON MAYO

Sometimes, recipes include an editor's note stating that reduced-fat or fat-free mayonnaise may not be substituted for the regular kind. That's because lighter mayo can break down when heated and leave an unpleasant texture. Also, eggs in mayonnaise may be needed for leavening in baked goods, and not all lighter mayo contains eggs. In the Veggie Pockets recipe here, reduced-fat mayo is perfect.

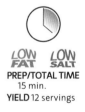

LOW **FAT** LOW **SALT**
PREP/TOTAL TIME
15 min.
YIELD 12 servings

NUTRITION FACTS
One serving
(1 pocket) equals:
143 calories
4 g fat
0 g saturated fat
1 mg cholesterol
218 mg sodium
24 g carbohydrate
0 g fiber
4 g protein

DIABETIC EXCHANGES
1 starch
1 vegetable
1 fat

PREP/TOTAL TIME
30 min.
YIELD 4 servings

NUTRITION FACTS
One serving
(3 patties and
1/4 cup sauce)
equals:
209 calories
10 g fat
1 g saturated fat
1 mg cholesterol
955 mg sodium
14 g carbohydrate
3 g fiber
14 g protein

DIABETIC
EXCHANGES
2 lean meat
1 vegetable
1 fat
1/2 starch

Egg Foo Yong with Sauce

These fried patties are quick to make...and reheat nicely in the microwave, too.

Rochelle Higgins, Fredericksburg, Virginia

4 teaspoons cornstarch

1 tablespoon sugar

2 teaspoons grated fresh gingerroot

1 cup reduced-sodium chicken broth

2 tablespoons reduced-sodium soy sauce

2 tablespoons sherry *or* apple juice

EGG FOO YONG:

1-1/2 cups egg substitute

1/4 cup chopped green onions

2 cups canned bean sprouts, rinsed and drained

1 can (8 ounces) water chestnuts, drained and chopped

1 can (4 ounces) mushroom stems and pieces, drained

1/4 teaspoon salt

1/8 teaspoon Chinese five spice

2 tablespoons canola oil

1. In a small saucepan, combine the cornstarch, sugar and ginger. Stir in the broth until smooth. Add soy sauce and sherry or apple juice. Bring to a boil; cook and stir for 2-3 minutes or until thickened. Remove from the heat; set aside.

2. In a bowl, combine egg substitute and onions; let stand for 10 minutes. Add bean sprouts, water chestnuts, mushrooms, salt and Chinese five spice; mix well.

3. In a nonstick skillet, heat the oil. Drop batter by 1/4 cupfuls into oil. Cook until golden brown, about 2 to 2-1/2 minutes on each side. Serve with sauce.

THE SLIMMING FACTS

Egg substitutes without yolks are light on calories. A 1/4 cup of egg substitute, which is the equivelant to 1 egg, has about 30 calories while the egg has about 78 calories. In addition this product has no fat or cholesterol.

PREP/TOTAL TIME
Prep: 20 min.
Bake: 20 min.
YIELD 6 servings

NUTRITION FACTS
One serving
(1 burrito) equals:
262 calories
9 g fat
0 g saturated fat
25 mg cholesterol
550 mg sodium
31 g carbohydrate
0 g fiber
17 g protein

DIABETIC
EXCHANGES
1-1/2 starch
1-1/2 meat
1 vegetable

Spinach Burritos

I made up this recipe a couple of years ago after trying a similar dish in a restaurant. Our oldest son tells me these saucy burritos are "awesome!" Plus, they're simple to fix.

Dolores Zornow, Poynette, Wisconsin

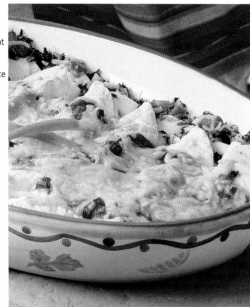

1/2 cup chopped onion

2 garlic cloves, minced

2 teaspoons margarine

1 package (10 ounces) frozen chopped spinach, thawed and squeezed dry

1/8 teaspoon pepper

6 fat-free flour tortillas (10 inches)

3/4 cup picante sauce, *divided*

2 cups (8 ounces) shredded reduced-fat cheddar cheese, *divided*

1. In a skillet, saute the onion and garlic in margarine until tender. Add the spinach and pepper; cook for 2-3 minutes or until heated through. Place about 3 tablespoonfuls on each tortilla; top with 1 tablespoon of picante sauce and 2 tablespoons of cheese.

2. Roll up and place seam side down in a 13-in. x 9-in. x 2-in. baking dish coated with cooking spray. Top with remaining picante sauce and cheese. Bake, uncovered, at 350° for 20-25 minutes or until sauce is bubbly and cheese is melted.

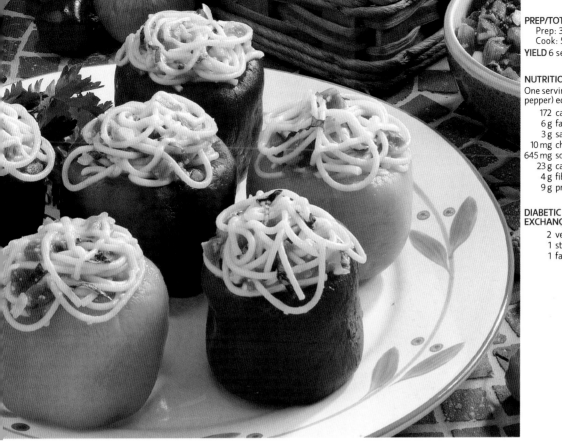

PREP/TOTAL TIME
Prep: 30 min.
Cook: 5 min.
YIELD 6 servings

NUTRITION FACTS
One serving (1 filled
pepper) equals:
172 calories
6 g fat
3 g saturated fat
10 mg cholesterol
645 mg sodium
23 g carbohydrate
4 g fiber
9 g protein

DIABETIC
EXCHANGES
2 vegetable
1 starch
1 fat

Pasta-Filled Peppers

Whole bell peppers can make a rainbow of colorful "cups," perfect for serving this fresh-tasting tomato-herb pasta.

Conni Krause, Virginia Beach, Virginia

- 6 medium green, sweet red *and/or* yellow peppers
- 6 ounces uncooked spaghetti
- 3/4 cup diced onion
- 2 garlic cloves, minced
- 2 teaspoons canola oil
- 1-3/4 cups diced fresh tomatoes
- 1 tablespoon all-purpose flour
- 3/4 teaspoon salt
- 1-1/4 cups vegetable broth
- 3/4 cup shredded part-skim mozzarella cheese
- 1/4 cup minced fresh basil
- 3 tablespoons grated Parmesan cheese

1. Place whole peppers on a broiler pan; broil 6 in. from the heat for 10-15 minutes or until skins are blistered and blackened, turning often. Immediately place peppers in a bowl; cover and let stand for 10 minutes. Peel off and discard charred skins. Carefully cut tops off peppers and discard; remove seeds. Set peppers aside.

2. Cook spaghetti according to package directions. Meanwhile, in a large nonstick skillet, saute onion and garlic in oil until tender. Add tomatoes; cook for 1 minute. In a small bowl, combine the flour, salt and broth until smooth. Gradually stir into tomato mixture. Bring to a boil; cook and stir for 1 minute or until slightly thickened.

3. Drain spaghetti; add to the tomato mixture and toss to coat. Sprinkle with mozzarella cheese, basil and Parmesan; toss. Spoon into peppers. Place in a 3-qt. microwave-safe baking dish. Cover and microwave on high for 1-3 minutes or until heated through.

Editor's Note: This recipe was tested in a 1,100-watt microwave.

Roasted Garlic and Pepper Pizza

Years ago, I found the recipe for this tasty pizza, lightened it up and added some of our favorite ingredients. It can be prepared ahead and baked as your guests arrive.

Bonnie Matherly, Buckingham, Illinois

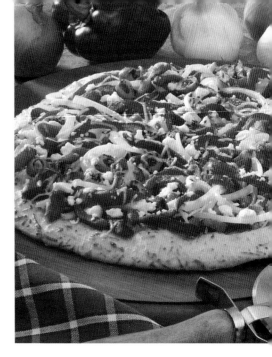

PREP/TOTAL TIME
Prep: 35 min. +
cooling
Bake: 15 min.
YIELD 12 servings

NUTRITION FACTS
One serving
(1 slice) equals:
  138 calories
  7 g fat
  2 g saturated fat
  10 mg cholesterol
  321 mg sodium
  14 g carbohydrate
  1 g fiber
  5 g protein

DIABETIC EXCHANGES
  1 starch
  1 fat

- 1 large garlic bulb
- 1 teaspoon plus 2 tablespoons olive oil, *divided*
- 2 large sweet red peppers
- 1/2 cup sliced pimiento-stuffed olives
- 2 tablespoons red wine vinegar
- 1 teaspoon dried oregano
- 1/2 teaspoon dried basil
- 1/8 teaspoon white pepper
- 1 prebaked thin Italian bread shell crust (10 ounces)
- 3/4 cup sweet onion slices
- 3/4 cup crumbled feta cheese
- 1/3 cup shredded Parmesan cheese

1. Remove papery outer skin from garlic (do not peel or separate cloves). Cut top off garlic head; brush with 1 teaspoon oil. Wrap bulb in heavy-duty foil. Bake at 425° for 20-25 minutes or until softened. Cool for 10-15 minutes; squeeze softened garlic out of skins. Cut garlic into slices.

2. Cut red peppers in half; remove and discard seeds. Place cut side down on a baking sheet. Broil 4 in. from the heat until skins are blistered and blackened. Immediately place peppers in a bowl; cover and let stand for 15-20 minutes. Peel off and discard charred skin; cut peppers into julienne strips.

3. In a bowl, combine the olives, vinegar, oregano, basil, pepper and remaining oil. Place crust on a 12-in. pizza pan. Spoon oil mixture over crust. Top with garlic, peppers, onion and cheeses. Bake at 350° for 15-20 minutes or until cheese is melted.

Baked Macaroni and Cheese

This recipe proves that you can watch your diet and still enjoy down-home cooking. The herbs make it deliciously different.

Lois McAtee, Oceanside, California

PREP/TOTAL TIME
Prep: 10 min.
Bake: 30 min.
YIELD 4 servings

NUTRITION FACTS
One serving
(1 cup) equals:
  372 calories
  9 g fat
  0 g saturated fat
  50 mg cholesterol
  615 mg sodium
  50 g carbohydrate
  0 g fiber
  23 g protein

DIABETIC EXCHANGES
  3 starch
  2 meat

- 1 tablespoon margarine
- 3 tablespoons all-purpose flour
- 2 cups fat-free milk
- 3/4 to 1 teaspoon dried marjoram
- 1/2 teaspoon dried thyme
- 1/8 teaspoon ground nutmeg
- 1/8 teaspoon paprika
- 1 tablespoon Dijon mustard
- 1/2 cup grated Parmesan cheese, *divided*
- 1 package (7 ounces) elbow macaroni, cooked and drained
- 1 cup reduced-fat cottage cheese

1. In a large saucepan, melt margarine. Stir in flour until smooth. Gradually add milk, stirring constantly. Bring to a boil over medium heat; boil for 2 minutes or until thickened. Add marjoram, thyme, nutmeg and paprika; stir until blended. Remove from the heat. Stir in mustard and 1/3 cup Parmesan cheese; mix well. Add macaroni and cottage cheese; stir until coated.

2. Pour into an 8-in. square baking dish coated with cooking spray. Bake, uncovered, at 350° for 30 minutes or until top is golden brown.

Sweet Pepper Sandwiches

We love this recipe because it's easy and meatless. Family members assemble their own sandwiches to their liking.

Cara Neth, Fort Collins, Colorado

- 1 *each* small green, sweet red and yellow pepper, thinly sliced
- 1 small onion, thinly sliced
- 1 garlic clove, minced
- 1 tablespoon olive oil
- 1 tablespoon balsamic vinegar
- 2 ounces fresh mozzarella cheese
- 1/4 cup fat-free mayonnaise
- 1/2 teaspoon prepared horseradish
- 4 hard rolls, split and toasted
- 8 fresh basil leaves
- 1 plum tomato, thinly sliced

1. In a large nonstick skillet, saute peppers, onion and garlic in oil until crisp-tender. Drizzle with vinegar; toss to coat.

2. Cut mozzarella cheese into four slices. Combine the mayonnaise and horseradish; spread over cut sides of rolls. Spoon vegetable mixture onto bottom halves; top with cheese. Broil 4-6 in. from the heat for 2-4 minutes or until cheese is melted. Top with basil leaves, tomato and roll tops.

PREP/TOTAL TIME
25 min.
YIELD 4 servings

NUTRITION FACTS
One serving
(1 sandwich) equals:
278 calories
10 g fat
3 g saturated fat
13 mg cholesterol
456 mg sodium
39 g carbohydrate
3 g fiber
9 g protein

DIABETIC EXCHANGES
2 starch
1-1/2 fat
1 vegetable

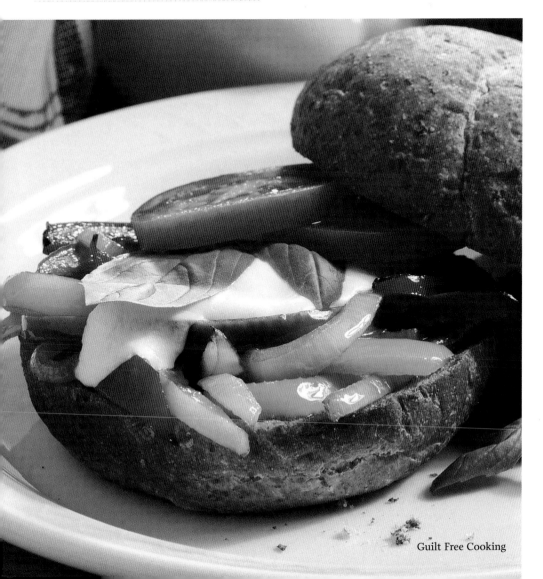

PREP/TOTAL TIME
Prep: 45 min. +
chilling
Cook: 30 min.
YIELD 12 servings

NUTRITION FACTS
One serving
(1 patty) equals:
126 calories
4 g fat
2 g saturated fat
8 mg cholesterol
286 mg sodium
15 g carbohydrate
2 g fiber
7 g protein

DIABETIC EXCHANGES
1 starch
1 lean meat

Great Grain Burgers

I've experimented with many ingredients to make a good meatless burger. This version cooks up golden brown and crispy.

Pat Whitaker, Lebanon, Oregon

1/2 cup uncooked brown rice
1/2 cup uncooked bulgur
1 tablespoon salt-free seasoning blend
1/4 teaspoon poultry seasoning
2 cups water
2 cups finely chopped fresh mushrooms
3/4 cup old-fashioned oats
1 cup (4 ounces) shredded part-skim mozzarella cheese
1/4 cup shredded reduced-fat cheddar cheese
1/3 cup finely chopped onion
1/2 cup fat-free cottage cheese
1/4 cup egg substitute
2 tablespoons minced fresh parsley
1 teaspoon salt
1/2 teaspoon dried basil
1/8 teaspoon celery seed
3 teaspoons canola oil, *divided*
12 sandwich rolls, optional
Lettuce leaves and tomato slices, optional

1. In a saucepan, combine the rice, bulgur, seasoning blend, poultry seasoning and water; bring to a boil. Reduce heat; cover and simmer for 30 minutes or until rice is tender. Remove from the heat; cool completely. Refrigerate.

2. In a large bowl, combine the mushrooms, oats, mozzarella cheese, cheddar cheese and onion. In a blender or food processor, process cottage cheese and egg substitute until smooth; add to the mushroom mixture. Stir in the parsley, salt, basil, celery seed and chilled rice mixture. Shape 1/2 cupfuls into patties.

3. In a large nonstick skillet, cook four patties in 1 teaspoon oil for 5 minutes on each side or until lightly browned and crisp. Repeat with remaining patties and oil. Serve on rolls with lettuce and tomato if desired.

PREP/TOTAL TIME
Prep: 20 min.
Bake: 35 min.
YIELD 8 servings

NUTRITION FACTS
One serving
(1 lasagna roll) equals:
259 calories
6 g fat
3 g saturated fat
23 mg cholesterol
648 mg sodium
31 g carbohydrate
6 g fiber
15 g protein

DIABETIC EXCHANGES
2 starch
1 lean meat
1 vegetable

Southwest Lasagna Rolls

We love this south-of-the-border lasagna. The cheesy dish comes together fast with a carton of vegetarian chili, and makes a great entree served with a green salad and baked tortilla chips.

Trisha Kruse, Eagle, Idaho

1 can (15 ounces) fat-free vegetarian chili
1 carton (15 ounces) reduced-fat ricotta cheese
1 cup (4 ounces) shredded reduced-fat Mexican cheese blend
1 can (4 ounces) chopped green chilies
1 teaspoon taco seasoning
1/4 teaspoon salt
8 lasagna noodles, cooked and drained
1 jar (16 ounces) salsa

1. In a large bowl, combine the chili, cheeses, chilies, taco seasoning and salt. Spread about 1/2 cup on each noodle; carefully roll up. Place seam side down in a 13-in. x 9-in. x 2-in. baking dish coated with cooking spray.

2. Cover and bake at 350° for 25 minutes. Uncover; top with salsa. Bake 10 minutes longer or until heated through.

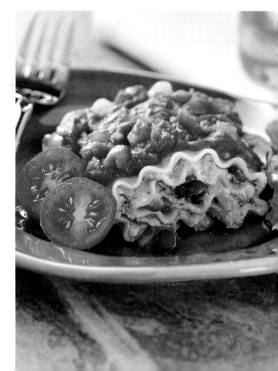

Spinach Manicotti

This meatless entree is so good. Plus, I don't have to cook the pasta before assembling it.

Mary Steiner, West Bend, Wisconsin

- 1 carton (15 ounces) fat-free ricotta cheese
- 2 cups (8 ounces) shredded part-skim mozzarella cheese, *divided*
- 1 package (10 ounces) frozen chopped spinach, thawed and squeezed dry
- 1/2 cup reduced-fat sour cream
- 1/4 cup dry bread crumbs
- 1 tablespoon Italian seasoning
- 1 teaspoon garlic powder
- 1 teaspoon onion powder
- 2 cups tomato juice
- 1 cup chunky salsa
- 1 can (15 ounces) crushed tomatoes
- 14 uncooked manicotti shells

1. In a large bowl, combine the ricotta, 1-1/2 cups mozzarella cheese, spinach, sour cream, bread crumbs, Italian seasoning, garlic powder and onion powder.

2. Combine juice, salsa and crushed tomatoes; spread 1 cup sauce in an ungreased

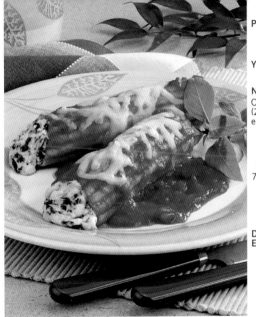

13-in. x 9-in. x 2-in. baking dish. Stuff manicotti with spinach mixture; arrange over sauce. Pour remaining sauce over manicotti.

3. Cover and bake at 350° for 55 minutes. Uncover; sprinkle with remaining mozzarella cheese. Bake 15 minutes longer or until noodles are tender.

PREP/TOTAL TIME
Prep: 15 min.
Bake: 1 hour 10 min.
YIELD 7 servings

NUTRITION FACTS
One serving
(2 stuffed manicotti) equals:

345 calories
8 g fat
5 g saturated fat
34 mg cholesterol
782 mg sodium
45 g carbohydrate
4 g fiber
22 g protein

DIABETIC EXCHANGES
2 starch
2 lean meat
2 vegetable

Italian Zucchini Bake

Kids of all ages are guaranteed to like this fun spin on pizza. You can't even tell there's zucchini in this cheesy casserole.

Carol Mieske, Red Bluff, California

- 3-1/2 cups shredded zucchini
- 1/2 teaspoon salt
- 3/4 cup egg substitute
- 1/2 cup dry bread crumbs
- 1/4 cup all-purpose flour
- 2 teaspoons Italian seasoning
- 1/2 pound fresh mushrooms, sliced
- 2 teaspoons olive oil
- 1 can (15 ounces) pizza sauce, *divided*
- 3/4 cup chopped green pepper
- 1/4 cup sliced ripe olives, drained
- 1-1/2 cups (6 ounces) shredded part-skim mozzarella cheese, *divided*

1. Place zucchini in a colander over a plate; sprinkle with salt and toss. Let stand for 15 minutes. Rinse and drain well. In a bowl, combine the zucchini, egg substitute, bread crumbs, flour and Italian seasoning. Spread in an 11-in. x 7-in. x 2-in. baking dish coated with cooking spray. Bake, uncovered, at 350° for 25 minutes.

2. In a nonstick skillet, saute mushrooms in oil. Spread half of the pizza sauce over zucchini mixture; sprinkle with the mushrooms, green pepper, olives and half of the cheese. Top with remaining pizza sauce and cheese. Bake 15 minutes longer or until hot and bubbly.

PREP/TOTAL TIME
Prep: 20 min. + standing
Bake: 40 min.
YIELD 6 servings

NUTRITION FACTS
One serving
(1 cup) equals:

226 calories
8 g fat
4 g saturated fat
17 mg cholesterol
818 mg sodium
24 g carbohydrate
3 g fiber
10 g protein

DIABETIC EXCHANGES
2 vegetables
1 starch
1 lean meat
1 fat

Zucchini Crepes

I frequently keep a batch of these tender, well-stuffed crepes in the freezer. Then when unexpected guests drop by, I simply pull out a few and reheat them.

Patricia Moyer, Island Pond, Vermont

NUTRITION FACTS
One serving
(2 filled crepes)
equals:

264 calories
7 g fat
2 g saturated fat
78 mg cholesterol
900 mg sodium
33 g carbohydrate
3 g fiber
18 g protein

DIABETIC
EXCHANGES
2 lean meat
1-1/2 starch
1 vegetable

- 1 cup all-purpose flour
- 2 eggs
- 1/2 cup egg substitute
- 1-1/2 cups fat-free milk
- 3/4 teaspoon salt

FILLING:

- 1 large onion, chopped
- 1 medium green pepper, chopped
- 1 cup sliced fresh mushrooms
- 1 tablespoon canola oil
- 1 medium zucchini, shredded and squeezed dry
- 2 medium tomatoes, chopped and seeded
- 1-1/2 cups (6 ounces) shredded reduced-fat cheddar cheese, *divided*
- 1/4 teaspoon salt
- 1/4 teaspoon dried oregano
- 1/8 teaspoon pepper
- 1-1/2 cups meatless spaghetti sauce

1. In a large bowl, whisk together the flour, eggs, egg substitute, milk and salt until smooth. Cover and refrigerate for 1 hour.

2. Heat an 8-in. nonstick skillet coated with cooking spray; pour about 1/4 cup batter into center of skillet. Lift and tilt pan to evenly coat bottom. Cook until top appears dry; turn and cook 15-20 seconds longer. Remove to a wire rack. Repeat with remaining batter, coating with spray as needed. When cool, stack crepes with waxed paper or paper towels in between.

3. In a large skillet, saute the onion, green pepper and mushrooms in oil until tender. Add zucchini; saute 2-3 minutes longer. Remove from the heat; stir in tomatoes, 1 cup cheese, salt, oregano and pepper.

4. Spoon onto crepes and roll up. Arrange in a 13-in. x 9-in. x 2-in. baking dish coated with cooking spray. Spread spaghetti sauce over crepes. Cover and bake at 350° for 15-20 minutes. Sprinkle with remaining cheese. Bake, uncovered, 5 minutes longer or until cheese is melted.

Spaghetti Casserole

I often get requests for this family-pleasing recipe. The hearty, meatless main course features spaghetti and lasagna ingredients.

Kathy Bence, Edmonds, Washington

- 6 ounces uncooked spaghetti
- 1 tablespoon butter
- 1/3 cup shredded Parmesan cheese
- 1 jar (26 ounces) meatless spaghetti sauce
- 2 cups chopped green pepper
- 1 can (14-1/2 ounces) diced tomatoes, drained
- 1 carton (8 ounces) part-skim ricotta cheese
- 1 can (8 ounces) mushroom stems and pieces, drained
- 1 small onion, chopped
- 3 garlic cloves, minced
- 12 fresh basil leaves, thinly sliced
- 1/2 teaspoon dried oregano
- 3 cups (12 ounces) shredded part-skim mozzarella cheese, *divided*

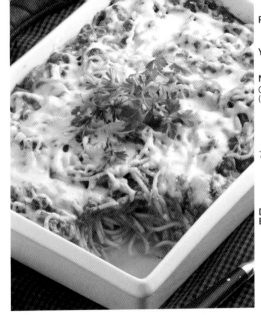

1. Cook spaghetti according to package directions; drain. Add butter and Parmesan cheese; toss to coat. In a large bowl, combine the spaghetti sauce, green pepper and tomatoes. In a blender, process the ricotta cheese until pureed. Add to the spaghetti sauce mixture. Stir in the mushrooms, onion, garlic, basil, oregano and 1-1/2 cups mozzarella cheese. Add the spaghetti; toss to coat.

2. Transfer to a 13-in. x 9-in. x 2-in. baking dish coated with cooking spray. Sprinkle with remaining mozzarella. Cover; bake at 350° for 40-45 minutes or until heated through.

PREP/TOTAL TIME
Prep: 20 min.
Bake: 40 min.
YIELD 9 servings

NUTRITION FACTS
One serving
(1-1/2 cups) equals:
301 calories
12 g fat
7 g saturated fat
41 mg cholesterol
774 mg sodium
31 g carbohydrate
4 g fiber
18 g protein

DIABETIC EXCHANGES
2 starch
2 fat
1 lean meat

Three-Bean Cassoulet

Brimming with a trio of bean varieties, this recipe is as easy as one, two, three. Serve it as a main dish or even as a side.

Carol Berigan, Golden, Colorado

- 2 cans (14-1/2 ounces *each*) stewed tomatoes
- 1 can (15-1/2 ounces) great northern beans, rinsed and drained
- 1 can (15 ounces) garbanzo beans *or* chickpeas, rinsed and drained
- 1 can (15 ounces) butter beans, rinsed and drained
- 1 cup finely chopped carrots
- 1 cup finely chopped onion
- 2 garlic cloves, minced
- 1 bay leaf
- 2 teaspoons dried parsley flakes
- 1 teaspoon dried basil
- 1/2 teaspoon dried thyme
- 1/2 teaspoon salt
- 1/8 teaspoon pepper

1. In an ungreased 3-qt. baking dish, combine all ingredients. Cover and bake at 350° for 60-70 minutes or until the vegetables are tender, stirring occasionally. Discard the bay leaf before serving.

CASSOULET CLUE

A cassoulet is a classic, hearty, French country meal. The traditional variety contains beans, meat and sausage. Packed with three kinds of beans, lots of veggies and seasonings, the Three-Bean Cassoulet recipe here is a great meatless alternative.

LOW FAT

PREP/TOTAL TIME
Prep: 5 min.
Bake: 60 min.
YIELD: 9 servings

NUTRITION FACTS
One serving
(3/4 cup) equals:
197 calories
1 g fat
1 g saturated fat
0 g cholesterol
687 mg sodium
41 g carbohydrate
9 g fiber
10 g protein

DIABETIC EXCHANGES
2 starch
2 vegetable

Mushroom Broccoli Pizza

I enjoy vegetable gardening and often cook with my homegrown harvest. This pizza is a delicious way to put that bounty to use.

Kathleen Kelly, Days Creek, Oregon

1 package (1/4 ounce) active dry yeast
3/4 cup warm water (110° to 115°)
1 teaspoon olive oil
1/2 teaspoon sugar
1/2 cup whole wheat flour
1/2 teaspoon salt
1-1/2 cups all-purpose flour

TOPPINGS:

3 cups broccoli florets
1 cup sliced fresh mushrooms
1/4 cup chopped onion
4 garlic cloves, minced
1 tablespoon olive oil
1/2 cup pizza sauce
4 plum tomatoes, sliced lengthwise
1/4 cup chopped fresh basil
1-1/2 cups (6 ounces) shredded part-skim mozzarella cheese
1/3 cup shredded Parmesan cheese

1. In a large bowl, dissolve the yeast in warm water. Add oil and sugar; mix well. Combine whole wheat flour and salt; stir into yeast mixture until smooth. Stir in enough all-purpose flour to form a soft dough.

2. Turn onto a floured surface; knead until smooth and elastic, about 6-8 minutes. Place in a bowl coated with cooking spray, turning once to coat top. Cover and let rise in a warm place until doubled, about 1-1/2 hours.

3. Punch dough down. Press onto the bottom and 1 in. up the sides of a 12-in. pizza pan coated with cooking spray. Prick dough several times with a fork. Bake at 425° for 6-8 minutes.

4. Place the broccoli in a steamer basket; place in a saucepan over 1 in. of water. Bring to a boil; cover and steam for 5-6 minutes or until crisp-tender. Transfer to a colander. Rinse with cold water; drain and set aside.

5. In a nonstick skillet, saute mushrooms, onion and garlic in oil until mushrooms are tender. Spread pizza sauce over crust. Top with mushroom mixture, tomatoes, broccoli, basil and cheeses. Bake at 425° for 12-14 minutes or until crust is golden and cheese is melted.

Baked Lentils with Cheese

Onions, garlic, tomatoes, green pepper and several herbs and spices give a hearty punch to this cheesy and filling lentil dish.

Pamela Ulrich, Charlottesville, Virginia

2-1/4 cups water
1-3/4 cups dried lentils, rinsed
1 cup chopped onion
2 medium carrots, thinly sliced
1/2 cup thinly sliced celery
2 garlic cloves, minced
1 teaspoon salt
1/4 teaspoon pepper
1/8 teaspoon dried marjoram
1/8 teaspoon rubbed sage
1/8 teaspoon dried thyme
1 bay leaf
2 cups chopped fresh tomatoes
1/2 cup finely chopped green pepper
2 tablespoons minced fresh parsley
2-1/2 cups (10 ounces) shredded reduced-fat cheddar cheese

1. In a 13-in. x 9-in. x 2-in. baking dish, combine the water, lentils, onion, carrots, celery, garlic and seasonings. Cover and bake at 350° for 45 minutes.

2. Stir in the tomatoes and green pepper. Cover and bake 15 minutes longer. Sprinkle with parsley and cheese. Bake, uncovered, for 5-10 minutes or until cheese is melted. Discard bay leaf before serving.

HIGH-FIBER LENTILS

Lentils are seeds that are grown in pods and are part of the legume family. Unlike most other legumes, lentils don't need to be soaked before using. The most commonly available lentils are brown, but red, yellow and green are available in specialty markets. Lentils are low in calories and fat, and they're a good source of fiber, folic acid and iron.

PREP/TOTAL TIME
Prep: 10 min.
Bake: 65 min.
YIELD 8 servings

NUTRITION FACTS
One serving
(1 cup) equals:
289 calories
7 g fat
4 g saturated fat
21 mg cholesterol
535 mg sodium
34 g carbohydrate
15 g fiber
26 g protein

DIABETIC EXCHANGES
2 starch
2 lean meat
1/2 fat

Five-Veggie Stir-Fry

This satisfying main course bursts with a medley of flavors. Orange juice lends a hint of citrus to the mildly seasoned sauce.

Rachel Thompson, Midlothian, Virginia

2 tablespoons cornstarch
2 tablespoons sugar
1/2 teaspoon ground ginger
1 cup orange juice
1/4 cup reduced-sodium soy sauce
2 garlic cloves, minced
2 large carrots, sliced
2 cups broccoli florets
2 cups cauliflowerets
4 teaspoons olive oil, *divided*
1 cup quartered fresh mushrooms
1 cup fresh *or* frozen snow peas
4 cups hot cooked rice

1. In a small bowl, combine the cornstarch, sugar and ginger. Stir in orange juice, soy sauce and garlic until blended; set aside.

2. In a nonstick skillet or wok, stir-fry the carrots, broccoli and cauliflower in 3 teaspoons oil for 4-5 minutes. Add mushrooms, peas and remaining oil; stir-fry for 3 minutes. Stir orange juice mixture and add to the pan. Bring to a boil; cook and stir until thickened. Serve over rice.

LOW FAT

PREP/TOTAL TIME
20 min.
YIELD: 4 servings

NUTRITION FACTS
One serving
(1 cup) equals:
382 calories
5 g fat
1 g saturated fat
0 mg cholesterol
648 mg sodium
74 g carbohydrate
3 g fiber
9 g protein

DIABETIC EXCHANGES
3 starch
2 vegetable
1 lean meat
1 fat

LOW FAT

PREP/TOTAL TIME
Prep: 25 min.
Cook: 25 min.
YIELD: 10 servings
(about 3-1/2 quarts)

NUTRITION FACTS
One serving
(1-1/2 cups) equals:
247 calories
3 g fat
1 g saturated fat
0 cholesterol
836 mg sodium
46 g carbohydrate
11 g fiber
11 g protein

DIABETIC EXCHANGES
2 starch
2 vegetable
1 very lean meat
1/2 fat

Mexican Bean 'n' Barley Chili

Chili powder adds just the right amount of heat to this filling, fast and fabulous vegetarian meal. It's one easy, cold-weather recipe the whole family will warm to...and it feeds a bunch!

Lana Day, Bloomington, Indiana

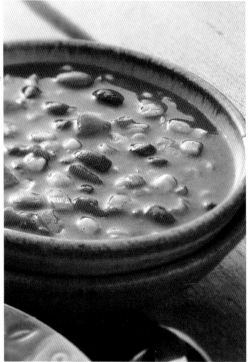

1 large onion, chopped
1 garlic clove, minced
1 tablespoon olive oil
1 *each* medium green and sweet red pepper, chopped
2 cups frozen corn, thawed
3/4 cup quick-cooking barley
2 cups water
1 can (16 ounces) chili beans in chili sauce, undrained
1 can (15 ounces) pinto beans, rinsed and drained
1 can (15 ounces) black beans, rinsed and drained
1 can (15 ounces) tomato sauce
1 can (14-1/2 ounces) diced tomatoes, undrained
1 can (14-1/2 ounces) vegetable broth
2 cans (4 ounces *each*) chopped green chilies
2 tablespoons chili powder
1/2 teaspoon pepper

1. In a Dutch oven coated with cooking spray, saute the onion and garlic in oil for 2 minutes. Stir in peppers; cook 3-4 minutes longer or until tender.

2. Stir in the remaining ingredients; bring to a boil. Reduce heat; cover and simmer for 15-20 minutes or until barley is tender.

PREP/TOTAL TIME
10 min.
YIELD 1 serving

NUTRITION FACTS
One serving
(1 sandwich) equals:
290 calories
9 g fat
5 g saturated fat
19 mg cholesterol
727 mg sodium
37 g carbohydrate
5 g fiber
15 g protein

DIABETIC EXCHANGES
2 starch
1 lean meat
1 vegetable
1 fat

Toasted Veggie Sandwich

Best when assembled with fresh garden ingredients, this sandwich is wholesome and a meal all by itself.

Gail Nonamaker, Saluda, North Carolina

1 teaspoon fat-free mayonnaise
1 teaspoon spicy brown *or* horseradish mustard
2 slices rye bread
1 slice (1 ounce) reduced-fat Swiss cheese, cut in half
3 tablespoons grated carrot
1 tablespoon finely chopped onion
2 tablespoons sauerkraut, well drained and chopped
1/2 cup thinly sliced fresh spinach
Refrigerated butter-flavored spray

1. Spread mayonnaise and mustard on each slice of bread. On one piece of bread, layer a half slice of cheese, carrot, onion, sauerkraut, spinach and remaining cheese. Cover with second piece of bread.

2. Spray both sides of the sandwich with refrigerated butter-flavored spray. In a small nonstick skillet, toast sandwich over medium heat until bread is browned on both sides.

Editor's Note: This recipe was tested in a 1,100-watt microwave.

Refried Bean Enchiladas

These crowd-pleasing bundles are so fast and easy to prepare. The recipe, which came from my sister-in-law, is a family favorite.

Carolyn Sykora, Bloomer, Wisconsin

2	cups vegetarian refried beans
1	cup (8 ounces) 1% cottage cheese
1-1/2	cups (6 ounces) shredded reduced-fat cheddar cheese, *divided*
1	tablespoon olive oil
4-1/2	teaspoons all-purpose flour
1	tablespoon chili powder
1/2	teaspoon garlic powder
1/4	teaspoon salt
1-1/2	cups water
1	teaspoon cider vinegar
1/2	teaspoon dried minced onion
12	flour tortillas (6 inches)

1. In a large bowl, combine the beans, cottage cheese and 1 cup cheddar cheese; set aside. For sauce, in a large nonstick skillet, whisk the oil, flour, chili powder, garlic powder and salt until smooth. Gradually stir in the water, vinegar and onion. Bring to a boil; cook and stir for 2 minutes or until thickened. Remove from the heat.

2. Dip both sides of each tortilla into sauce. Place about 1/2 cup bean mixture down the center of each tortilla. Roll up and place seam side down in a 13-in. x 9-in. x 2-in. baking dish coated with cooking spray. Pour remaining sauce over top; sprinkle with remaining cheese. Cover and bake at 350° for 20-25 minutes or until heated through.

PREP/TOTAL TIME
Prep: 20 min.
Bake: 20 min.
YIELD 6 servings

NUTRITION FACTS
One serving
(2 enchiladas)
equals:

384	calories
11 g	fat
5 g	saturated fat
22 mg	cholesterol
729 mg	sodium
48 g	carbohydrate
7 g	fiber
24 g	protein

DIABETIC EXCHANGES
3 starch
2 lean meat
1 fat

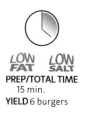

LOW FAT **LOW SALT**

PREP/TOTAL TIME
15 min.
YIELD 6 burgers

NUTRITION FACTS
One serving
(1 burger calculated
without bread)
equals:
   57 calories
   1 g fat
   0 g saturated fat
   Trace cholesterol
   63 mg sodium
   8 g carbohydrate
   1 g fiber
   5 g protein

DIABETIC EXCHANGES
   1 vegetable
   1/2 lean meat

Veggie Burgers

We created these delicious patties with our garden bounty in mind. To suit your family, experiment with different vegetables...or use more of your favorite ones.

Mary James, Port Orchard, Washington

  1 small zucchini, grated
  1 medium uncooked potato, peeled and grated
  1 medium carrot, grated
  1/4 cup grated onion
  3/4 cup egg substitute
Pepper to taste
  12 slices whole wheat bread, toasted
Sliced red onion and lettuce leaves, optional

1. In a bowl, combine the first six ingredients; mix well. Pour about 1/2 cup batter onto a hot griddle lightly coated with cooking spray. Fry for 2-3 minutes on each side or until golden brown. Serve on toasted bread with onion and lettuce if desired.

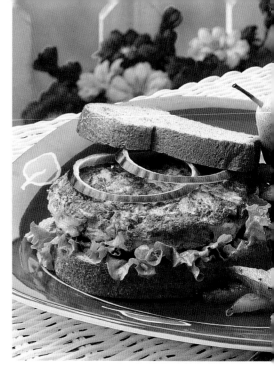

PREP/TOTAL TIME
Prep: 15 min.
Bake: 35 min.
YIELD 6 servings

NUTRITION FACTS
One serving
(1 slice) equals:
   218 calories
   12 g fat
   5 g saturated fat
   15 mg cholesterol
   459 mg sodium
   10 g carbohydrate
   2 g fiber
   19 g protein

DIABETIC EXCHANGES
   2 lean meat
   1 vegetable
   1 fat
   1/2 starch

Crustless Mushroom Spinach Tart

With no crust, this delicious veggie dish is so easy to prepare. The aroma alone will be enough to bring your family to the table.

Mary Lopez, Willow Creek, California

  2 tablespoons seasoned bread crumbs
  1/2 pound fresh mushrooms, sliced
  1/2 cup chopped onion
  2 tablespoons olive oil

  1 package (10 ounces) frozen chopped spinach, thawed and squeezed dry
  1 cup 2% milk
  1 cup egg substitute
  1/4 teaspoon salt
  1/4 teaspoon pepper
  1-1/4 shredded reduced-fat Mexican cheese blend, *divided*
  1/3 cup grated Parmesan cheese

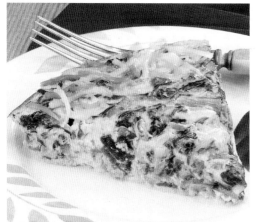

1. Coat a 9-in. pie plate with cooking spray. Sprinkle bottom and sides with crumbs; shake out the excess. Set plate aside.

2. In a nonstick skillet, saute mushrooms and onion in oil for 12-14 minutes or until all of the liquid has evaporated. Remove from the heat; stir in spinach.

3. In a bowl, combine the milk, egg substitute, salt and pepper. Stir in the spinach mixture, 1 cup Mexican cheese blend and Parmesan cheese. Pour into prepared pie plate. Bake at 350° for 35-40 minutes or until a knife inserted near the center comes out clean. Sprinkle remaining Mexican cheese blend around edge of tart. Let stand for 5 minutes before slicing.

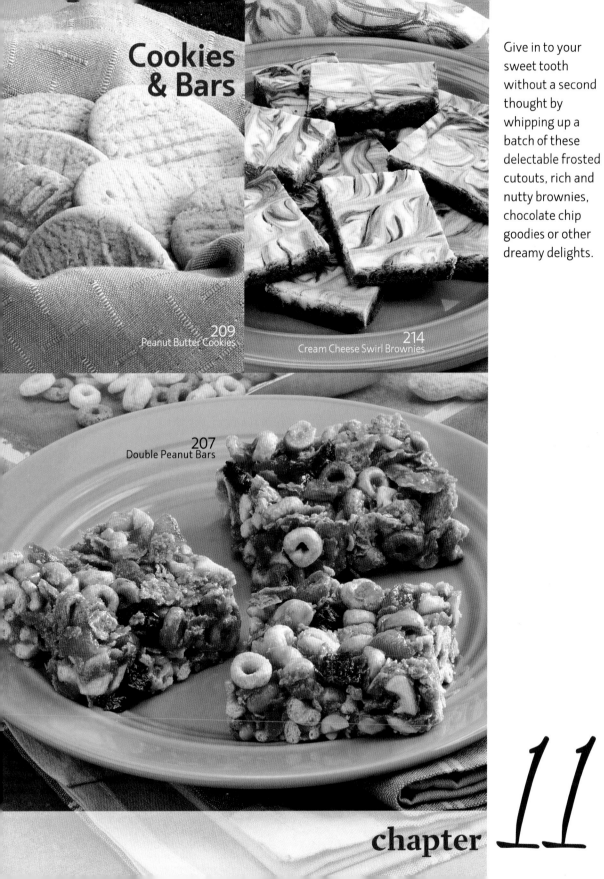

Cookies & Bars

Give in to your sweet tooth without a second thought by whipping up a batch of these delectable frosted cutouts, rich and nutty brownies, chocolate chip goodies or other dreamy delights.

209
Peanut Butter Cookies

214
Cream Cheese Swirl Brownies

207
Double Peanut Bars

chapter 11

Chocolate Cappuccino Cookies

These chocolaty cookies have a mild coffee flavor that makes them a hit with everyone who tries them, especially java fans.

Eleanor Senske, Rock Island, Illinois

PREP/TOTAL TIME
Prep: 20 min.
Bake: 10 min.
per batch
YIELD 3-1/2 dozen

NUTRITION FACTS
One serving
(1 cookie) equals:
43 calories
1 g fat
Trace saturated fat
0 mg cholesterol
15 mg sodium
8 g carbohydrate
Trace fiber
1 g protein

DIABETIC EXCHANGE
1/2 starch

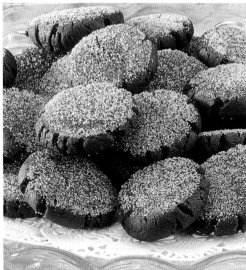

1 tablespoon instant coffee granules
1 tablespoon hot water
1 egg white
3/4 cup plus 1 tablespoon sugar, *divided*
1/4 cup canola oil
2 tablespoons corn syrup
2 teaspoons vanilla extract
1-1/4 cups all-purpose flour
1/2 cup baking cocoa
1/4 teaspoon salt

1. In a small bowl, dissolve coffee granules in hot water. In a large mixing bowl, combine the egg white, 3/4 cup sugar, oil, corn syrup, vanilla and coffee; beat until well blended. Combine the flour, cocoa and salt; gradually add to coffee mixture.

2. Roll into 1-in. balls. Place 2 in. apart on ungreased baking sheets. Flatten to 1/4-in. thickness with a glass dipped in the remaining sugar. Bake at 350° for 5-7 minutes or until center is set. Remove to wire racks to cool. Store in an airtight container.

Frosted Pumpkin Bars

PREP/TOTAL TIME
Prep: 15 min.
Bake: 25 min.
YIELD 15 servings

NUTRITION FACTS
One serving
(1 bar) equals:
185 calories
6 g fat
1 g saturated fat
18 mg cholesterol
146 mg sodium
32 g carbohydrate
1 g fiber
3 g protein

DIABETIC EXCHANGES
2 starch
1 fat

My granddaughter, Jennifer, gave me the recipe for spiced pumpkin bars with a cream cheese frosting. It's hard to eat just one!

Dovie Sears, Shepherdsville, Kentucky

1 cup all-purpose flour
1 cup sugar
1 teaspoon ground cinnamon
1 teaspoon baking powder
1/2 teaspoon salt
1/2 teaspoon ground cloves
1 egg
2 egg whites
1 cup canned pumpkin
1/4 cup canola oil
2 tablespoons water
4 ounces reduced-fat cream cheese
1-1/2 cups confectioners' sugar
1 teaspoon vanilla extract
1/4 teaspoon grated lemon peel

1. In a mixing bowl, combine the flour, sugar, cinnamon, baking powder, salt and cloves. Add the egg, egg whites, pumpkin, oil and water; mix well.

2. Transfer to an 11-in. x 7-in. x 2-in. baking pan coated with cooking spray. Bake at 350° for 25-30 minutes or until a toothpick inserted near center comes out clean. Cool on a wire rack.

3. In a mixing bowl, beat cream cheese. Beat in the confectioners' sugar, vanilla and lemon peel. Frost bars. Chill for 15 minutes, then cut. Refrigerate leftovers.

CUT FAT WITH PUMPKIN

Pumpkin adds flavor and color to these tender Frosted Pumpkin Bars. Pumpkin also adds moistness which allows this recipe to use less oil than is needed in a typical bar.

Double Peanut Bars

These sweet, no-bake snacks are terrific energy bars. Any dried fruit works well, but I prefer cranberries. Lots of nuts and peanut butter make the bars popular at my house.

Kim Rocker, LaGrange, Georgia

1-1/2 cups Wheaties
1 cup Multi Grain Cheerios
1/2 cup unsalted dry roasted peanuts
1/2 cup chopped dried mixed fruit
1/3 cup packed brown sugar
1/3 cup honey
3 tablespoons peanut butter

1. In a bowl, combine the cereals, peanuts and mixed fruit. In a small saucepan, combine the brown sugar, honey and peanut butter. Cook and stir until brown sugar and peanut butter are melted and mixture is smooth. Pour over the cereal mixture; gently stir to coat evenly.

2. Transfer to an 8-in. square dish coated with cooking spray; gently press down. Cool and cut into bars. Store in the refrigerator.

LOW SALT

PREP/TOTAL TIME
15 min.
YIELD 9 servings

NUTRITION FACTS
One serving
(1 bar) equals:
201 calories
7 g fat
1 g saturated fat
0 mg cholesterol
65 mg sodium
34 g carbohydrate
3 g fiber
5 g protein

DIABETIC EXCHANGES
2 starch
1 fat

Pineapple Coconut Squares

LOW SALT

PREP/TOTAL TIME
Prep: 15 min.
Bake: 35 min. +
cooling
YIELD 16 servings

NUTRITION FACTS
One serving
(1 square) equals:
192 calories
7 g fat
5 g saturated fat
46 mg cholesterol
79 mg sodium
30 g carbohydrate
1 g fiber
3 g protein

**DIABETIC
EXCHANGES**
2 starch
1 fat

I don't remember where I got this recipe, but I'm glad I did! I make these goodies often.

Elaine Anderson, Aliquippa, Pennsylvania

2 tablespoons butter, melted

3 tablespoons sugar

1 egg

1 cup all-purpose flour

1 teaspoon baking powder

2 cans (8 ounces *each*) unsweetened crushed pineapple, drained

TOPPING:

1 tablespoon butter, melted

1 cup sugar

2 eggs

2 cups flaked coconut

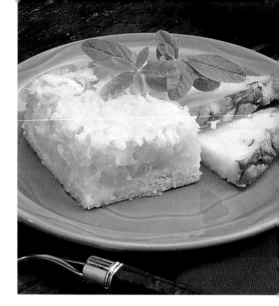

1. In a mixing bowl, beat the butter and sugar. Beat in egg. Combine flour and baking powder; stir into egg mixture. Press into a 9-in. square baking dish coated with cooking spray. Spread pineapple over the crust; set aside.

2. For topping, in a mixing bowl, beat the butter and sugar. Beat in eggs. Stir in coconut. Spread over pineapple. Bake at 325° for 35-40 minutes or until golden brown. Cool before cutting into squares.

Honey Spice Cookies

LOW FAT   **LOW SALT**

PREP/TOTAL TIME
Prep: 20 min. +
chilling
Bake: 10 min.
per batch
YIELD 12-1/2 dozen

NUTRITION FACTS
One serving
(1 cookie) equals:
54 calories
Trace fat
Trace saturated fat
4 mg cholesterol
43 mg sodium
13 g carbohydrate
Trace fiber
1 g protein

**DIABETIC
EXCHANGE**
1/2 starch

With four children, I bake a lot of cookies. These nicely spiced sweets are a favorite, and the recipe makes a big batch.

Joan Gerber, Bluffton, Indiana

2 cups honey

2 cups sugar

3 eggs

7-1/2 cups all-purpose flour

3 teaspoons baking soda

3 teaspoons ground cinnamon

1 teaspoon salt

1 teaspoon ground allspice

1 teaspoon ground cloves

2 cups confectioners' sugar

3 tablespoons fat-free milk

1. In a mixing bowl, beat the honey and sugar. Add eggs, one at a time, beating well after each addition. Combine the flour, baking soda, cinnamon, salt, allspice and cloves; gradually add to honey mixture. Shape dough into five 10-in. rolls; wrap in plastic wrap. Refrigerate for 2 hours or until firm.

2. Unwrap dough and cut into 1/4-in. slices. Place 2 in. apart on baking sheets coated with cooking spray. Combine confectioners' sugar and milk; lightly brush over cookies. Bake at 350° for 8-10 minutes or until lightly browned. Remove to wire racks to cool.

Peanut Butter Cookies

When folks bite into one of these yummy cookies, they never guess it's low in fat.

Maria Regakis, Somerville, Massachusetts

- 3 tablespoons butter, softened
- 2 tablespoons reduced-fat peanut butter
- 1/2 cup packed brown sugar
- 1/4 cup sugar
- 1 egg white
- 1 teaspoon vanilla extract
- 1 cup all-purpose flour
- 1/4 teaspoon baking soda
- 1/8 teaspoon salt

1. In a large mixing bowl, cream the butter, peanut butter and sugars. Add egg white; beat until blended. Beat in vanilla. Combine flour, baking soda and salt; gradually add to the creamed mixture. Shape into an 8-in. roll; wrap in plastic wrap. Freeze for 2 hours or until firm.

2. Unwrap and cut into slices, about 1/4 in. thick. Place 2 in. apart on baking sheets coated with cooking spray. Flatten with a fork. Bake at 350° for 6-8 minutes for chewy cookies or 8-10 minutes for crisp cookies. Cool for 1-2 minutes before removing to wire racks; cool completely.

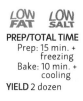

LOW FAT LOW SALT

PREP/TOTAL TIME
Prep: 15 min. + freezing
Bake: 10 min. + cooling

YIELD 2 dozen

NUTRITION FACTS
One serving
(1 cookie) equals:
- 62 calories
- 2 g fat
- 1 g saturated fat
- 4 mg cholesterol
- 64 mg sodium
- 11 g carbohydrate
- 1 g fiber
- 1 g protein

DIABETIC EXCHANGES
1/2 starch
1/2 fat

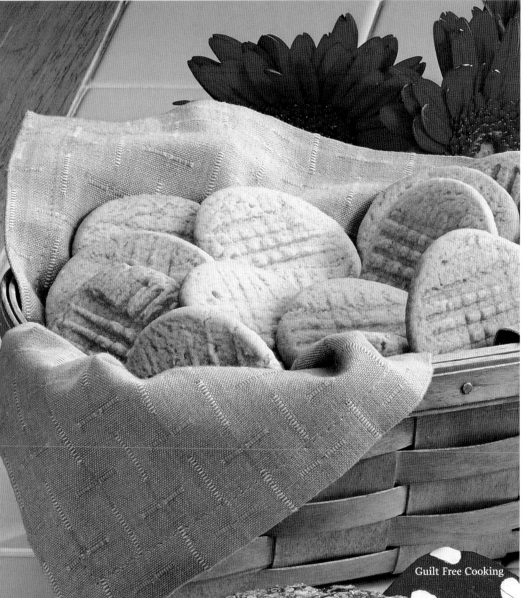

Gingerbread Cookies

When your friends reach into a tin of these old-fashioned cookies, they're sure to think Grandma baked them! We came up with this lighter recipe for crunchy cutouts with simple icing accents.

Taste of Home Test Kitchen

PREP/TOTAL TIME
Prep: 25 min. + chilling
Bake: 5 min. per batch
YIELD 6-1/2 dozen

NUTRITION FACTS
One serving (1 cookie) equals:
81 calories
1g fat
1g saturated fat
5 mg cholesterol
39 mg sodium
18 g carbohydrate
49 g fiber
1g protein

DIABETIC EXCHANGE
1 starch

- 6 tablespoons butter, softened
- 1 cup sugar
- 1 cup molasses
- 1 egg
- 2 tablespoons white vinegar
- 4 cups all-purpose flour
- 2 teaspoons ground ginger
- 1-1/4 teaspoons baking soda
- 1 teaspoon ground cinnamon
- 1/2 teaspoon ground cloves
- 1/4 teaspoon salt
- 5 cups confectioners' sugar
- 5 to 6 tablespoons fat-free milk
- Assorted paste food coloring, optional

1. In a mixing bowl, beat butter and sugar until crumbly, about 2 minutes. Beat in the molasses, egg and vinegar. Combine the flour, ginger, baking soda, cinnamon, cloves and salt; gradually add to the creamed mixture. Cover and refrigerate for 4 hours or until easy to handle (dough will be sticky).

2. On a lightly floured surface, roll out dough to 1/8-in. thickness. Cut with 4-in. cookie cutters dipped in flour. Using a floured spatula, place cookies 1 in. apart on baking sheets coated with cooking spray. Bake at 375° for 5-6 minutes or until set. Remove to wire racks to cool.

3. For icing, combine confectioners' sugar and milk in a bowl. Spread over cooled cookies; let dry completely. If desired, combine paste food coloring and a few drops of water; using a fine brush or the blunt end of a wooden skewer, decorate cookies.

Raspberry Nut Bars

Raspberry jam adds sweetness to these pretty bars. I revised the original recipe to reduce fat and calories. The end result is a treat so yummy, it's hard to resist.

Beth Ask, Ulster, Pennsylvania

- 1/2   cup stick margarine
- 1/4   cup reduced-fat stick margarine
- 1/3   cup packed brown sugar
- 1/4   cup sugar
- 1   egg
- 1   teaspoon vanilla extract
- 2   cups all-purpose flour
- 1   teaspoon baking powder
- 1/4   teaspoon baking soda
- 1/4   teaspoon salt
- 3/4   cup chopped pecans, *divided*
- 2/3   cup raspberry jam
- 2   tablespoons lemon juice

GLAZE:
- 1/2   cup confectioners' sugar
- 2   teaspoons fat-free milk

1. In a large bowl, cream margarines and sugars. Beat in the egg and vanilla. Combine the flour, baking powder, baking soda and salt; add to the creamed mixture. Stir in 1/2 cup pecans.

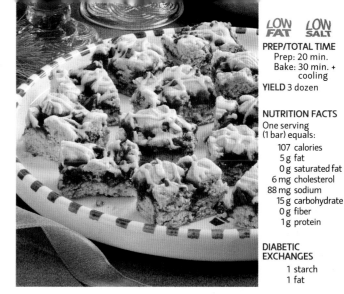

2. Spread half of the dough into a 13-in. x 9-in. x 2-in. baking pan coated with cooking spray. Combine jam and lemon juice; spread over dough. Dollop remaining dough over top. Sprinkle with remaining pecans.

3. Bake at 325° for 30-35 minutes or until lightly browned. Cool on a wire rack. Combine glaze ingredients; drizzle over bars.

Editor's Note: This recipe was tested with Parkay Light stick margarine.

PREP/TOTAL TIME
Prep: 20 min.
Bake: 30 min. + cooling
YIELD 3 dozen

NUTRITION FACTS
One serving
(1 bar) equals:
- 107 calories
- 5 g fat
- 0 g saturated fat
- 6 mg cholesterol
- 88 mg sodium
- 15 g carbohydrate
- 0 g fiber
- 1 g protein

DIABETIC EXCHANGES
- 1 starch
- 1 fat

Pecan Cookies

Around our house, we especially enjoy these slightly sweet cookies as a midday snack. They're also nice as a breakfast treat.

Bonnie Jolly, Bailey, Colorado

- 1-1/2 cups whole wheat flour
- 1/2   cup all-purpose flour
- 1   teaspoon baking powder
- 2   tablespoons quick-cooking oats
- 1/2   cup margarine
- 3/4   cup finely chopped pecans
- 1/2   cup packed brown sugar
- 1/4   to 1/2 cup fat-free milk

1. In a large bowl, combine the flours and baking powder; stir in oats. Cut margarine into pieces; cut into flour mixture until well mixed. Add pecans and sugar; mix well. Stir in enough milk with a fork to form a stiff dough.

2. Turn onto a floured surface; knead lightly until smooth. Roll out dough onto a floured surface to 1/4-in. to 1/8-in. thickness. Cut with 1-1/2-in. round cookie cutter. Place on baking sheets coated with cooking spray. Bake at 375° for 10 minutes or until lightly browned. Cool on wire racks.

PREP/TOTAL TIME
Prep: 20 min.
Bake: 10 min.
per batch
YIELD about 7-1/2 dozen

NUTRITION FACTS
One serving
(2 cookies) equals:
- 60 calories
- 3 g fat
- 0 g saturated fat
- Trace cholesterol
- 36 mg sodium
- 7 g carbohydrate
- 0 g fiber
- 1 g protein

DIABETIC EXCHANGES
- 1/2 starch
- 1/2 fat

Cocoa Chip Cookies

PREP/TOTAL TIME
Prep: 15 min.
Bake: 10 min.
per batch
YIELD 2-1/2 dozen

NUTRITION FACTS
One serving
(1 cookie) equals:
64 calories
2 g fat
1 g saturated fat
10 mg cholesterol
79 mg sodium
11 g carbohydrate
Trace fiber
1 g protein

DIABETIC EXCHANGE
1 starch

We whipped up these soft, airy cookies using a double dose of chocolate flavor from baking cocoa and semisweet chips. The lower-in-sugar goodies are sure to please any chocoholic!

Taste of Home Test Kitchen

2 tablespoons butter, softened
2 ounces reduced-fat cream cheese, cubed
6 tablespoons sugar
6 tablespoons brown sugar
1 egg
1 egg white
1 cup all-purpose flour
3 tablespoons baking cocoa
1/2 teaspoon baking soda
1/2 teaspoon salt
1/2 cup miniature semisweet chocolate chips

1. In a large bowl, cream the butter, cream cheese and sugars. Add the egg and egg white; mix well. Combine the flour, cocoa, baking soda and salt; gradually add to the creamed mixture. Stir in chocolate chips.

2. Drop by rounded tablespoonfuls 2 in. apart onto baking sheets coated with cooking spray. Bake at 375° for 7-10 minutes or until edges are set. Cool for 2 minutes before removing to wire racks. Store in an airtight container.

Oatmeal Raisin Cookies

PREP/TOTAL TIME
Prep: 15 min.
Bake: 10 min.
per batch
YIELD 44 cookies

NUTRITION FACTS
One serving
(1 cookie) equals:
77 calories
Trace fat
Trace saturated fat
Trace cholesterol
24 mg sodium
18 g carbohydrate
1 g fiber
1 g protein

DIABETIC EXCHANGE
1 starch

The first time I made these old-fashioned cookies, I didn't tell my family that the treats were lower in fat and calories. Their reaction when they found out? "No way!"

Julie Hauser, Sheridan, California

1 cup raisins
1/4 cup water
3 egg whites
1 tablespoon molasses
1 cup sugar
1 cup packed brown sugar
1-1/2 teaspoons vanilla extract
1 cup all-purpose flour
1/2 cup nonfat dry milk powder
1-1/2 teaspoons baking powder
1-1/2 teaspoons ground cinnamon
2-1/2 cups quick-cooking oats

1. In a food processor or blender, combine the raisins, water, egg whites and molasses. Cover and process for 10-15 seconds or until the raisins are finely chopped. Transfer to a mixing bowl. Beat in sugars and vanilla. Combine the flour, milk powder, baking powder and cinnamon; gradually add to raisin mixture. Stir in oats.

2. Drop by tablespoonfuls 2 in. apart onto baking sheets coated with cooking spray. Bake at 350° for 8-10 minutes or until edges are golden brown. Remove to wire racks to cool.

Cranberry Oat Cookies

You'll delight everyone with these goodies. The irresistible cookies are crunchy on the outside, chewy on the inside and dotted with plenty of dried cranberries.

Heather Breen, Chicago, Illinois

- 1/2 cup plus 2 tablespoons packed brown sugar
- 1/4 cup sugar
- 1/3 cup canola oil
- 1 egg
- 1 tablespoon fat-free milk
- 3/4 teaspoon vanilla extract
- 1-1/4 cups quick-cooking oats
- 3/4 cup plus 2 tablespoons all-purpose flour
- 1/2 teaspoon baking soda
- 1/2 teaspoon salt
- 1/2 cup dried cranberries

1. In a large mixing bowl, combine the sugars and oil. Beat in the egg, milk and vanilla. Combine the oats, flour, baking soda and salt; gradually add to the sugar mixture. Stir in the cranberries.

2. Drop by tablespoonfuls onto baking sheets coated with cooking spray. Bake at 375° for 10-12 minutes or until lightly browned. Remove to wire racks.

VERY VANILLA

Next to the pure vanilla extract and regular imitation vanilla extract on grocery store shelves, you'll see double-strength imitation vanilla. This variety is double the strength of both pure and imitation vanilla. If you're using double-strength, add half of the amount called for in the recipe.

LOW FAT **LOW SALT**

PREP/TOTAL TIME
Prep: 15 min.
Bake: 10 min.
per batch
YIELD 2-1/2 dozen

NUTRITION FACTS
One serving
(1 cookie) equals:
79 calories
3 g fat
Trace saturated fat
7 mg cholesterol
64 mg sodium
13 g carbohydrate
1 g fiber
1 g protein

DIABETIC EXCHANGE
1 starch

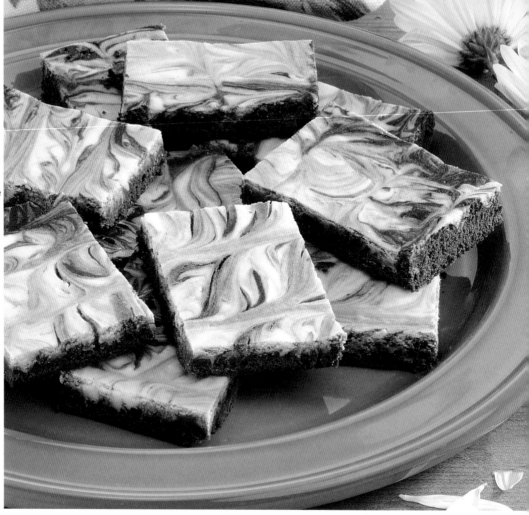

PREP/TOTAL TIME
Prep: 20 min.
Bake: 25 min.
YIELD 1 dozen

NUTRITION FACTS
One serving
(1 brownie) equals:

167 calories
7 g fat
3 g saturated fat
28 mg cholesterol
108 mg sodium
23 g carbohydrate
Trace fiber
4 g protein

DIABETIC EXCHANGES
1-1/2 starch
1 fat

Cream Cheese Swirl Brownies

I'm a chocolate lover, and this recipe has satisfied my cravings many times. No one guesses the brownies are light because their chewy texture and rich taste can't be beat.

Heidi Johnson, Worland, Wyoming

3 eggs

6 tablespoons reduced-fat stick margarine

1 cup sugar, *divided*

3 teaspoons vanilla extract

1/2 cup all-purpose flour

1/4 cup baking cocoa

1 package (8 ounces) reduced-fat cream cheese

1. Separate two eggs, putting each white in a separate bowl (discard yolks or save for another use); set aside. In a small mixing bowl, beat margarine and 3/4 cup sugar until crumbly. Add the whole egg, one egg white and vanilla; mix well.

2. Combine flour and cocoa; add to egg mixture and beat until blended. Pour into a 9-in. square baking pan coated with cooking spray; set aside.

3. In a mixing bowl, beat cream cheese and remaining sugar until smooth. Beat in the second egg white. Drop by rounded tablespoonfuls over batter; cut through batter with a knife to swirl. Bake at 350° for 25-30 minutes or until set and edges pull away from sides of pan. Cool on a wire rack.

Editor's Note: This recipe was tested with Parkay Light stick margarine.

Apple Nut Bars

For big apple flavor packed into a chunky bar, consider these treats. They're fuss-free because you don't have to peel the apples.

Karen Nelson, Sullivan, Wisconsin

2	egg whites
2/3	cup sugar
1/2	teaspoon vanilla extract
1/2	cup all-purpose flour
1	teaspoon baking powder
2	cups chopped unpeeled tart apples
1/4	cup chopped pecans

1. In a bowl, whisk egg whites, sugar and vanilla for about 1-1/2 minutes. Add flour and baking powder; whisk for 1 minute. Fold in the apples and pecans.

2. Pour into an 8-in. square baking pan coated with cooking spray. Bake at 350° for 25-30 minutes or until a toothpick inserted near the center comes out clean. Cool.

EGG WHITE EASE

If you often cook with egg whites, an egg separator is a handy gadget to have. To use it, hold the separator over a custard cup and crack the egg into the separator. As each egg is separated, place the yolk in another bowl and empty the egg whites into a mixing bowl. Keep in mind that it's easier to separate eggs if you use them directly from the refrigerator.

PREP/TOTAL TIME
Prep: 15 min.
Bake: 25 min.
YIELD 1 dozen

NUTRITION FACTS
One serving
(1 bar) equals:
73 calories
2 g fat
0 g saturated fat
0 mg cholesterol
50 mg sodium
14 g carbohydrate
0 g fiber
1 g protein

DIABETIC EXCHANGE
1 starch

Pineapple Almond Bars

Almonds are a crunchy complement to the sweet fruit filling in these yummy treats. They're pretty enough for special occasions.

Janice Smith, Cynthiana, Kentucky

3/4	cup all-purpose flour
3/4	cup quick-cooking oats
1/3	cup packed brown sugar
5	tablespoons reduced-fat butter
1/2	teaspoon almond extract
3	tablespoons sliced almonds
1	cup pineapple preserves

1. In a food processor, combine the flour, oats and brown sugar; cover and process until blended. Add butter and extract; cover and pulse until crumbly. Remove 1/2 cup crumb mixture to a bowl; stir in sliced almonds.

2. Press the remaining crumb mixture into a 9-in. square baking pan coated with cooking spray. Spread the preserves over crust. Sprinkle with reserved crumb mixture.

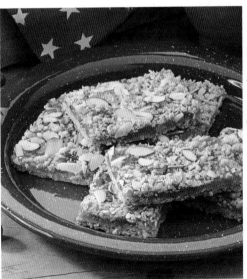

3. Bake at 350° for 25-30 minutes or until golden. Cool on a wire rack.

Editor's Note: This recipe was tested with Land O'Lakes light stick butter.

PREP/TOTAL TIME
Prep: 10 min.
Bake: 25 min.
YIELD 1 dozen

NUTRITION FACTS
One serving
(1 bar) equals:
166 calories
4 g fat
1 g saturated fat
0 mg cholesterol
39 mg sodium
34 g carbohydrate
1 g fiber
2 g protein

DIABETIC EXCHANGES
1 starch
1 fruit
1/2 fat

Walnut Oat Brownies

Oatmeal and wheat germ add a nutritious touch to these fudgy brownies dotted with walnuts and sprinkled with confectioners' sugar. They seem too good to be true!

Marilyn Yates, Roanoke, Virginia

PREP/TOTAL TIME
Prep: 15 min.
Bake: 25 min. + cooling
YIELD 1 dozen

NUTRITION FACTS
One serving
(1 brownie) equals:
180 calories
10 g fat
5 g saturated fat
11 mg cholesterol
145 mg sodium
19 g carbohydrate
2 g fiber
5 g protein

DIABETIC EXCHANGES
2 fat
1 starch

1/3 cup quick-cooking oats

1/3 cup nonfat dry milk powder

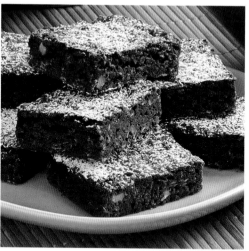

1/4 cup toasted wheat germ

1/4 cup packed brown sugar

2 tablespoons sugar

1/2 teaspoon baking powder

1/4 teaspoon salt

6 squares (1 ounce *each*) semisweet chocolate

1/4 cup butter

1/2 cup egg substitute

1/4 cup chopped walnuts

1 teaspoon vanilla extract

Confectioners' sugar, optional

1. In a large bowl, combine the first seven ingredients. In a microwave-safe bowl, melt chocolate and butter; cool slightly. Stir in the egg substitute, walnuts and vanilla. Stir into the dry ingredients.

2. Pour into an 8-in. square baking dish coated with cooking spray. Bake at 350° for 25-30 minutes or until a toothpick inserted near the center comes out clean. Cool on a wire rack. Dust with confectioners' sugar if desired. Cut into bars.

Soft Gingersnaps

These soft, cake-like gingersnap cookies are delightfully old-fashioned, which makes it hard to believe they're low in fat. Give them a try, and I'm sure you'll agree!

Shonna Lee Leonard, Lower Sackville, Nova Scotia

PREP/TOTAL TIME
Prep: 20 min.
Bake: 10 min.
per batch
YIELD 3 dozen

NUTRITION FACTS
One serving
(2 cookies) equals:
62 calories
2 g fat
0 g saturated fat
1 mg cholesterol
93 mg sodium
11 g carbohydrate
0 g fiber
1 g protein

DIABETIC EXCHANGES
1/2 starch
1/2 fat

1-1/2 cups all-purpose flour

1/2 cup whole wheat flour

2 teaspoons baking soda

1 teaspoon ground cinnamon

1 teaspoon ground cloves

1 teaspoon ground ginger

1/4 teaspoon salt

1/2 cup egg substitute

1/2 cup sugar

1/4 cup packed brown sugar

1/4 cup canola oil

1/4 cup molasses

1. In a mixing bowl, combine the flours, baking soda, cinnamon, cloves, ginger and salt. Combine the egg substitute, sugars, oil and molasses; mix well. Add to dry ingredients; mix well.

2. Drop by teaspoonfuls 2 in. apart onto baking sheets coated with cooking spray. Bake at 350° for 8-10 minutes or until cookies spring back when lightly touched. Cool for 5 minutes; remove from pans to wire racks to cool completely.

Cranberry Cheesecake Bars

I came across this recipe several years ago, and it's become a family favorite. A crumbly oat topping and crust sandwich the smooth cream cheese and cranberry fillings.

Rhonda Lund, Laramie, Wyoming

- 2 cups plus 2 tablespoons all-purpose flour, *divided*
- 1 cup quick-cooking oats
- 3/4 cup packed brown sugar
- 1/2 cup butter, melted
- 1 package (8 ounces) reduced-fat cream cheese
- 1 can (14 ounces) fat-free sweetened condensed milk
- 4 egg whites
- 1 teaspoon vanilla extract
- 1 can (16 ounces) whole-berry cranberry sauce
- 2 tablespoons cornstarch

1. In a bowl, combine 2 cups flour, oats, brown sugar and butter; mix until crumbly. Press 2-1/2 cups of the crumb mixture into a greased 13-in. x 9-in. x 2-in. baking dish. Bake at 350° for 10 minutes.

2. In a large bowl, beat cream cheese until smooth. Beat in the milk, egg whites, vanilla and remaining flour. Spoon over prepared crust.

3. In a small bowl, combine the cranberry sauce and cornstarch. Spoon over cream cheese mixture. Sprinkle with the remaining crumb mixture.

4. Bake at 350° for 30-35 minutes or until the center is almost set. Cool on a wire rack before cutting.

LOW FAT   LOW SALT

PREP/TOTAL TIME
Prep: 15 min.
Bake: 30 min.
YIELD 3 dozen

NUTRITION FACTS
One serving
(1 bar) equals:
142 calories
4 g fat
2 g saturated fat
11 mg cholesterol
67 mg sodium
24 g carbohydrate
1 g fiber
3 g protein

DIABETIC EXCHANGES
1-1/2 starch
1/2 fat

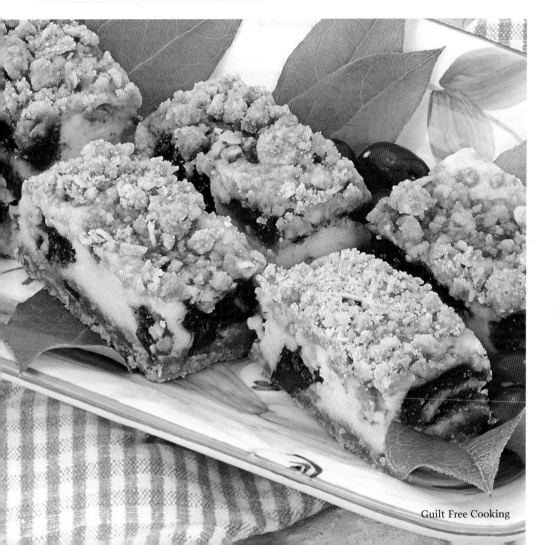

Blondies with Chips

My friends and family love my pared-down version of this classic snack...and never suspect that I add whole wheat flour.

Kai Kupinski, Canton, Michigan

PREP/TOTAL TIME
Prep: 5 min.
Bake: 20 min. +
cooling
YIELD 1 dozen

NUTRITION FACTS
One serving
(1 bar) equals:
133 calories
7 g fat
2 g saturated fat
18 mg cholesterol
67 mg sodium
17 g carbohydrate
1 g fiber
2 g protein

DIABETIC EXCHANGES
1 starch
1 fat

1/3 cup all-purpose flour
1/3 cup whole wheat flour
1/4 cup packed brown sugar
1/2 teaspoon baking powder
1/4 teaspoon salt
1 egg
1/4 cup canola oil
2 tablespoons honey
1 teaspoon vanilla extract
1/2 cup semisweet chocolate chips

1. In a small bowl, combine the flours, sugar, baking powder and salt. In another bowl, whisk the egg, oil, honey and vanilla; stir into dry ingredients until blended. Stir in chocolate chips (batter will be thick).

2. Spread into an 8-in. square baking dish coated with cooking spray. Bake at 350° for 20-22 minutes or until a toothpick inserted near the center comes out clean. Cool on a wire rack. Cut into bars.

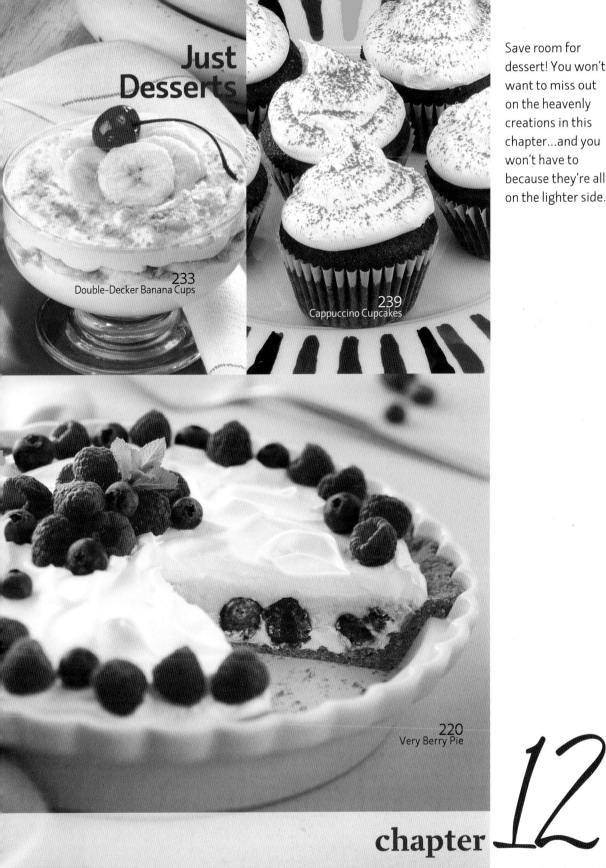

Just Desserts

Save room for dessert! You won't want to miss out on the heavenly creations in this chapter...and you won't have to because they're all on the lighter side.

233
Double-Decker Banana Cups

239
Cappuccino Cupcakes

220
Very Berry Pie

chapter 12

Very Berry Pie

LOW FAT LOW SALT

PREP/TOTAL TIME
Prep: 20 min. +
chilling
Bake: 10 min. +
cooling
YIELD 8 servings

NUTRITION FACTS
One serving
(1 piece) equals:
206 calories
9 g fat
6 g saturated fat
16 mg cholesterol
377 mg sodium
30 g carbohydrate
2 g fiber
3 g protein

**DIABETIC
EXCHANGES**
2 starch
1-1/2 fat

This light pie is the perfect dessert for a get-together. The tangy fresh berries are a pleasant contrast to the smooth, creamy vanilla filling.

Taste of Home Test Kitchen

1-1/2 cups reduced-fat graham cracker crumbs

1 tablespoon sugar

1 egg white

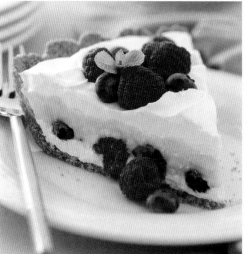

1/4 cup butter, melted

2 cups reduced-fat whipped topping, *divided*

1 cup fresh raspberries

1 cup fresh blueberries

Sugar substitute equivalent to 1 tablespoon sugar

1-1/2 cups cold fat-free milk

1 package (1-1/2 ounces) sugar-free instant vanilla pudding mix

1. In a small bowl, combine cracker crumbs and sugar; stir in egg white and butter. Press onto the bottom and up the sides of a 9-in. pie plate coated with cooking spray. Bake at 375° for 8-10 minutes or until set. Cool completely on a wire rack.

2. Spread 1/2 cup whipped topping over crust. Combine berries and sugar substitute; spoon 1-1/2 cups over topping.

3. In a bowl, whisk the milk and pudding mix for 2 minutes; let stand for 2 minutes or until soft-set. Spoon over berries. Spread with remaining whipped topping. Top with remaining berries. Refrigerate for 45 minutes or until set.

Editor's Note: This recipe was tested with Splenda No Calorie Sweetener.

Chocolate Angel Food Cake

LOW FAT

PREP/TOTAL TIME
Prep: 15 min.
Bake: 35 min. +
cooling
YIELD 12 servings

NUTRITION FACTS
One serving
(1 slice) equals:
184 calories
2 g fat
1 g saturated fat
0 mg cholesterol
329 mg sodium
38 g carbohydrate
2 g fiber
4 g protein

**DIABETIC
EXCHANGE**
2-1/2 starch

When I needed a light dessert for guests on a restricted diet, I combined two of my favorite recipes to make this chocolate cake with raspberry sauce. Everyone enjoyed it.

Lana Drum, Maryville, Tennessee

1 package (16 ounces) angel food cake mix

1-1/4 cups cold water

1/2 cup baking cocoa

RASPBERRY SAUCE:

Sugar substitute equivalent to 1/4 cup sugar

2 teaspoons cornstarch

1 package (12 ounces) frozen unsweetened raspberries, thawed

1-1/4 cups reduced-fat whipped topping

1. In a large mixing bowl, beat cake mix and water on low speed for 30 seconds. Beat on high for 45 seconds. Add cocoa; beat on high 15 seconds longer.

2. Gently spoon into an ungreased 10-in. tube pan. Cut through the batter with a knife to remove air pockets. Bake on the lowest oven rack at 350° for 35-40 minutes or until lightly browned and entire tops appear dry. Immediately invert pan; cool completely, about 1 hour.

3. In a saucepan, combine the sugar substitute and cornstarch. Add raspberries; stir until blended. Bring to a boil; cook and stir for 2 minutes or until the mixture is thickened. Remove saucepan from the heat; cool.

4. Run a knife around side and center tube of pan; remove the cake. Strain the raspberry sauce; spoon over cake slices. Dollop with whipped topping.

Editor's Note: This recipe was tested with Splenda No Calorie Sweetener.

Banana Split Cheesecake

This fruity dessert makes a light and festive treat that's sure to dazzle friends and family. Topped off with chocolate syrup, caramel and pecans, this no-bake cheesecake has an ooey-gooey look and mouthwatering taste.

Cherie Sweet, Evansville, Indiana

- 1 can (8 ounces) unsweetened crushed pineapple, *divided*
- 2 medium firm bananas, sliced
- 1 reduced-fat graham cracker crust (8 inches)
- 1 package (8 ounces) fat-free cream cheese
- 1-1/2 cups pineapple sherbet, softened
- 1 package (1 ounce) sugar-free instant vanilla pudding mix
- 1 carton (8 ounces) frozen reduced-fat whipped topping, thawed, *divided*
- 4 maraschino cherries, *divided*
- 1 tablespoon chocolate syrup
- 1 tablespoon caramel ice cream topping
- 1 tablespoon chopped pecans

1. Drain pineapple, reserving juice. In a small bowl, combine bananas and 2 tablespoons reserved juice; let stand for 5 minutes. Drain bananas, discarding juice. Arrange bananas over bottom of crust; set aside.

2. In a large bowl, beat the cream cheese and 2 tablespoons reserved pineapple juice. Gradually beat in sherbet. Gradually beat in pudding mix; beat 2 minutes longer. Refrigerate 1/3 cup pineapple until serving; fold remaining pineapple into cream cheese mixture. Fold in 2 cups whipped topping; spread evenly over banana slices. Cover and freeze until firm.

3. Remove from the freezer 10-15 minutes before serving. Chop three maraschino cherries and pat dry; arrange cherries and reserved pineapple around edge of pie. Drizzle with chocolate syrup and caramel topping. Dollop remaining whipped topping onto center of pie. Sprinkle with pecans; top with remaining cherry.

PREP/TOTAL TIME
35 min. + freezing
YIELD 10 servings

NUTRITION FACTS
One serving
(1 piece) equals:
247 calories
6 g fat
4 g saturated fat
3 mg cholesterol
336 mg sodium
41 g carbohydrate
1 g fiber
5 g protein

DIABETIC EXCHANGES
2 starch
1/2 fruit
1 fat

Blueberry Crumb Pie

LOW SALT

PREP/TOTAL TIME
Prep: 25 min. +
    freezing
Bake: 50 min.
YIELD 8 servings

NUTRITION FACTS
One serving
(1 piece) equals:
  313 calories
  9 g fat
  3 g saturated fat
  9 mg cholesterol
  164 mg sodium
  55 g carbohydrate
  2 g fiber
  4 g protein

DIABETIC EXCHANGES
  2 starch
  1-1/2 fruit
  1-1/2 fat

Treating yourself to this indulgent dessert won't give you the blues later on! This light recipe keeps fat and calories to a minimum.

Taste of Home Test Kitchen

1-1/4 cups all-purpose flour, *divided*
    5 tablespoons cold water
1-1/4 teaspoons lemon juice
1-1/4 teaspoons sugar
  1/4 teaspoon salt
    3 tablespoons plus 2 teaspoons shortening

FILLING:

4-1/2 cups fresh or frozen blueberries
    1 cup (8 ounces) reduced-fat vanilla yogurt
  1/2 cup packed brown sugar
    3 tablespoons all-purpose flour
1-1/2 teaspoons vanilla extract
  1/4 teaspoon grated lemon peel
  1/2 cup graham cracker crumbs (about 12 squares)
    2 tablespoons sugar
    2 tablespoons butter, melted

1. In a bowl, whisk together 1/4 cup flour, water and lemon juice; set aside. In a large bowl, combine sugar, salt and remaining flour; cut in shortening until crumbly. Gradually add flour mixture, tossing with a fork until moistened.

2. On a piece of plastic wrap, press dough into a 4-in. circle. Cover with a second sheet of plastic wrap; roll into a 12-in. circle. Freeze for 10 minutes. Let stand for 1 minute; remove plastic wrap.

3. Transfer pastry to pie plate; trim to 1/2 in. beyond edge of plate. Flute edges. Prick bottom and sides of pastry with a fork. Line shell with a double thickness of heavy-duty foil. Bake at 375° for 8 minutes. Remove foil; bake 5 minutes longer.

4. Place blueberries in crust. In a bowl, combine the yogurt, brown sugar, flour, vanilla and peel; spread over berries. Combine graham cracker crumbs, sugar and butter; sprinkle over yogurt mixture. Bake at 375° for 35-40 minutes or until crumbs are lightly browned and filling is bubbly.

Editor's Note: If using frozen blueberries, do not thaw before adding to batter.

Peanut Butter Chocolate Pudding

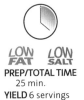

LOW FAT   LOW SALT

PREP/TOTAL TIME
25 min.
YIELD 6 servings

NUTRITION FACTS
One serving equals:
  102 calories
  3 g fat
  0 g saturated fat
  1 mg cholesterol
  144 mg sodium
  13 g carbohydrate
  0 g fiber
  5 g protein

DIABETIC EXCHANGES
  1 starch
  1/2 fat

Being a diabetic with dietary restrictions, I was so pleased to discover the recipe for this cool, pretty, satisfying dessert.

Shirlye Price, Hartford, Kentucky

    2 cups cold fat-free milk, *divided*
    2 tablespoons reduced-fat chunky peanut butter
    1 cup reduced-fat whipped topping, *divided*
    1 package (1.4 ounces) sugar-free instant chocolate (fudge) pudding mix

1. In a small bowl, mix 2 tablespoons milk and peanut butter until smooth. Fold in 3/4 cup whipped topping; set aside. In a mixing bowl, beat pudding mix and remaining milk until blended, about 2 minutes. Let stand for 5 minutes.

2. Spoon half of the pudding into six parfait glasses or bowls; top with peanut butter mixture and remaining pudding. Garnish with remaining whipped topping.

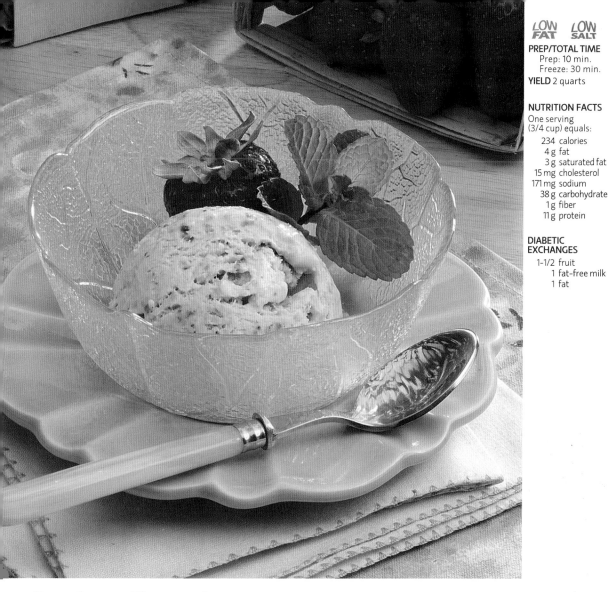

LOW FAT   LOW SALT

PREP/TOTAL TIME
Prep: 10 min.
Freeze: 30 min.
YIELD 2 quarts

NUTRITION FACTS
One serving
(3/4 cup) equals:
234 calories
4 g fat
3 g saturated fat
15 mg cholesterol
171 mg sodium
38 g carbohydrate
1 g fiber
11 g protein

DIABETIC EXCHANGES
1-1/2 fruit
1 fat-free milk
1 fat

Strawberry Cheesecake Ice Cream

This special, rich ice cream is wonderful for family gatherings. We love how it tastes like a fabulous berry-topped cheesecake.

Karen Maubach, Fairbury, Illinois

- 3 cups sliced fresh strawberries
- 6 ounces reduced-fat cream cheese
- 2 cans (12 ounces *each*) fat-free evaporated milk
- 1 can (14 ounces) fat-free sweetened condensed milk
- 1 teaspoon vanilla extract
- 1 cup reduced-fat whipped topping

1. Place the strawberries in a blender or food processor; cover and process until smooth. In a large mixing bowl, beat cream cheese until smooth. Add evaporated milk and condensed milk, vanilla and pureed strawberries; mix well. Fold in whipped topping.

2. Fill the cylinder of ice cream freezer two-thirds full; freeze according to manufacturer's directions. Refrigerate remaining mixture until ready to freeze. Allow to ripen in ice cream freezer or firm up in your refrigerator freezer for 2-4 hours before serving.

PREP/TOTAL TIME
Prep: 45 min. + chilling
Bake: 35 min. + cooling

YIELD 12 servings

NUTRITION FACTS
One serving
(1 piece) equals:
259 calories
7 g fat
0 g saturated fat
14 mg cholesterol
272 mg sodium
42 g carbohydrate
0 g fiber
8 g protein

DIABETIC EXCHANGES
2 starch
1-1/2 fat
1 fruit

Rhubarb-Topped Cheesecake

No one believes that this creamy cheesecake topped with tangy rhubarb is actually light.

Ruth Eisenreich, Catonsville, Maryland

3/4 cup graham cracker crumbs (about 10 squares)

1/2 teaspoon ground cinnamon

3 tablespoons reduced-fat margarine, melted

2 packages (8 ounces *each*) reduced-fat cream cheese, softened

3/4 cup sugar

1 cup egg substitute

1 cup (8 ounces) fat-free vanilla yogurt

1/4 cup lemon juice

1 teaspoon grated lemon peel

TOPPING:

3 cups diced fresh *or* frozen rhubarb

1 cup sugar

2 tablespoons plus 1/2 cup cold water, *divided*

1 tablespoon cornstarch

Red food coloring, optional

1. In a small bowl, combine the cracker crumbs and cinnamon; stir in margarine. Press onto the bottom of a 9-in. springform pan; place pan on a baking sheet and set aside.

2. In a large bowl, beat cream cheese and sugar until smooth. Slowly add egg substitute; beat on low just until combined. Beat in the yogurt, lemon juice and peel just until combined. Pour over crust.

3. Bake at 350° for 35-40 minutes or until center is almost set. Cool on a wire rack for 10 minutes. Carefully run a knife around edge of pan to loosen; cool 1 hour longer. Cover and refrigerate overnight.

4. In a large saucepan, combine the rhubarb, sugar and 2 tablespoons water. Bring to a boil. Reduce heat; simmer until rhubarb is tender, about 10 minutes. Combine cornstarch and remaining water until smooth; gradually stir into rhubarb mixture. Bring to a boil; cook and stir for 2 minutes or until thickened. Add food coloring if desired. Cover and refrigerate until cool. Spoon over slices of cheesecake.

Editor's Note: If using frozen rhubarb, measure rhubarb while still frozen, then thaw completely. Drain in a colander, but do not press liquid out. This recipe was tested with Parkay Light stick margarine.

Light Tiramisu

I call this my skinny dessert. It tastes very much like the traditional Italian dessert but uses low-fat and sugar-free ingredients.

Jackie Newell, Roanoke, Virginia

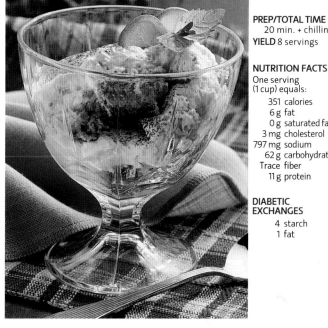

1 prepared angel food cake (8 inches), cut into 1-inch cubes

1/2 cup instant sugar-free cappuccino mix, *divided*

2 cups cold fat-free milk, *divided*

1 package (8 ounces) fat-free cream cheese, softened

1 package (1 ounce) sugar-free instant vanilla pudding mix

2 cups reduced-fat whipped topping

1/2 teaspoon baking cocoa

1. Place cake cubes in an ungreased 13-in. x 9-in. x 2-in. dish. In a small bowl, combine 1/4 cup cappuccino mix and 1/2 cup milk until dissolved. Pour over cake.

2. In a mixing bowl, beat cream cheese. In another bowl, combine pudding mix and remaining cappuccino mix and milk; whisk until smooth and thickened. Add to the cream cheese; mix well. Fold in the whipped topping; spoon over cake mixture. Refrigerate for 3 hours or overnight. Sprinkle with cocoa just before serving.

PREP/TOTAL TIME
20 min. + chilling
YIELD 8 servings

NUTRITION FACTS
One serving
(1 cup) equals:
351 calories
6 g fat
0 g saturated fat
3 mg cholesterol
797 mg sodium
62 g carbohydrate
Trace fiber
11 g protein

DIABETIC EXCHANGES
4 starch
1 fat

Chocolate Marvel Cake

This chocolaty cake featuring fluffy mocha frosting is deliciously moist. It's a treat I'm proud to prepare for family and guests alike.

Pearl Watts, Cincinnati, Ohio

1 cup strong brewed coffee

1 cup fat-free milk

2 jars (4 ounces *each*) pureed prune baby food

4 egg whites

2 teaspoons vanilla extract

2 cups all-purpose flour

2 cups sugar

3/4 cup baking cocoa

2 teaspoons baking soda

1 teaspoon baking powder

1/4 teaspoon salt

FROSTING:

6 tablespoons margarine, softened

2-2/3 cups confectioners' sugar

1/4 cup baking cocoa

2 tablespoons fat-free milk

2 tablespoons strong brewed coffee

1 teaspoon vanilla extract

1. In a large bowl, combine coffee, milk, baby food, egg whites and vanilla; beat until well blended. Combine flour, sugar, cocoa, baking soda, baking powder and salt; add to coffee mixture. Beat for 2 minutes or until well blended (batter will be thin).

2. Pour into two 9-in. round baking pans coated with cooking spray and lightly floured. Bake at 350° for 30-35 minutes or until the cake pulls away from the sides of pan. Cool for 10 minutes; remove from pans to wire racks to cool completely.

3. For frosting, in a large bowl, cream the margarine, confectioners' sugar and cocoa. Gradually add milk, coffee and vanilla; beat well. Frost between layers and over top and sides of cake.

LOW FAT

PREP/TOTAL TIME
Prep: 20 min.
Bake: 30 min. + cooling
YIELD 16 servings

NUTRITION FACTS
One serving
(1 slice) equals:
306 calories
5 g fat
0 g saturated fat
Trace cholesterol
614 mg sodium
64 g carbohydrate
0 g fiber
4 g protein

DIABETIC EXCHANGES
3 starch
1 fruit
1 fat

Frosted Spice Cake

PREP/TOTAL TIME
Prep: 15 min.
Bake: 25 min.
YIELD 20 servings

NUTRITION FACTS
One serving
(1 piece) equals:
283 calories
11 g fat
2 g saturated fat
0 mg cholesterol
261 mg sodium
45 g carbohydrate
1 g fiber
2 g protein

DIABETIC EXCHANGES
2 starch
2 fat
1 fruit

This spice cake is moist and flavorful. I stir a little cinnamon into the prepared frosting.

Lorraine Darocha, Berkshire, Massachusetts

- 3 cups all-purpose flour
- 2 cups sugar
- 2 teaspoons baking soda
- 1 teaspoon salt
- 1-1/8 teaspoons ground cinnamon, *divided*
- 1/2 teaspoon ground cloves
- 1/2 teaspoon ground nutmeg
- 2 cups water
- 2/3 cup canola oil
- 2 tablespoons white vinegar
- 2 teaspoons vanilla extract
- 1 can (12 ounces) whipped vanilla frosting

1. In a large mixing bowl, combine the flour, sugar, baking soda, salt, 1 teaspoon cinnamon, cloves and nutmeg. Combine the water, oil, vinegar and vanilla; add to the dry ingredients and beat until smooth (the batter will be thin).

2. Pour into a 13-in. x 9-in. x 2-in. baking pan coated with cooking spray. Bake at 350° for 25-30 minutes or until a toothpick inserted near the center comes out clean. Cool on a wire rack. Stir the remaining cinnamon into the frosting; spread over cake.

Editor's Note: This recipe does not use eggs.

Creamy Apple Crumb Pie

PREP/TOTAL TIME
Prep: 20 min.
Bake: 50 min. + cooling
YIELD 8 servings

NUTRITION FACTS
One serving
(1 piece) equals:
299 calories
11 g fat
6 g saturated fat
22 mg cholesterol
126 mg sodium
49 g carbohydrate
2 g fiber
4 g protein

DIABETIC EXCHANGES
2 starch
2 fat
1 fruit

I revised this classic apple pie recipe from one I discovered in a church cookbook. I knew for sure that my version was a keeper when my mother-in-law asked for a copy!

Linda Pawelski, Milwaukee, Wisconsin

- 1 pastry for single-crust pie (9 inches)
- 6 cups cubed peeled tart apples (about 6 medium)
- 1/3 cup sugar
- 3 tablespoons cornstarch
- 1 teaspoon ground cinnamon
- 1/4 teaspoon ground allspice
- 1 cup (8 ounces) reduced-fat sour cream
- 1 teaspoon vanilla extract

TOPPING:
- 1/2 cup all-purpose flour
- 1/4 cup packed brown sugar
- 1/2 teaspoon ground cinnamon
- 2 tablespoons cold butter

1. Line a 9-in. deep-dish pie plate with pastry; flute edges. In a large bowl, combine the apples, sugar, cornstarch, cinnamon and allspice. Combine sour cream and vanilla; stir into apple mixture. Spoon into pastry shell.

2. For topping, combine the flour, brown sugar and cinnamon in a bowl; cut in butter until mixture resembles coarse crumbs. Sprinkle over filling.

3. Bake at 400° for 25 minutes. Reduce heat to 350°; bake 25-30 minutes longer or until filling is bubbly and topping is golden. Cool on a wire rack. Refrigerate leftovers.

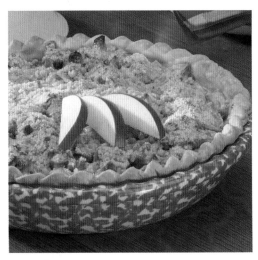

Orange Pineapple Torte

Special family dinners wouldn't be complete without this beautiful, impressive cake. It's surprisingly rich-tasting and not too sweet.

Karen Mellinger Baker, Dover, Ohio

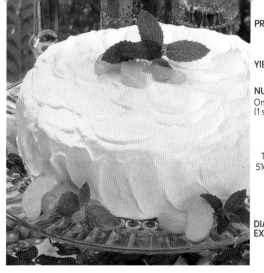

- 1 package (18-1/4 ounces) yellow cake mix
- 2 packages (1 ounce *each*) sugar-free instant vanilla pudding mix, *divided*
- 4 egg whites
- 1 cup water
- 1/4 cup canola oil
- 1/4 teaspoon baking soda
- 1 cup cold fat-free milk
- 1 carton (8 ounces) frozen reduced-fat whipped topping, thawed
- 1 can (20 ounces) unsweetened crushed pineapple, well drained
- 1 can (11 ounces) mandarin oranges, drained, *divided*

Fresh mint, optional

1. In a large bowl, combine cake mix, one package of pudding mix, egg whites, water, oil and baking soda. Beat on low speed for 1 minute; beat on medium for 4 minutes.

2. Pour into two greased and floured 9-in. round baking pans. Bake at 350° for 25-30 minutes or until a toothpick insert-ed near the center comes out clean. Cool for 10 minutes; remove from pans to a wire rack to cool completely.

3. For filling, combine milk and remaining pudding mix. Whisk for 2 minutes; let stand for 2 minutes. Fold in whipped topping. In a medium bowl, combine 1-1/2 cups pudding mixture with pineapple and half of the oranges.

4. Slice each cake layer in half horizon-tally. Spread pineapple mixture between the layers. Frost top and sides of cake with remaining pudding mixture. Garnish with remaining oranges and mint if desired. Store in the refrigerator.

PREP/TOTAL TIME
Prep: 25 min.
Bake: 25 min. + cooling
YIELD 12 servings

NUTRITION FACTS
One serving
(1 slice) equals:
335 calories
9 g fat
0 g saturated fat
Trace cholesterol
516 mg sodium
58 g carbohydrate
0 g fiber
4 g protein

DIABETIC EXCHANGES
2 starch
2 fruit
2 fat

Blueberry Crisp

The use of frozen blueberries allows me to make this fruity crisp with a sweet golden topping any time of year. A dollop of vanilla frozen yogurt adds to its great homemade taste.

Betty Geiger, Marion, Michigan

- 2 packages (12 ounces *each*) frozen unsweetened blueberries, thawed
- 2 tablespoons plus 1/2 cup all-purpose flour, *divided*
- 2 tablespoons brown sugar
- 1/4 teaspoon ground cinnamon
- 3 tablespoons cold margarine

TOPPING:

- 1 cup (8 ounces) fat-free plain yogurt
- 1/2 teaspoon vanilla extract

Sugar substitute equivalent to 2 teaspoons sugar

1. Place the blueberries in an 8-in. baking dish coated with cooking spray. Sprinkle with 2 tablespoons flour. In a bowl, com-bine brown sugar, cinnamon and remain-ing flour; cut in margarine until crumbly. Sprinkle over berries.

2. Bake at 350° for 25-30 minutes or until bubbly and golden brown. For top-ping, combine yogurt, vanilla and sugar substitute; serve with the crisp.

Editor's Note: This recipe was tested with Splenda No Calorie Sweetener.

PREP/TOTAL TIME
Prep: 15 min.
Bake: 25 min.
YIELD 6 servings

NUTRITION FACTS
One serving equals:
198 calories
7 g fat
0 g saturated fat
1 mg cholesterol
99 mg sodium
31 g carbohydrate
3 g fiber
5 g protein

DIABETIC EXCHANGES
1-1/2 fat
1 starch
1 fruit

Fudgy Brownie Dessert

PREP/TOTAL TIME
Prep: 20 min. + chilling
Bake: 20 min. + cooling
YIELD 15 servings

NUTRITION FACTS
One serving
(1 brownie) equals:

220 calories
8 g fat
0 g saturated fat
1 mg cholesterol
106 mg sodium
33 g carbohydrate
0 g fiber
7 g protein

DIABETIC EXCHANGES
2 starch
1-1/2 fat

I came up with this recipe when searching for a low-fat dessert for my chocolate-loving family. My husband's and son's eyes light up whenever I serve these fudgy brownies topped with a fluffy mousse.

Karen Yoder, Bremerton, Washington

- 1/2 cup sugar
- 1/4 cup cornstarch
- 1/4 cup baking cocoa
- 1 can (12 ounces) fat-free evaporated milk
- 1/2 cup egg substitute

BROWNIE CRUST:

- 1-1/4 cups baking cocoa
- 1 cup sugar
- 3/4 cup all-purpose flour
- 1 teaspoon baking powder
- 1 cup unsweetened applesauce
- 1 cup egg substitute
- 1/4 cup canola oil
- 2 teaspoons vanilla extract
- 1 carton (8 ounces) frozen reduced-fat whipped topping, thawed

1. In a saucepan, combine the sugar, cornstarch and cocoa. Stir in milk until smooth. Cook and stir over low heat just until boiling. Remove from heat; stir a small amount into egg substitute. Return all to pan; cook for 1 minute or until thickened. Refrigerate.

2. Meanwhile, for crust, combine cocoa, sugar, flour and baking powder in a bowl. Combine applesauce, egg substitute, oil and vanilla; add to the dry ingredients and mix just until blended. Pour into a 13-in. x 9-in. x 2-in. baking pan coated with cooking spray. Bake at 350° for 20 minutes or until a toothpick inserted near the center comes out clean. Cool on a wire rack.

3. In a mixing bowl, beat the chilled chocolate mixture until light. Fold in whipped topping; carefully spread over crust. Refrigerate for 2 hours before serving. Store in the refrigerator.

Lemon Chiffon Cake

This fluffy, citrusy cake is a real treat drizzled with the sweet-tart lemon glaze.

Rebecca Baird, Salt Lake City, Utah

- 1/2 cup fat-free evaporated milk
- 1/2 cup reduced-fat sour cream
- 1/4 cup lemon juice
- 2 tablespoons canola oil
- 2 teaspoons vanilla extract
- 1 teaspoon grated lemon peel
- 1 teaspoon lemon extract
- 2 cups cake flour
- 1-1/2 cups sugar
- 1 tablespoon baking powder
- 1/2 teaspoon salt
- 1 cup egg whites (about 7)
- 1/2 teaspoon cream of tartar

LEMON GLAZE:
- 1-3/4 cups confectioners' sugar
- 3 tablespoons lemon juice

1. In a large mixing bowl, combine the first seven ingredients. Sift together the flour, sugar, baking powder and salt; gradually beat into lemon mixture until smooth.

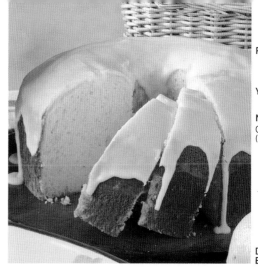

LOW FAT LOW SALT

PREP/TOTAL TIME
Prep: 15 min.
Bake: 45 min. + cooling
YIELD 16 servings

NUTRITION FACTS
One serving
(1 slice) equals:
228 calories
3 g fat
0 g saturated fat
3 mg cholesterol
157 mg sodium
47 g carbohydrate
0 g fiber
4 g protein

DIABETIC EXCHANGES
1 starch
1 fruit
1/2 fat

2. In a small mixing bowl, beat egg whites until foamy. Add cream of tartar; beat until stiff peaks form. Gently fold into the lemon mixture.

3. Pour into an ungreased 10-in. tube pan with removable bottom. Bake at 325° for 45-55 minutes or until cake springs back when lightly touched. Immediately invert pan; cool completely. Remove cake to a serving platter. Combine glaze ingredients; drizzle over cake.

Raspberry Pear Crisp

If you want a change of pace from the usual pie or cake, give this honey of a dessert a try. It's tart, crispy and just plain good.

Ruby Williams, Bogalusa, Louisiana

- 2 medium ripe pears, peeled and thinly sliced
- 3 cups fresh raspberries
- 2 tablespoons sugar
- 1 cup quick-cooking oats
- 1/4 cup honey
- 3 tablespoons stick margarine, melted
- 1 teaspoon ground cinnamon
- 1/2 teaspoon ground nutmeg

1. Place pears in an 8-in. square baking dish coated with cooking spray. Sprinkle with raspberries and sugar.

2. In a bowl, combine the oats, honey, margarine, cinnamon and nutmeg. Sprinkle over raspberries. Bake, uncovered, at 350° for 30-35 minutes or until pears are tender and mixture is bubbly.

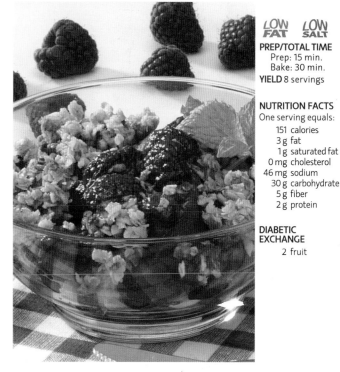

LOW FAT LOW SALT

PREP/TOTAL TIME
Prep: 15 min.
Bake: 30 min.
YIELD 8 servings

NUTRITION FACTS
One serving equals:
151 calories
3 g fat
1 g saturated fat
0 mg cholesterol
46 mg sodium
30 g carbohydrate
5 g fiber
2 g protein

DIABETIC EXCHANGE
2 fruit

Tart Cherry Pie

PREP/TOTAL TIME
Prep: 15 min. + cooling
YIELD 8 servings

NUTRITION FACTS
One serving
(1 piece) equals:
  176 calories
  8 g fat
  0 g saturated fat
  0 mg cholesterol
  293 mg sodium
  24 g carbohydrate
  0 g fiber
  3 g protein

DIABETIC EXCHANGES
  1 starch
  1/2 fruit
  1/2 fat

My aunt and I are diabetic, and we both like this yummy, sweet-tart pie. Our friends even request this dessert when they come to visit.

Bonnie Johnson, DeKalb, Illinois

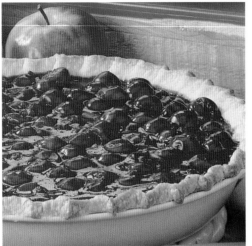

2 cans (14-1/2 ounces *each*) pitted tart cherries
1 package (.8 ounce) sugar-free cook-and-serve vanilla pudding mix
1 package (.3 ounce) sugar-free cherry gelatin
Sugar substitute equivalent to 4 teaspoons sugar
1 pastry shell (9 inches), baked

1. Drain cherries, reserving juice; set the cherries aside. In a saucepan, combine cherry juice and dry pudding mix. Cook and stir until mixture comes to a boil and is thickened and bubbly.

2. Remove from the heat; stir in gelatin powder and sweetener until dissolved. Stir in cherries; transfer to pastry shell. Cool completely. Store in the refrigerator.

Editor's Note: This recipe was tested with Splenda No Calorie Sweetener.

Caramel-Pecan Cheese Pie

PREP/TOTAL TIME
Prep: 20 min. + chilling
YIELD 8 servings

NUTRITION FACTS
One serving
(1 piece) equals:
  270 calories
  12 g fat
  6 g saturated fat
  6 mg cholesterol
  186 mg sodium
  31 g carbohydrate
  1 g fiber
  7 g protein

DIABETIC EXCHANGES
  2 starch
  2 fat

Summers get quite hot where I live, so when the weather is warm, I try to use my oven as little as possible. Family and friends love this no-bake pie drizzled with caramel topping.

Patsy Mullins, Taft, Tennessee

1 envelope unflavored gelatin
1/3 cup water
1/4 cup lemon juice
3 ounces reduced-fat cream cheese, cubed
1 cup nonfat dry milk powder
Sugar substitute equivalent to 2 tablespoons sugar
1 carton (8 ounces) frozen reduced-fat whipped topping, thawed
5 tablespoons chopped pecans, toasted, *divided*
1 reduced-fat graham cracker crust (9 inches)
2 tablespoons fat-free caramel ice cream topping

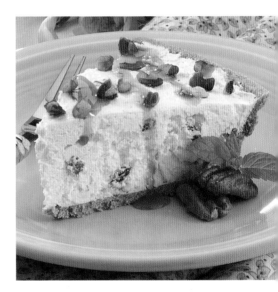

1. In a small saucepan, sprinkle gelatin over water; let stand for 1 minute. Bring to a boil, stirring until gelatin is completely dissolved. Cool slightly.

2. In a blender or food processor, combine the lemon juice, cream cheese and gelatin mixture; cover and process until smooth. Add milk powder and sugar substitute; cover and process for 1 minute.

3. Transfer to a large bowl; fold in whipped topping. Stir in 3 tablespoons pecans. Pour into crust. Sprinkle with remaining pecans. Drizzle with the caramel topping. Cover and refrigerate for 2-3 hours or until set.

Editor's Note: This recipe was tested with Splenda No Calorie Sweetener.

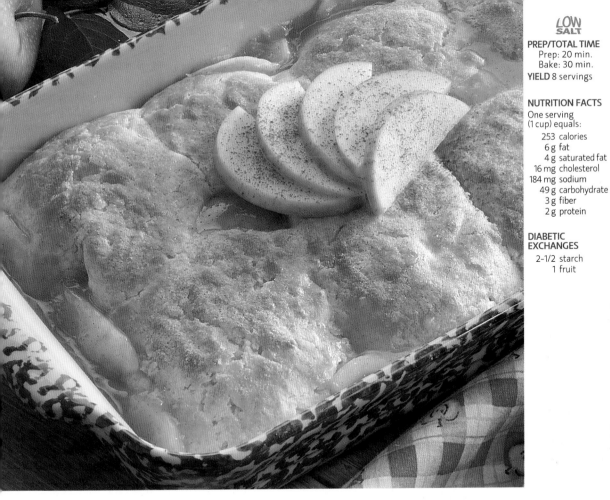

LOW SALT

PREP/TOTAL TIME
Prep: 20 min.
Bake: 30 min.
YIELD 8 servings

NUTRITION FACTS
One serving
(1 cup) equals:
253 calories
6 g fat
4 g saturated fat
16 mg cholesterol
184 mg sodium
49 g carbohydrate
3 g fiber
2 g protein

DIABETIC EXCHANGES
2-1/2 starch
1 fruit

Apple Cobbler

The fragrant aroma of apples and cinnamon wafting from the kitchen will whet your appetite for this yummy fall favorite.

Vivian Haen, Menomonee Falls, Wisconsin

1/3 cup sugar

1 tablespoon cornstarch

1/2 teaspoon ground cinnamon

1/4 teaspoon ground nutmeg

4 cups sliced peeled tart apples (about 4 large)

1/3 cup orange juice

TOPPING:

1 cup all-purpose flour

1/3 cup plus 2 teaspoons sugar, *divided*

1-1/2 teaspoons baking powder

1/4 teaspoon salt

1/4 cup cold butter, cubed

1/2 cup fat-free milk

1. In a large bowl, combine the sugar, cornstarch, cinnamon and nutmeg. Add apples and orange juice; toss to coat. Transfer to an 11-in. x 7-in. x 2-in. baking dish coated with cooking spray.

2. Combine flour, 1/3 cup sugar, baking powder and salt. Cut in butter until mixture resembles coarse crumbs. Stir in milk just until moistened. Drop eight mounds onto apple mixture. Sprinkle with remaining sugar.

3. Bake at 375° for 30-35 minutes or until a toothpick inserted into topping comes out clean. Serve warm if desired.

Chocolate Macaroon Cupcakes

A coconut and ricotta cheese center is the sweet surprise inside these treats. They're the perfect cure for a chocolate craving!

Dolores Skrout, Summerhill, Pennsylvania

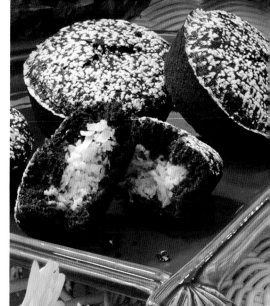

PREP/TOTAL TIME
Prep: 20 min.
Bake: 30 min. +
cooling
YIELD 1-1/2 dozen

NUTRITION FACTS
One serving
(1 cupcake) equals:
121 calories
1 g fat
1 g saturated fat
14 mg cholesterol
75 mg sodium
24 g carbohydrate
1 g fiber
4 g protein

DIABETIC EXCHANGE
1-1/2 starch

2 egg whites
1 egg
1/3 cup unsweetened applesauce
1 teaspoon vanilla extract
1-1/4 cups all-purpose flour
1 cup sugar
1/3 cup baking cocoa
1/2 teaspoon baking soda
3/4 cup buttermilk

FILLING:
1 cup fat-free ricotta cheese
1/4 cup sugar
1 egg white
1/3 cup flaked coconut
1/2 teaspoon coconut *or* almond extract
2 teaspoons confectioners' sugar

1. In a large bowl, combine egg whites, egg, applesauce and vanilla. Combine flour, sugar, cocoa and baking soda; gradually add to the egg mixture alternately with buttermilk. Spoon half of batter into 18 muffin cups coated with cooking spray.

2. In another bowl, beat ricotta cheese, sugar and egg white until smooth. Stir in the coconut and extract. Spoon 1 tablespoonful in the center of each muffin cup.

3. Fill muffin cups two-thirds full with remaining batter. Bake at 350° for 28-33 minutes or until a toothpick inserted in the cupcake comes out clean. Cool for 5 minutes before removing from pans to wire racks to cool completely. Dust with the confectioners' sugar.

Refreshing Lime Pie

Even folks watching their diet can savor a slice of this fluffy dessert. It's so good, especially after a summer barbecue.

Mildred Baker, Youngstown, Ohio

PREP/TOTAL TIME
Prep: 15 min. +
chilling
YIELD 8 servings

NUTRITION FACTS
One serving
(1 piece) equals:
172 calories
6 g fat
0 g saturated fat
1 mg cholesterol
183 mg sodium
24 g carbohydrate
0 g fiber
6 g protein

DIABETIC EXCHANGES
1 starch
1 fat
1/2 fat-free milk

1 envelope unflavored gelatin
1/2 cup cold water
1 package (.3 ounce) sugar-free lime gelatin
1/2 cup boiling water
3 cartons (8 ounces *each*) fat-free reduced-sugar key lime pie yogurt *or* lemon yogurt
1-1/2 cups reduced-fat whipped topping
1 shortbread crust (8 inches)

1. In a small bowl, sprinkle unflavored gelatin over cold water; let stand for 1 minute. In another bowl, dissolve lime gelatin in boiling water; stir in unflavored gelatin until dissolved. Refrigerate for 10 minutes.

2. Stir in yogurt. Chill until partially set. Fold in whipped topping. Pour into crust. Chill until firm.

Double-Decker Banana Cups

I prepare these petite parfaits by layering a vanilla pudding mixture with sliced bananas and graham cracker crumbs. They make a speedy dessert or even a delightful snack.

Patricia Kinsella, Calgary, Alberta

- 1 cup cold fat-free milk
- 1 package (3.4 ounces) instant vanilla pudding mix
- 1 cup reduced-fat whipped topping
- 1 cup thinly sliced firm bananas
- 4 teaspoons graham cracker crumbs
- 4 maraschino cherries with stems

1. In a bowl, whisk together milk and pudding mix for 2 minutes. Fold in whipped topping. Refrigerate for at least 5 minutes.

2. Divide half of pudding mixture among four dessert dishes. Top with half of the banana slices and remaining pudding mixture. Sprinkle with crumbs. Top each with the remaining banana slices and garnish with a cherry. Serve immediately.

LOW FAT

PREP/TOTAL TIME
20 min.
YIELD 4 servings

NUTRITION FACTS
One serving
(3/4 cup) equals:
193 calories
2 g fat
2 g saturated fat
1 mg cholesterol
350 mg sodium
40 g carbohydrate
1 g fiber
3 g protein

DIABETIC EXCHANGES
2 starch
1/2 fruit

PREP/TOTAL TIME
Prep: 20 min. +
chilling
Bake: 30 min. +
cooling
YIELD 8 servings

NUTRITION FACTS
One serving
(1 piece) equals:
268 calories
12 g fat
6 g saturated fat
21 mg cholesterol
119 mg sodium
34 g carbohydrate
2 g fiber
5 g protein

DIABETIC EXCHANGES
2 fat
1 starch
1 fruit

Strawberry Cream Cheese Pie

Cheesecake lovers will savor every bite of this light and pretty pie, even if they don't have to watch their diets.

Kim Marie Van Rheenen, Mendota, Illinois

Pastry for a single-crust pie (9 inches)

- 1 package (8 ounces) reduced-fat cream cheese
- 1/2 cup egg substitute
- 3 tablespoons honey
- 1 teaspoon vanilla extract
- 3-1/2 cups sliced fresh strawberries
- 1 tablespoon cornstarch
- 1/2 cup cold water
- 1/2 cup reduced-sugar strawberry preserves

Fat-free whipped topping, optional

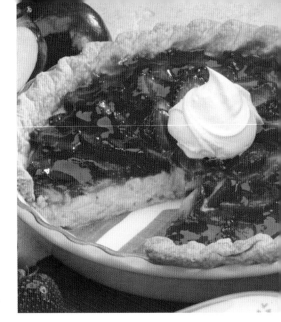

1. Roll out pastry to fit a 9-in. pie plate; transfer pastry to plate. Trim pastry to 1/2 in. beyond edge of plate; flute edges. Prick bottom and sides of crust with a fork. Bake at 350° for 13-15 minutes or until lightly browned.

2. Meanwhile, in a large bowl, beat the cream cheese, egg substitute, honey and vanilla until smooth. Pour into the crust. Bake 15-18 minutes longer or until the center is almost set. Cool on a wire rack to room temperature.

3. Arrange strawberries over filling. In a saucepan, combine cornstarch and water until smooth. Stir in preserves. Bring to a boil; cook and stir for 2 minutes or until thickened. Spoon or brush over the strawberries. Refrigerate for 2 hours before cutting. Garnish with whipped topping if desired. Refrigerate leftovers.

PREP/TOTAL TIME
Prep: 10 min.
Bake: 25 min.
YIELD 10 servings

NUTRITION FACTS
One serving
(1 slice) equals:
158 calories
1 g fat
0 g saturated fat
Trace cholesterol
282 mg sodium
27 g carbohydrate
0 g fiber
7 g protein

DIABETIC EXCHANGE
2 starch

Pineapple Upside-Down Cake

I like to dole out slices of this sunny-colored dessert while it's still warm from the oven. The light cake gets fruity flavor from crushed pineapple and lemon gelatin.

Anne Polhemus, North Merrick, New York

- 1 can (20 ounces) unsweetened crushed pineapple
- 1 package (.3 ounce) sugar-free lemon gelatin
- 1/2 cup egg substitute
- 1 egg white
- 3/4 cup sugar
- 1 teaspoon vanilla extract
- 3/4 cup all-purpose flour
- 1 teaspoon baking powder

1. Drain pineapple, reserving 1/3 cup juice. Line a 9-in. round baking pan with waxed paper; coat with cooking spray. Spread pineapple over waxed paper; sprinkle with gelatin.

2. In a bowl, beat egg substitute and egg white. Beat in sugar, reserved pineapple juice and vanilla. Combine flour and baking powder; add to egg mixture and stir well. Pour over gelatin.

3. Bake at 350° for 25-30 minutes or until a toothpick inserted near the center comes out clean. Cool for 5 minutes; invert onto a serving plate. Carefully remove waxed paper and serve warm.

Cream Cheese Bonbons

These pretty, coconut-speckled candies are rolled in grated chocolate, but you could also coat them in finely chopped nuts, chocolate sprinkles or brightly colored jimmies.

Beverly Coyde, Gasport, New York

1 package (8 ounces) reduced-fat cream cheese

Sugar substitute equivalent to 1/3 cup sugar

1 tablespoon sugar

1/2 teaspoon vanilla extract

1 cup flaked coconut

1 square (1 ounce) unsweetened chocolate, grated

1. In a small mixing bowl, beat the cream cheese, sugar substitute, sugar and vanilla until smooth. Stir in the coconut until combined. Refrigerate for 30 minutes or until easy to handle.

2. Shape cream cheese mixture into 1-in. balls; roll in grated chocolate. Refrigerate for at least 1 hour. Store in an airtight container in the refrigerator.

Editor's Note: This recipe was tested with Splenda No Calorie Sweetener.

LOW SALT

PREP/TOTAL TIME
Prep: 20 min.
+ chilling

YIELD 1-1/2 dozen

NUTRITION FACTS
One serving
(1 bonbon) equals:
73 calories
6 g fat
4 g saturated fat
10 mg cholesterol
64 mg sodium
5 g carbohydrate
Trace fiber
2 g protein

DIABETIC EXCHANGES
1 fat
1/2 starch

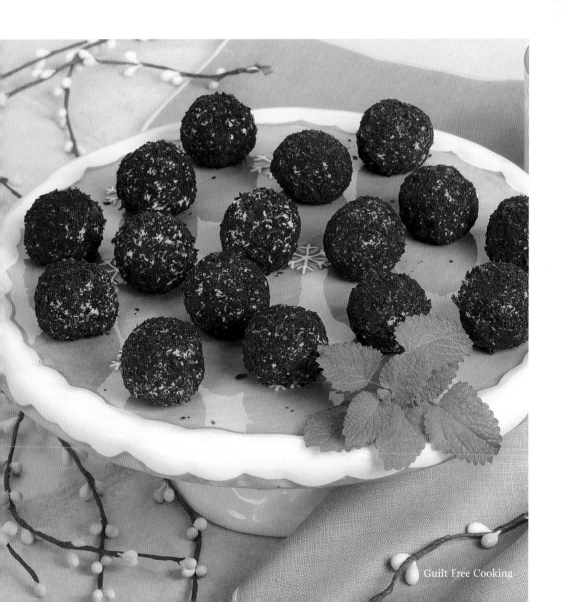

Strawberry Lemon Trifle

PREP/TOTAL TIME
Prep: 20 min. + chilling
YIELD 14 servings

NUTRITION FACTS
One serving
(1/2 cup) equals:
180 calories
1 g fat
0 g saturated fat
2 mg cholesterol
378 mg sodium
39 g carbohydrate
0 g fiber
6 g protein

DIABETIC EXCHANGES
2 starch
1/2 fruit

Layered in a glass bowl, this refreshingly fruity dessert looks so lovely that people will think you fussed. The secret is to start with a purchased angel food cake.

Lynn Marie Frucci, Pullman, Washington

4 ounces fat-free cream cheese, softened

1 cup fat-free vanilla yogurt

2 cups cold fat-free milk

1 package (3.4 ounces) instant lemon pudding mix

2 teaspoons grated lemon peel

2-1/2 cups sliced fresh strawberries, *divided*

1 tablespoon white grape juice *or* water

1 prepared angel food cake (10 inches)

1. In a mixing bowl, beat cream cheese and yogurt. Add the milk, pudding mix and lemon peel; beat until smooth. In a blender, process 1/2 cup strawberries and grape juice until smooth.

2. Tear cake into 1-in. cubes; place a third in a trifle bowl or 3-qt. serving bowl. Top with a third of the pudding mixture and half of the remaining strawberries. Drizzle with half of the strawberry sauce. Repeat. Top with the remaining cake and pudding mixture. Cover and refrigerate for at least 2 hours.

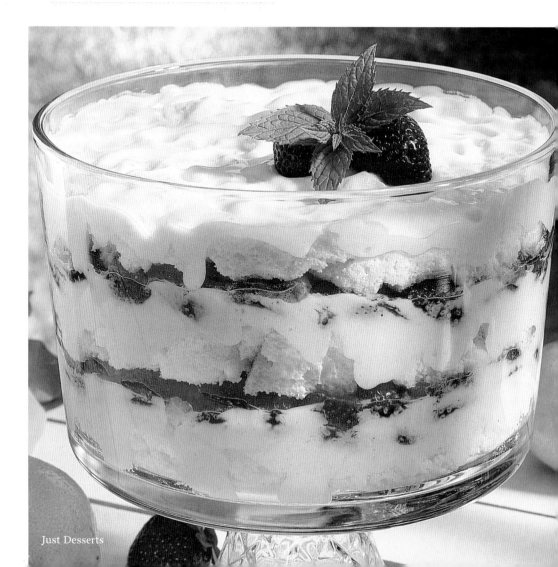

Raisin Carrot Cake

This lightened-up, moist cake is popular with my husband and son. I'm happy to make it for them every time they ask!

Joyce Donald, Star City, Saskatchewan

2	egg whites
3/4	cup sugar
1/2	cup unsweetened applesauce
1/4	cup canola oil
1-1/2	cups finely shredded carrots
1/2	cup reduced-fat vanilla yogurt
1/4	cup water
1	cup all-purpose flour, *divided*
1	cup whole wheat flour
2	teaspoons ground cinnamon
1-1/2	teaspoons baking soda
1/4	teaspoon salt
1/4	teaspoon ground nutmeg
1/4	teaspoon ground cloves
3/4	cup raisins
1-1/2	teaspoons confectioners' sugar

1. In a large bowl, beat egg whites until foamy. Add the sugar, applesauce and oil; mix well. Stir in the carrots, yogurt and water. Set aside 1 tablespoon all-purpose flour. Combine the whole wheat flour, cinnamon, baking soda, salt, nutmeg, cloves and remaining all-purpose flour; add to batter and mix just until moistened. Toss raisins with reserved flour; stir into batter.

2. Pour into a 9-in. square baking pan coated with cooking spray. Bake at 325° for 50-55 minutes or until a toothpick inserted near the center comes out clean. Cool on a wire rack. Sprinkle with confectioners' sugar.

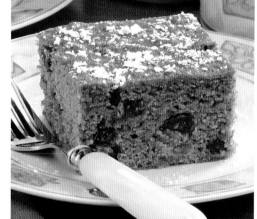

PREP/TOTAL TIME
Prep: 15 min.
Bake: 50 min. +
cooling
YIELD 9 servings

NUTRITION FACTS
One serving
(1 piece) equals:
279 calories
7 g fat
1 g saturated fat
1 mg cholesterol
306 mg sodium
52 g carbohydrate
4 g fiber
5 g protein

DIABETIC EXCHANGES
2-1/2 starch
1 fruit
1 fat

Peach-Topped Cake

With tender yellow cake on the bottom and a refreshing peach-filled gelatin on top, this bright orange dessert is perfect for summer.

Chris Lafser, Richmond, Virginia

2	tablespoons butter, softened
1/2	cup sugar
1	egg
1/2	teaspoon vanilla extract
3/4	cup cake flour
3/4	teaspoon baking powder
1/4	teaspoon salt
1/4	cup fat-free milk

TOPPING:

1	envelope unflavored gelatin
1-3/4	cups cold water, *divided*
1/4	cup sugar
1	envelope sugar-free orange soft drink mix
2	medium ripe peaches, thinly sliced or 1 can (15 ounces) sliced peaches
1/2	cup reduced-fat whipped topping

1. In a small bowl, beat butter and sugar until crumbly. Beat in egg and vanilla. Combine flour, baking powder and salt; add to sugar mixture alternately with milk.

2. Spread into a 9-in. springform pan coated with cooking spray. Bake at 350° for 10-15 minutes or until a toothpick inserted near the center comes out clean. Cool on a wire rack.

3. In a small saucepan, sprinkle gelatin over 1/2 cup cold water. Let stand for 1 minute. Stir in sugar and soft drink mix; cook and stir over low heat until gelatin is dissolved. Transfer to a large bowl; stir in remaining cold water. Refrigerate until partially set, about 1-1/2 hours.

4. Line outside of springform pan with foil. Arrange peaches over top of cake. Pour gelatin over peaches. Chill overnight. Just before serving, remove foil and sides of pan. Garnish with whipped topping. Refrigerate leftovers.

PREP/TOTAL TIME
Prep: 20 min. +
chilling
Bake: 10 min.
YIELD 12 servings

NUTRITION FACTS
One serving
(1 slice) equals:
121 calories
3 g fat
2 g saturated fat
23 mg cholesterol
103 mg sodium
22 g carbohydrate
Trace fiber
2 g protein

DIABETIC EXCHANGES
1 fruit
1/2 starch
1/2 fat

Double Chocolate Pie

PREP/TOTAL TIME
15 min. + chilling
YIELD 8 servings

If you thought your days of enjoying rich chocolate pies were over, think again! This pudding pie is a creamy, decadent delight.

Carol LaNaye Burnette, Sylvan Springs, Alabama

NUTRITION FACTS
One serving
(1 piece) equals:
191 calories
3 g fat
1 g saturated fat
1 mg cholesterol
426 mg sodium
34 g carbohydrate
Trace fiber
3 g protein

DIABETIC EXCHANGES
2 starch
1 fat

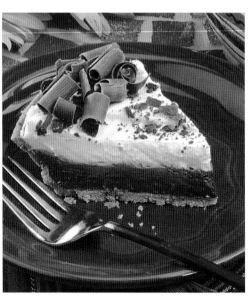

1-1/2 cups cold fat-free milk, *divided*

1 package (1.4 ounces) sugar-free instant chocolate fudge pudding mix

1 carton (8 ounces) frozen fat-free whipped topping, thawed, *divided*

1 reduced-fat graham cracker crust (8 inches)

1 package (1 ounce) sugar-free instant white chocolate *or* vanilla pudding mix

Semisweet chocolate curls and shavings, optional

1. In a bowl, whisk 3/4 cup milk and chocolate pudding mix for 2 minutes or until thickened. Fold in 1-3/4 cups whipped topping. Spread into crust.

2. In another bowl, whisk the remaining milk and white chocolate pudding mix for 2 minutes or until slightly thickened. Fold in remaining whipped topping. Spread over chocolate layer. Refrigerate for 4 hours or until set. Garnish with chocolate if desired.

Banana Split Ice Cream

PREP/TOTAL TIME
Prep: 20 min. + chilling
Freeze: overnight
YIELD about 2-1/2 quarts

This lightened-up ice cream dessert has all of the flavors of a classic banana split. I've been experimenting with ice cream recipes for years, and this one is a real treat.

Carol Dale, Greenville, Texas

NUTRITION FACTS
One serving
(1/2 cup) equals:
193 calories
3 g fat
0 g saturated fat
4 mg cholesterol
111 mg sodium
35 g carbohydrate
1 g fiber
8 g protein

DIABETIC EXCHANGES
1-1/2 fruit
1 milk
1 fat

5 cups fat-free milk, *divided*

1 cup egg substitute

2 cans (14 ounces *each*) fat-free sweetened condensed milk

2 medium ripe bananas, mashed

2 tablespoons lime juice

1 tablespoon vanilla extract

3/4 cup fat-free chocolate ice cream topping

1/2 cup chopped pecans

1/4 cup chopped maraschino cherries

1. In a heavy saucepan, combine 2-1/2 cups fat-free milk and egg substitute. Cook and stir over low heat until mixture is thick enough to coat a metal spoon and reaches at least 160°, about 10 minutes. Remove from the heat; set pan in ice and stir to cool quickly. Pour into a large bowl; stir in condensed milk and remaining fat-free milk. Cover and refrigerate overnight.

2. Combine bananas, lime juice and vanilla; stir into milk mixture. Fill ice cream freezer two-thirds full; freeze according to manufacturer's directions. Refrigerate remaining mixture until ready to freeze. Spoon each batch into a large freezer-safe container; gently fold in chocolate topping, pecans and cherries. Store in refrigerator freezer.

HERE'S THE SCOOP

When homemade ice cream has been in the freezer for more than 2 to 3 hours, it may need to stand at room temperature for 5 to 10 minutes for easier scooping.

Cappuccino Cupcakes

With fluffy whipped topping and a dusting of cocoa, these cupcakes are irresistible. Coffee flavor makes them even more special.

Carol Forcum, Marion, Illinois

- 2 cups all-purpose flour
- 1-1/2 cups sugar
- 1/2 cup baking cocoa
- 1 teaspoon baking soda
- 1/2 teaspoon salt
- 1/4 cup instant coffee granules
- 1/2 cup hot water
- 2 eggs
- 1/2 cup prune baby food
- 1/4 cup canola oil
- 2 teaspoons vanilla extract
- 1-1/2 cups reduced-fat whipped topping

Additional baking cocoa

1. In a bowl, combine flour, sugar, cocoa, baking soda and salt. Dissolve coffee granules in hot water. In another bowl, whisk the eggs, baby food, oil, vanilla and coffee mixture. Stir into dry ingredients just until moistened.

2. Fill paper-lined muffin cups two-thirds full. Bake at 350° for 18-20 minutes or until a toothpick comes out clean. Cool for 10 minutes before removing from pans to wire racks to cool completely. Just before serving, frost cupcakes with whipped topping and sprinkle with additional cocoa.

LOW FAT LOW SALT

PREP/TOTAL TIME
Prep: 15 min.
Bake: 20 min. + cooling
YIELD 17 cupcakes

NUTRITION FACTS
One serving
(1 cupcake) equals:
190 calories
5 g fat
1 g saturated fat
25 mg cholesterol
152 mg sodium
34 g carbohydrate
1 g fiber
3 g protein

DIABETIC EXCHANGES
2 starch
1 fat

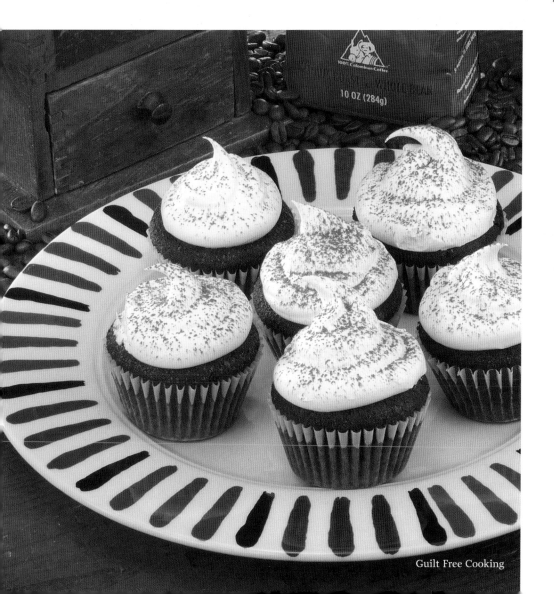

PREP/TOTAL TIME
Prep: 25 min. +
chilling
YIELD 12 servings

NUTRITION FACTS
One serving
(1 slice) equals:
227 calories
7 g fat
4 g saturated fat
7 mg cholesterol
457 mg sodium
30 g carbohydrate
2 g fiber
13 g protein

**DIABETIC
EXCHANGES**
2 starch
1 very lean
meat
1 fat

No-Bake Chocolate Cheesecake

Your family will fall in love with this sweet treat. Each silky, smooth slice is topped with juicy raspberries and a drizzle of white chocolate.

Taste of Home Test Kitchen

3/4 cup graham cracker crumbs

2 tablespoons reduced-fat margarine, melted

1 envelope unflavored gelatin

1 cup cold water

4 squares (1 ounce *each*) semisweet chocolate, coarsely chopped

4 packages (8 ounces *each*) fat-free cream cheese

Sugar substitute equivalent to 1 cup sugar

1/2 cup sugar

1/4 cup baking cocoa

2 teaspoons vanilla extract

TOPPING:

2 cups fresh raspberries

1 ounce white candy coating

1. In a bowl, combine cracker crumbs and margarine; press onto the bottom of a 9-in. springform pan. Place pan on a baking sheet. Bake at 375° for 8-10 minutes or until lightly browned. Cool on a wire rack.

2. For filling, in a small saucepan, sprinkle gelatin over cold water; let stand for 1 minute. Heat over low heat, stirring until gelatin is completely dissolved. Add the semisweet chocolate; stir until melted.

3. In a large bowl, beat the cream cheese, sugar substitute and sugar until smooth. Gradually add the chocolate mixture and cocoa. Beat in vanilla. Pour into the crust; refrigerate for 2-3 hours or until firm.

4. Arrange raspberries on top of cheesecake. In a heavy saucepan or microwave, melt the white candy coating; stir until smooth. Drizzle or pipe over the berries. Carefully run a knife around edge of pan to loosen. Remove sides of pan. Refrigerate leftovers.

Editor's Note: This recipe was tested with Parkay Light stick margarine and Splenda No Calorie Sweetener.

Gran's Apple Cake

Our grandmother occasionally brought over this wonderful cake warm from the oven. Its spicy apple flavor combined with the sweet cream cheese frosting was always a welcome treat. I've lightened up this recipe a bit since then, but it's still a family favorite.

Lauris Conrad, Turlock, California

1-2/3 cups sugar

2 eggs

1/2 cup unsweetened applesauce

2 tablespoons canola oil

2 teaspoons vanilla extract

2 cups all-purpose flour

2 teaspoons baking soda

2 teaspoons ground cinnamon

3/4 teaspoon salt

6 cups chopped peeled tart apples (about 5 medium)

1/2 cup chopped pecans

FROSTING:

4 ounces reduced-fat cream cheese

2 tablespoons butter, softened

1 teaspoon vanilla extract

1 cup confectioners' sugar

1. In a large bowl, combine the sugar, eggs, applesauce, oil and vanilla. Beat for 2 minutes on medium speed. Combine the flour, baking soda, cinnamon and salt; add to applesauce mixture and beat until combined. Fold in apples and pecans.

2. Transfer to a 13-in. x 9-in. x 2-in. baking dish coated with cooking spray. Bake at 350° for 35-40 minutes or until top is golden brown and a toothpick inserted near the center comes out clean. Cool on a wire rack.

3. For frosting, combine cream cheese, butter and vanilla in a small mixing bowl until smooth. Gradually beat in confectioners' sugar (mixture will be soft). Spread over cooled cake.

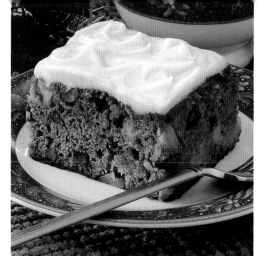

PREP/TOTAL TIME
Prep: 30 min.
Bake: 35 min.
YIELD 18 servings

NUTRITION FACTS
One serving
(1 piece) equals:
241 calories
8 g fat
2 g saturated fat
32 mg cholesterol
283 mg sodium
42 g carbohydrate
2 g fiber
3 g protein

DIABETIC EXCHANGES
2 starch
1-1/2 fat
1 fruit

Banana Cupcakes

This recipe came from my mother-in-law more than 40 years ago. The banana treats taste as good today as they did back then!

Arloia Lutz, Sebewaing, Michigan

1/3 cup shortening

2/3 cup sugar

1 egg

1 teaspoon vanilla extract

3/4 cup mashed ripe bananas (about 2 small)

1-1/3 cups cake flour

1 teaspoon baking powder

1/2 teaspoon salt

1/2 teaspoon baking soda

1/2 teaspoon ground cinnamon

1/2 teaspoon ground cloves

1/4 teaspoon ground nutmeg

1 tablespoon confectioners' sugar

1. In a mixing bowl, cream shortening and sugar. Add egg, vanilla and banana; mix well. Combine the flour, baking powder, salt, baking soda, cinnamon, cloves and nutmeg; add to the creamed mixture just until combined.

2. Fill paper-lined muffin cups two-thirds full. Bake at 375° for 18-20 minutes or until a toothpick comes out clean. Cool for 10 minutes before removing from pan to a wire rack to cool completely. Dust with confectioners' sugar.

PREP/TOTAL TIME
Prep: 15 min.
Bake: 20 min. + cooling
YIELD 1 dozen

NUTRITION FACTS
One serving
(1 cupcake) equals:
154 calories
6 g fat
2 g saturated fat
18 mg cholesterol
175 mg sodium
24 g carbohydrate
1 g fiber
2 g protein

DIABETIC EXCHANGES
1-1/2 starch
1 fat

Maple Pumpkin Pie

PREP/TOTAL TIME
Prep: 15 min. + chilling
Bake: 55 min.
YIELD 8 servings

NUTRITION FACTS
One serving
(1 piece) equals:
282 calories
10 g fat
1 g saturated fat
3 mg cholesterol
245 mg sodium
42 g carbohydrate
3 g fiber
8 g protein

DIABETIC EXCHANGES
2-1/2 starch
2 fat

Since I have to watch my saturated fat, I was happy to find this recipe for a good pumpkin pie. We love its mild maple flavor.

Betty Leonard, Steinhatchee, Florida

1-1/2 cups all-purpose flour
1 tablespoon sugar
1/2 teaspoon salt
1/4 teaspoon baking powder
1/3 cup canola oil
1 teaspoon cider vinegar
2 to 4 tablespoons cold water

FILLING:
1 can (15 ounces) solid-pack pumpkin
3/4 cup egg substitute
1/2 cup maple syrup
1 teaspoon ground cinnamon
1/2 teaspoon ground ginger
1/2 teaspoon maple flavoring
1/4 teaspoon ground nutmeg
1 cup fat-free evaporated milk

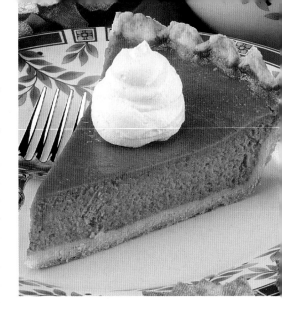

1. In a small bowl, combine the flour, sugar, salt and baking powder. Stir in oil and vinegar. Gradually add water, tossing with a fork until a ball forms. Shape into a 6-in. circle. Roll out between two pieces of plastic wrap to fit a 9-in. pie plate.

2. Remove top piece of plastic wrap; invert pastry into a 9-in. pie plate coated with cooking spray. Remove remaining plastic wrap. Trim pastry to 1/2 in. beyond edge of plate; flute edges. Refrigerate for 20 minutes or until chilled.

3. In a large bowl, combine the pumpkin, egg substitute, syrup, cinnamon, ginger, maple flavoring and nutmeg; mix just until blended. Gradually stir in milk. Pour into pastry shell.

4. Bake at 450° for 10 minutes. Reduce heat to 350°; bake for 45-50 minutes or until a knife inserted near center comes out clean. Cool on a wire rack. Store in refrigerator.

Cherry Meringue Dessert

PREP/TOTAL TIME
Prep: 35 min.
Bake: 1 hour + cooling
YIELD 15 servings

NUTRITION FACTS
One serving
(1 piece) equals:
108 calories
1 g fat
1 g saturated fat
0 mg cholesterol
18 mg sodium
23 g carbohydrate
Trace fiber
1 g protein

DIABETIC EXCHANGES
1 fruit
1/2 starch

A delicate meringue crust is filled with whipped topping and cherry pie filling for this pretty dessert. It looks impressive, but it couldn't be simpler to make.

Roberta Moellenberg, Idalia, Colorado

4 egg whites
1/4 teaspoon cream of tartar
1 teaspoon vanilla extract
1 cup sugar
2 cups reduced-fat whipped topping
1 can (20 ounces) reduced-sugar cherry pie filling

1. Place egg whites in a large mixing bowl; let stand at room temperature for 30 minutes. Add cream of tartar and vanilla; beat on medium speed until soft peaks form. Gradually beat in sugar, 1 tablespoon at a time, on high until stiff glossy peaks form and sugar is dissolved.

2. Spread onto the bottom and up the sides of a greased 13-in. x 9-in. x 2-in. baking dish. Bake at 275° for 1 hour; turn oven off (do not open door). Let meringue cool in oven for at least 8 hours or overnight. Just before serving, spread with whipped topping and top with pie filling.

Cran-Apple Crisp

Cranberries, walnuts, brown sugar and orange peel help give this apple-packed crowd-pleaser its delightful flavor. After the first taste, guests will be asking for the recipe...and a second helping.

Diane Everett, Newtown, Connecticut

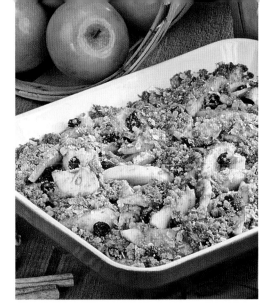

LOW SALT
PREP/TOTAL TIME
Prep: 15 min.
Bake: 40 min.
YIELD 15 servings

8 cups sliced peeled Granny Smith *or* other tart apples (about 5 large)

3/4 cup sugar

1/2 cup dried cranberries

1/2 cup chopped walnuts

1/4 cup all-purpose flour

1-1/2 to 2 teaspoons grated orange peel

1/2 cup packed brown sugar

1/3 cup whole wheat flour

1/3 cup nonfat dry milk powder

1 teaspoon ground cinnamon

1/4 to 1/2 teaspoon cloves

5 tablespoons cold butter

1/3 cup quick-cooking oats

1. In a large bowl, combine the first six ingredients; toss to coat. Transfer to a 13-in. x 9-in. x 2-in. baking dish coated with cooking spray.

2. For topping, in a small bowl, combine the brown sugar, whole wheat flour, milk powder, cinnamon and cloves. Cut in butter until mixture resembles coarse crumbs. Stir in oats. Sprinkle over apples. Bake, uncovered, at 350° for 40-45 minutes or until golden brown.

NUTRITION FACTS
One serving equals:
202 calories
7 g fat
3 g saturated fat
11 mg cholesterol
51 mg sodium
35 g carbohydrate
2 g fiber
2 g protein

DIABETIC EXCHANGES
1-1/2 fat
1 starch
1 fruit

Banana Cream Pie

Being diabetic doesn't stop me from having dessert—this smooth pie that uses sugar-free instant vanilla pudding is simply luscious!

Lila Case, Bella Vista, Arkansas

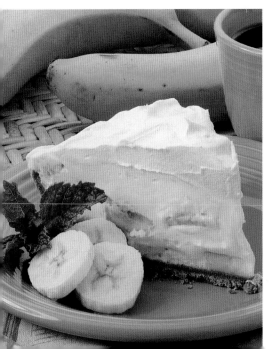

1-1/2 cups cold fat-free milk

1 package (1 ounce) sugar-free instant vanilla pudding mix

1/3 cup fat-free sour cream

1 carton (8 ounces) frozen reduced-fat whipped topping, thawed, *divided*

3 medium firm bananas, sliced

1 reduced-fat graham cracker crust (9 inches)

1. In a bowl, whisk milk and pudding mix for 2 minutes or until slightly thickened. Add sour cream; mix well. Fold in 1-1/2 cups whipped topping.

2. Place half of the banana slices in the crust; top with half of the pudding mixture. Repeat the layers. Spread with the remaining whipped topping. Refrigerate for 4-6 hours before serving (pie will be soft set). Refrigerate leftovers.

LOW SALT
PREP/TOTAL TIME
20 min. + chilling
YIELD 8 servings

NUTRITION FACTS
One serving
(1 piece) equals:
260 calories
7 g fat
5 g saturated fat
1 mg cholesterol
284 mg sodium
42 g carbohydrate
1 g fiber
4 g protein

DIABETIC EXCHANGES
2 starch
1 fruit

Chocolate Swirl Cake

This yummy chocolate cake won't ruin your waistline. Pretty swirls of cream cheese dress it up while cherry pie filling makes it moist.

Gail Maki, Marquette, Michigan

PREP/TOTAL TIME
Prep: 20 min.
Bake: 35 min. + cooling
YIELD 15 servings

NUTRITION FACTS
One serving
(1 slice) equals:
207 calories
5 g fat
2 g saturated fat
5 mg cholesterol
350 mg sodium
35 g carbohydrate
1 g fiber
5 g protein

DIABETIC EXCHANGES
1-1/2 starch
1 fat
1/2 fruit

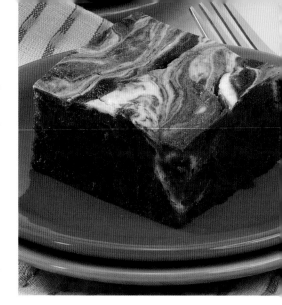

1 package (18-1/4 ounces) chocolate cake mix

1 can (20 ounces) reduced-sugar cherry pie filling

5 egg whites

1 teaspoon vanilla extract

TOPPING:

1 package (8 ounces) reduced-fat cream cheese

Sugar substitute equivalent to 1/3 cup sugar

1/2 teaspoon vanilla extract

2 egg whites

1. In a large bowl, combine the cake mix, pie filling, egg whites and vanilla just until moistened. Spread into a 13-in. x 9-in. x 2-in. baking dish coated with cooking spray; set aside.

2. In a small mixing bowl, beat the cream cheese, sugar substitute and vanilla. Add egg whites; beat on low speed just until combined. Spread over batter; cut through batter with a knife to swirl.

3. Bake at 350° for 35-40 minutes or until a toothpick inserted near the center comes out clean and topping is set. Cool on a wire rack. Store in the refrigerator.

Editor's Note: This recipe was tested with Splenda No Calorie Sweetener.

Marshmallow Fudge

It's nearly impossible to resist these rich chocolate squares chock-full of marshmallows and crunchy graham cracker pieces.

Holly Mann, Amherst, New Hampshire

PREP/TOTAL TIME
15 min. + chilling
YIELD 4 dozen

NUTRITION FACTS
One serving
(1 piece) equals:
41 calories
1 g fat
1 g saturated fat
1 mg cholesterol
10 mg sodium
7 g carbohydrate
1 g fiber
1 g protein

DIABETIC EXCHANGE
1/2 starch

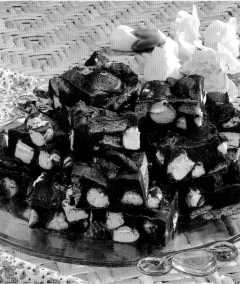

1-1/3 cups semisweet chocolate chips

2/3 cup fat-free sweetened condensed milk

1 teaspoon vanilla extract

1-1/3 cups miniature marshmallows

2 whole reduced-fat graham crackers, broken into bite-size pieces

1. Line an 8-in. square pan with foil and coat with cooking spray; set aside. In a heavy saucepan over low heat, melt chips with milk; stir until smooth. Remove from heat; cool for 2 minutes. Stir in vanilla. Fold in marshmallows and graham crackers.

2. Pour into prepared pan. Refrigerate for 1 hour or until firm. Lift out of the pan and remove foil; cut into 48 pieces.

Easy Cherry Cobbler

A warm and welcome ending to any meal, this cobbler tastes as comforting as it looks. Almond extract adds a flavor boost.

Sherry Craw, Mattoon, Illinois

- 1 can (20 ounces) reduced-sugar cherry pie filling
- 1/4 teaspoon almond extract
- 2 cups reduced-fat biscuit/baking mix
- 2 tablespoons plus 1 teaspoon sugar, *divided*
- 1/2 cup fat-free milk
- 2 tablespoons reduced-fat margarine, melted

1. In a large bowl, combine pie filling and extract; spread into a 9-in. deep-dish pie plate. Bake, uncovered, at 400° for 10 minutes. Meanwhile, in a bowl, combine the baking mix and 2 tablespoons sugar. In another bowl, combine the milk and margarine. Stir milk mixture into dry ingredients until a soft dough forms.

2. Drop the dough by spoonfuls over the warmed pie filling. Sprinkle with the remaining sugar. Bake, uncovered, at 400° for 20-25 minutes or until the topping is golden brown. Serve warm.

Editor's Note: This recipe was tested with Splenda No Calorie Sweetener.

LOW FAT

PREP/TOTAL TIME
Prep: 5 min.
Bake: 30 min.

YIELD 8 servings

NUTRITION FACTS
One serving
(1 cup) equals:
206 calories
4 g fat
1 g saturated fat
Trace cholesterol
393 mg sodium
40 g carbohydrate
1 g fiber
3 g protein

DIABETIC EXCHANGES
1-1/2 starch
1 fruit
1/2 fat

Sweet Potato Crisp

PREP/TOTAL TIME
Prep: 40 min.
Bake: 35 min.
YIELD 12 servings

NUTRITION FACTS
One serving equals:
180 calories
5 g fat
2 g saturated fat
9 mg cholesterol
140 mg sodium
29 g carbohydrate
3 g fiber
5 g protein

DIABETIC
EXCHANGES
2 starch
1 fat

This not-too-sweet potato and cranberry crisp has a buttery crumb topping. It's a nice change from candied sweet potatoes.

Kathy Hamsher, Moon Township, Pennsylvania

- 4 medium sweet potatoes, cooked, peeled and cubed
- 1 package (8 ounces) fat-free cream cheese
- 1/4 teaspoon ground cinnamon
- 2 medium apples, quartered
- 1 cup fresh *or* frozen cranberries
- 1/2 cup all-purpose flour
- 1/2 cup quick-cooking oats
- 1/2 cup packed brown sugar
- 3 tablespoons cold butter
- 1/4 cup chopped pecans

1. In a large mixing bowl, beat the sweet potatoes, cream cheese and cinnamon until smooth. Spread evenly into an 11-in. x 7-in. x 2-in. baking dish coated with cooking spray. Place apples and cranberries in a food processor; cover and process until chopped. Spread over sweet potato mixture.

2. In a small bowl, combine the flour, oats and brown sugar; cut in butter until mixture resembles coarse crumbs. Stir in pecans; sprinkle over filling. Bake, uncovered, at 350° for 35-40 minutes or until topping is golden brown and fruit is tender.

Caramel Chocolate Cheesecake Bites

PREP/TOTAL TIME
Prep: 15 min.
Bake: 15 min. + cooling
YIELD 3 dozen

NUTRITION FACTS
One serving (two mini cheesecakes) equals:
147 calories
8 g fat
3 g saturated fat
12 mg cholesterol
136 mg sodium
15 g carbohydrate
1 g fiber
5 g protein

DIABETIC
EXCHANGES
1-1/2 fat
1 starch

These tantalizing treats are the perfect size for people who like to try different desserts at parties. Baked in mini muffin cups, the caramel- and pecan-topped sweets offer a satisfying taste of rich cheesecake.

Barbara Nowakowski, North Tonawanda, New York

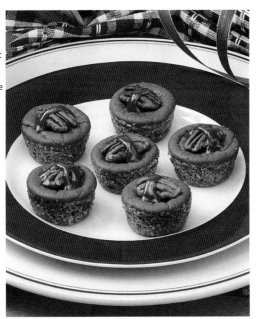

- 3/4 cup toasted wheat germ
- 2 packages (8 ounces *each*) reduced-fat cream cheese
- 3/4 cup sugar
- 1/3 cup baking cocoa
- 4 egg whites
- 1 teaspoon vanilla extract
- 36 pecan halves
- 3 tablespoons fat-free caramel ice cream topping

1. Coat 36 miniature muffin cups with cooking spray; generously coat each with wheat germ. Set aside. In a large bowl, beat cream cheese and sugar until smooth. Add cocoa; mix well. Beat in eggs and vanilla just until combined. Spoon 4 teaspoons into each muffin cup.

2. Bake at 350° for 13-16 minutes or until set. Cool in pans for 10 minutes before removing to wire racks. Cool for 30 minutes and refrigerate. (Cheesecake may sink in the center upon cooling.)

3. To serve, top each with a pecan. Microwave caramel topping on high for 10 seconds or until soft. Spoon 1/4 teaspoon over each.

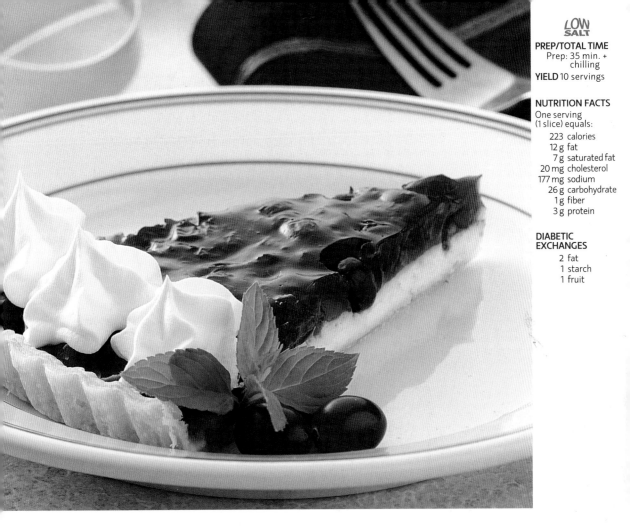

LOW SALT

PREP/TOTAL TIME
Prep: 35 min. +
chilling
YIELD 10 servings

NUTRITION FACTS
One serving
(1 slice) equals:
  223 calories
  12 g fat
  7 g saturated fat
20 mg cholesterol
177 mg sodium
26 g carbohydrate
1 g fiber
3 g protein

DIABETIC EXCHANGES
2 fat
1 starch
1 fruit

Cranberry Cheesecake Tart

If you need a dessert idea for Thanksgiving or Christmas dinner, consider this ruby-red tart. It looks gorgeous on the table and doesn't disappoint when you dig in.

Diane Halferty, Corpus Christi, Texas

Pastry for single-crust pie (9 inches)

- 1/3 cup sugar
- 2 tablespoons cornstarch
- 2/3 cup water
- 3 cups fresh or frozen cranberries

Sugar substitute equivalent to 1 tablespoon sugar

- 1 package (8 ounces) reduced-fat cream cheese
- 1-1/2 cups reduced-fat whipped topping, *divided*
- 1 teaspoon grated lemon peel

1. Press the pastry onto the bottom and up the sides of a 10-in. tart pan with removable bottom. Bake at 400° for 9-11 minutes or until lightly browned. Cool on a wire rack.

2. In a saucepan, combine sugar, cornstarch and water until smooth. Add cranberries. Bring to a boil over medium heat. Reduce heat to low; cook and stir for 3-5 minutes or until thickened and berries have popped. Remove from the heat; cool to room temperature. Stir in sugar substitute.

3. In a small mixing bowl, beat cream cheese and 1 cup whipped topping until smooth; add peel. Spread over pastry; top with berry mixture. Refrigerate for 2-4 hours or until set. Garnish with the remaining whipped topping.

LOW FAT **LOW SALT**

PREP/TOTAL TIME
Prep: 15 min. + chilling
YIELD 16 servings

Strawberry Banana Dessert

Like springtime on a plate, this eye-catching dessert has a bright cheery color and burst of refreshing fruit in every bite.

Margaret Kuntz, Bismarck, North Dakota

NUTRITION FACTS
One serving
(1 piece) equals:

138 calories
2 g fat
2 g saturated fat
0 mg cholesterol
168 mg sodium
27 g carbohydrate
1 g fiber
3 g protein

DIABETIC EXCHANGES
1 starch
1 fruit

3 medium firm bananas, sliced

1 prepared angel food cake (16 ounces), cut into 1-inch cubes

1 pint fresh strawberries, halved

1 package (.6 ounce) sugar-free strawberry gelatin

2 cups boiling water

1-1/2 cups cold water

1 carton (8 ounces) reduced-fat whipped topping, thawed

1. Layer banana slices and cake cubes in a 13-in. x 9-in. x 2-in. dish coated with nonstick cooking spray. Place strawberries over cake and press down gently.

2. In a bowl, dissolve gelatin in boiling water; stir in cold water. Pour over strawberries. Refrigerate for 3 hours or until set. Frost with whipped topping.

Alphabetical Index

A

Apple Cobbler, 231
Apple Cranberry Bread, 57
Apple Nut Bars, 215
Apricot Coffee Cake, 15
Asian Shrimp Soup, 53
Asparagus Ham Rolls, 144
Asparagus Tofu Stir-Fry, 189
Au Gratin Red Potatoes, 87
Autumn Pot Roast, 93

B

Bacon Ranch Dip, 32
Baked Basil Fries, 72
Baked Lentils with Cheese, 201
Baked Macaroni and Cheese, 194
Baked Pork Chimichangas, 156
Banana Cream Pie, 243
Banana Cupcakes, 241
Banana Split Cheesecake, 221
Banana Split Ice Cream, 238
Barbecued Turkey Pizza, 118
Barbecued Turkey Sandwiches, 126
Beef Fillets with Portobello Sauce, 101
Beef Minestrone, 40
Beef Noodle Casserole, 105
Bell Pepper Muffins, 58
Black Bean Fajitas, 188
Black Bean Soup, 44
Black Beans 'n' Rice, 152
Blondies with Chips, 218
BLT Tortillas, 146
Blueberry Crisp, 227
Blueberry Crumb Pie, 222
Blueberry Waffles, 20
Breaded Orange Roughy, 184
Breaded Pork Chops, 145
Breakfast Bake, 23
Brisket with Chunky Tomato Sauce, 100
Brisket with Gravy, 99
Broccoli Rice Hot Dish, 80
Broccoli Tuna Roll-Ups, 180
Broiled Parmesan Tomatoes, 90
Brown Rice 'n' Apple Stuffed Turkey, 119
Buttermilk Biscuits, 69
Buttermilk Blueberry Muffins, 13
Buttermilk Dill Bread, 65

C

Cabbage Rolls, 97
Canadian Bacon Potato Skins, 30
Cantonese Beef, 111
Cappuccino Cupcakes, 239
Cappuccino Shake, 31
Caramel Apple Dip, 36
Caramel Chocolate Cheesecake Bites, 246
Caramel-Pecan Cheese Pie, 230
Caramelized Pork Slices, 149
Catfish Jambalaya, 164
Cheese-Stuffed Potatoes, 89
Cheesy Potato Soup, 53
Cheesy Zucchini Medley, 86
Cherry Meringue Dessert, 242
Chicken 'n' Bean Tacos, 130
Chicken 'n' Biscuits, 139
Chicken Cacciatore, 132

Chicken Dressing Casserole, 138
Chicken-Fried Steak, 103
Chicken in Creamy Gravy, 132
Chicken Jambalaya, 122
Chicken Lasagna, 125
Chicken Noodle Casserole, 123
Chicken Pasta Primavera, 130
Chicken Pepper Fajitas, 136
Chicken Stew, 49
Chive Garden Rolls, 61
Chocolate Angel Food Cake, 220
Chocolate Banana Smoothies, 38
Chocolate Cappuccino Cookies, 206
Chocolate Macaroon Cupcakes, 232
Chocolate Marvel Cake, 225
Chocolate Swirl Cake, 244
Chuck Wagon Wraps, 110
Cilantro Lime Cod, 168
Cinnamon Buns, 22
Cinnamon Pecan Ring, 24
Cocoa Chip Cookies, 212
Confetti Barley Pilaf, 74
Confetti Potato Pancakes, 85
Confetti Salmon Steaks, 176
Country Raisin Rye Bread, 64
Crab Cakes, 165
Crab Rice Primavera, 183
Cran-Apple Crisp, 243
Cranberry Cheesecake Bars, 217
Cranberry Cheesecake Tart, 247
Cranberry-Mustard Pork Medallions, 162
Cranberry Oat Cookies, 213
Cream Cheese Bonbons, 235
Cream Cheese Ham Omelet, 19
Cream Cheese Swirl Brownies, 214
Creamy Apple Crumb Pie, 226
Creamy Broccoli Casserole, 88
Creamy Chicken Rice Soup, 43
Creamy Fruit Salad, 86
Creamy Guacamole, 35
Creamy Ham Turnovers, 158
Creole Catfish Fillets, 167
Creole Sausage and Vegetables, 160
Crispy Baked Cauliflower, 81
Crispy French Toast, 10
Crumb-Topped Scallops, 164
Crustless Mushroom Spinach Tart, 204
Crustless Spinach Quiche, 17

D

Dilly Potato Salad, 90
Double Chocolate Pie, 238
Double-Decker Banana Cups, 233
Double Peanut Bars, 207
Down-Home Pot Roast, 95

E

Easy Beef Goulash, 108
Easy Cherry Cobbler, 245
Egg Foo Yong with Sauce, 192
Eggs Florentine, 19

F

Fettuccine Italiana, 124
Five-Veggie Stir-Fry, 201
Flank Steak with Horseradish Sauce, 112
Flavorful Meat Loaf, 107

Fried Rice, 85
Frosted Pumpkin Bars, 206
Frosted Spice Cake, 226
Fruit Crepes, 10
Fruit Kabobs, 21
Fudgy Brownie Dessert, 228
Fudgy Fruit Dip, 36

G

Garden Frittata, 12
Garlic Cheese Breadsticks, 59
Garlic-Chive Mashed Potatoes, 75
Gingerbread Cookies, 210
Gingered Beef Stir-Fry, 101
Gran's Apple Cake, 241
Great Grain Burgers, 196
Green Bean Corn Casserole, 89
Grilled Breaded Chicken, 139
Grilled Halibut with Mustard Dill Sauce, 182

H

Ham and Apple Skillet, 11
Ham 'n' Cheese Muffins, 56
Ham and Lima Bean Soup, 50
Ham and Red Beans, 157
Ham Mushroom Fettuccine, 148
Ham Noodle Casserole, 161
Ham with Orange Sauce, 146
Harvest Soup, 42
Hash Brown Cheese Omelet, 20
Hearty Brunch Potatoes, 23
Hearty Oatmeal Pancakes, 18
Hearty Taco Casserole, 113
Herb-Stuffed Pork Loin, 161
Herbed Stuffed Green Peppers, 122
Homemade Fish Fingers, 170
Home-Style Coleslaw, 78
Home-Style Country Sausage, 17
Honey Spice Cookies, 208
Horseradish-Crusted Turkey Tenderloins, 116
Hot Cross Buns, 62
Hot Swiss Chicken Sandwiches, 136

I

Iced Coffee, 28
Irish Stew, 43
Italian Bread Wedges, 60
Italian-Sausage Pepper Sandwiches, 145
Italian Shepherd's Pie, 110
Italian Turkey and Noodles, 131
Italian Vegetable Soup, 52
Italian Zucchini Bake, 197

J

Jalapeno Corn Bread, 63

L

Lemon Chiffon Cake, 229
Lemon Dill Walleye, 173
Lemon Ginger Muffins, 11
Lentil Sausage Soup, 49
Light Chicken Cordon Bleu, 121
Light Sweet Potato Casserole, 76
Light Tiramisu, 225
Lime Fish Tacos, 181

M

Maple-Glazed Grilled Salmon, 178
Maple-Glazed Parsnips and Carrots, 79
Maple Oat Bread, 68
Maple Pumpkin Pie, 242
Marinated Barbecued Chicken, 137
Marshmallow Fudge, 244
Mashed Potato Bake, 78
Mediterranean Beef Toss, 100
Mediterranean Pork and Orzo, 154
Mediterranean Seafood Chowder, 46
Mediterranean-Style Red Snapper, 183
Mexican Bean 'n' Barley Chili, 202
Mexican Pork Stew, 41
Moist Ham Loaf, 159
Molded Cranberry Fruit Salad, 88
Mushroom Barley Soup, 44
Mushroom Broccoli Pizza, 200
Mushroom Cheese Chicken, 133
Mushroom Chicken Pizza, 135
Mushroom Pizza Burgers, 92
Mustard-Glazed Pork Chops, 153

N

No-Bake Chocolate Cheesecake, 240
No-Yolk Deviled Eggs, 34
Nostalgic Chicken and Dumplings, 120

O

Oatmeal Raisin Cookies, 212
Old-World Sauerbraten, 112
One-Pot Pork and Rice, 157
Onion Beef Stroganoff, 107
Onion Cheese Ball, 34
Onion-Garlic Bubble Bread, 70
Onion Herb Biscuits, 67
Open-Face Tuna Melts, 171
Open-Faced Meatball Sandwiches, 102
Orange Chocolate Chip Bread, 59
Orange-Cinnamon French Toast, 13
Orange Pineapple Torte, 227
Oven Fish 'n' Chips, 175
Oven-Fried Chicken, 125
Oven Swiss Steak, 104

P

Pasta-Filled Peppers, 193
Peach Scones, 60
Peach-Topped Cake, 237
Peanut Butter Chocolate Pudding, 222
Peanut Butter Cookies, 209
Pecan Cookies, 211
Pecan Waffles, 14
Penne Sausage Bake, 134
Pepper-Crusted Pork Tenderloin, 147
Perch with Cucumber Relish, 166
Pineapple Almond Bars, 215
Pineapple Coconut Squares, 208
Pineapple Iced Tea, 26
Pineapple Upside-Down Cake, 234
Polynesian Kabobs, 152
Pork 'n' Veggie Packets, 149
Pork Chops with Red Cabbage, 147
Pork Lo Mein, 143
Pork Picante, 142
Pork Soft-Shell Tacos, 155

R

Raisin Carrot Cake, 237
Ranch Tortilla Roll-Ups, 27
Raspberry Coffee Cake, 16
Raspberry Cream Smoothies, 29
Raspberry Nut Bars, 211
Raspberry Pear Crisp, 229
Refreshing Lime Pie, 232
Refried Bean Enchiladas, 203
Rhubarb-Topped Cheesecake, 224
Ribbon Pumpkin Bread, 66
Roasted Garlic and Pepper Pizza, 194
Root Vegetable Beef Stew, 51

S

Salisbury Steak with Gravy, 96
Salmon with Dill Sauce, 185
Salsa Chicken Skillet, 119
Salsa Potato Salad, 81
Salsa Red Beans 'n' Rice, 76
Salsa Tuna Salad, 178
Saucy Turkey Meatballs, 26
Sausage Bow Tie Salad, 151
Sausage Breakfast Wraps, 14
Sausage Corn Bread Dressing, 77
Savory 'n' Saucy Baked Beans, 75
Savory Roasted Chicken, 116
Scallops and Asparagus Stir-Fry, 171
Sea Scallops and Mushrooms, 174
Seasoned Scrambled Eggs, 16
Seasoned Snack Mix, 31
Seasoned Turkey Burgers, 120
Shredded Beef Barbecue, 104
Shrimp 'n' Veggie Pizza, 172
Shrimp Salad Bagels, 170
Shrimp Tartlets, 37
Shrimp with Creole Sauce, 29
Sirloin Veggie Kabobs, 94
Skillet Ole, 98
Skinny Crab Quiche, 177
Slow-Cooked Pork Roast, 154
Slow Cooker Beef Au Jus, 108
Smoked Salmon Spread, 33
Smoked Sausage with Pasta, 117
Snapper with Spicy Pineapple Glaze, 186
Soft Gingersnaps, 216
Southwest Lasagna Rolls, 196
Southwestern Broccoli Cheese Soup, 48
Southwestern Hominy, 79
Spaghetti Casserole, 199
Spaghetti with Italian Meatballs, 109
Spanish Chicken and Rice, 123
Spanish Rice with Bacon, 73
Spiced Beef Roast, 114
Spiced Pear Bread, 63
Spiced Tomato Drink, 35
Spiced Tomato Soup, 47
Spicy Haddock, 181
Spicy Shrimp Wraps, 179
Spinach Burritos, 192
Spinach Cheese Enchiladas, 188
Spinach Manicotti, 197
Steak Chili, 50
Steak Fajitas, 92
Stir-Fried Chicken Marinara, 126
Strawberry Banana Dessert, 248
Strawberry Cheesecake Ice Cream, 223

Strawberry Cream Cheese Pie, 234
Strawberry Lemon Trifle, 236
Strawberry Slush, 33
Stuffed Cornish Hens, 128
Stuffed Flank Steak, 103
Stuffed Mountain Trout, 174
Stuffed Mushrooms, 28
Superb Herb Bread, 69
Sweet 'n' Savory Apple Stuffing, 83
Sweet-and-Sour Chicken, 129
Sweet and Sour Ham, 150
Sweet Pepper Sandwiches, 195
Sweet Potato Apple Scallop, 72
Sweet Potato Crisp, 246
Sweet Potato Yeast Rolls, 56

T

Taco Fish, 184
Taco Soup, 47
Tangy Onion Flowers, 82
Tangy Pork Barbecue, 142
Tart Cherry Pie, 230
Tasty Lentil Tacos, 190
Tender Chicken Nuggets, 135
Teriyaki Pork, 150
Tex-Mex Lasagna, 106
Three-Bean Casserole, 84
Three-Bean Cassoulet, 199
Three-Bean Chili, 54
Three Grain Pan Rolls, 65
Toasted Veggie Sandwich, 202
Tomato Baked Haddock, 177
Tomato Ham Pasta, 158
Tomato-Topped Cod, 173
Tortellini Primavera, 191
Tortilla Pie, 98
Tropical Tenderloin Steaks, 96
Tuna Noodle Casserole, 167
Tuna Patties with Dill Sauce, 168
Turkey 'n' Beef Loaf, 138
Turkey Biscuit Potpie, 127
Turkey Dumpling Stew, 45
Turkey Noodle Soup, 40
Turkey Sloppy Joes, 129
Turkey Tetrazzini, 133

V

Veggie Burgers, 204
Veggie Macaroni Salad, 82
Veggie Pockets, 191
Very Berry Pie, 220

W

Walnut Oat Brownies, 216
Walnut Wheat Bread, 62
Wild Rice Chicken Bake, 140

Z

Zippy Burgers, 95
Zippy Shrimp Linguine, 169
Zippy White Chili, 46
Zucchini Beef Lasagna, 105
Zucchini Bread, 66
Zucchini Crepes, 198

General Index

APPLES
Apple Cobbler, 231
Apple Cranberry Bread, 57
Apple Nut Bars, 215
Brown Rice 'n' Apple Stuffed Turkey, 119
Caramel Apple Dip, 36
Cran-Apple Crisp, 243
Creamy Apple Crumb Pie, 226
Gran's Apple Cake, 241
Ham and Apple Skillet, 11
Sweet 'n' Savory Apple Stuffing, 83
Sweet Potato Apple Scallop, 72

ASPARAGUS
Asparagus Ham Rolls, 144
Asparagus Tofu Stir-Fry, 189
Scallops and Asparagus Stir-Fry, 171

BACON & CANADIAN BACON
Bacon Ranch Dip, 32
BLT Tortillas, 146
Canadian Bacon Potato Skins, 30
Spanish Rice with Bacon, 73

BANANAS
Banana Cream Pie, 243
Banana Cupcakes, 241
Banana Split Cheesecake, 221
Banana Split Ice Cream, 238
Chocolate Banana Smoothies, 38
Double-Decker Banana Cups, 233
Strawberry Banana Dessert, 248

BEANS & LENTILS
Baked Lentils with Cheese, 201
Black Bean Fajitas, 188
Black Bean Soup, 44
Black Beans 'n' Rice, 152
Chicken 'n' Bean Tacos, 130
Green Bean Corn Casserole, 89
Ham and Lima Bean Soup, 50
Ham and Red Beans, 157
Lentil Sausage Soup, 49
Mexican Bean 'n' Barley Chili, 202
Refried Bean Enchiladas, 203
Salsa Red Beans 'n' Rice, 76
Savory 'n' Saucy Baked Beans, 75
Tasty Lentil Tacos, 190
Tex-Mex Lasagna, 106
Three-Bean Casserole, 84
Three-Bean Cassoulet, 199
Three-Bean Chili, 54

BEEF (also see Ground Beef)
Autumn Pot Roast, 93
Beef Fillets with Portobello Sauce, 101
Brisket with Chunky Tomato Sauce, 100
Brisket with Gravy, 99
Cantonese Beef, 111
Chicken-Fried Steak, 103
Down-Home Pot Roast, 95
Easy Beef Goulash, 108
Flank Steak with Horseradish Sauce, 112
Gingered Beef Stir-Fry, 101
Old-World Sauerbraten, 112
Onion Beef Stroganoff, 107
Oven Swiss Steak, 104
Shredded Beef Barbecue, 104
Sirloin Veggie Kabobs, 94
Slow Cooker Beef Au Jus, 108
Spiced Beef Roast, 114
Steak Chili, 50

Steak Fajitas, 92
Stuffed Flank Steak, 103
Tropical Tenderloin Steaks, 96

BLUEBERRIES
Blueberry Crisp, 227
Blueberry Crumb Pie, 222
Blueberry Waffles, 20
Buttermilk Blueberry Muffins, 13
Very Berry Pie, 220

BREADS & ROLLS
Apple Cranberry Bread, 57
Apricot Coffee Cake, 15
Bell Pepper Muffins, 58
Buttermilk Biscuits, 69
Buttermilk Blueberry Muffins, 13
Buttermilk Dill Bread, 65
Chive Garden Rolls, 61
Cinnamon Buns, 22
Cinnamon Pecan Ring, 24
Country Raisin Rye Bread, 64
Garlic Cheese Breadsticks, 59
Ham 'n' Cheese Muffins, 56
Hot Cross Buns, 62
Italian Bread Wedges, 60
Jalapeno Corn Bread, 63
Lemon Ginger Muffins, 11
Maple Oat Bread, 68
Onion-Garlic Bubble Bread, 70
Onion Herb Biscuits, 67
Orange Chocolate Chip Bread, 59
Peach Scones, 60
Raspberry Coffee Cake, 16
Ribbon Pumpkin Bread, 66
Spiced Pear Bread, 63
Superb Herb Bread, 69
Sweet Potato Yeast Rolls, 56
Three Grain Pan Rolls, 65
Walnut Wheat Bread, 62
Zucchini Bread, 66

BREAKFAST & BRUNCH
Apricot Coffee Cake, 15
Blueberry Waffles, 20
Breakfast Bake, 23
Buttermilk Blueberry Muffins, 13
Cinnamon Buns, 22
Cinnamon Pecan Ring, 24
Cream Cheese Ham Omelet, 19
Crispy French Toast, 10
Crustless Spinach Quiche, 17
Eggs Florentine, 19
Fruit Crepes, 10
Fruit Kabobs, 21
Garden Frittata, 12
Ham and Apple Skillet, 11
Hash Brown Cheese Omelet, 20
Hearty Brunch Potatoes, 23
Hearty Oatmeal Pancakes, 18
Home-Style Country Sausage, 17
Lemon Ginger Muffins, 11
Orange-Cinnamon French Toast, 13
Pecan Waffles, 14
Raspberry Coffee Cake, 16
Sausage Breakfast Wraps, 14
Seasoned Scrambled Eggs, 16

BROCCOLI & CAULIFLOWER
Broccoli Rice Hot Dish, 80
Broccoli Tuna Roll-Ups, 180
Creamy Broccoli Casserole, 88
Crispy Baked Cauliflower, 81

Mushroom Broccoli Pizza, 200
Southwestern Broccoli Cheese Soup, 48

CABBAGE
Cabbage Rolls, 97
Home-Style Coleslaw, 78
Pork Chops with Red Cabbage, 147

CARROTS
Maple-Glazed Parsnips and Carrots, 79
Raisin Carrot Cake, 237

CHEESE
Au Gratin Red Potatoes, 87
Baked Lentils with Cheese, 201
Baked Macaroni and Cheese, 194
Banana Split Cheesecake, 221
Broiled Parmesan Tomatoes, 90
Caramel Chocolate Cheesecake Bites, 246
Caramel-Pecan Cheese Pie, 230
Cheese-Stuffed Potatoes, 89
Cheesy Potato Soup, 53
Cheesy Zucchini Medley, 86
Cranberry Cheesecake Bars, 217
Cranberry Cheesecake Tart, 247
Cream Cheese Bonbons, 235
Cream Cheese Ham Omelet, 19
Cream Cheese Swirl Brownies, 214
Garlic Cheese Breadsticks, 59
Ham 'n' Cheese Muffins, 56
Hash Brown Cheese Omelet, 20
Hot Swiss Chicken Sandwiches, 136
Light Chicken Cordon Bleu, 121
Mushroom Cheese Chicken, 133
No-Bake Chocolate Cheesecake, 240
Onion Cheese Ball, 34
Open-Face Tuna Melts, 171
Rhubarb-Topped Cheesecake, 224
Southwestern Broccoli Cheese Soup, 48
Spinach Cheese Enchiladas, 188
Strawberry Cheesecake Ice Cream, 223
Strawberry Cream Cheese Pie, 234

CHERRIES
Cherry Meringue Dessert, 242
Chocolate Swirl Cake, 244
Easy Cherry Cobbler, 245
Tart Cherry Pie, 230

CHICKEN
Main Dishes
Chicken 'n' Bean Tacos, 130
Chicken 'n' Biscuits, 139
Chicken Cacciatore, 132
Chicken Dressing Casserole, 138
Chicken in Creamy Gravy, 132
Chicken Jambalaya, 122
Chicken Lasagna, 125
Chicken Noodle Casserole, 123
Chicken Pasta Primavera, 130
Chicken Pepper Fajitas, 136
Grilled Breaded Chicken, 139
Hot Swiss Chicken Sandwiches, 136
Light Chicken Cordon Bleu, 121
Marinated Barbecued Chicken, 137
Mushroom Cheese Chicken, 133
Mushroom Chicken Pizza, 135
Nostalgic Chicken and Dumplings, 120
Oven-Fried Chicken, 125
Salsa Chicken Skillet, 119
Savory Roasted Chicken, 116
Spanish Chicken and Rice, 123
Stir-Fried Chicken Marinara, 126

CHICKEN
Main Dishes *(continued)*
Sweet-and-Sour Chicken, 129
Tender Chicken Nuggets, 135
Wild Rice Chicken Bake, 140
Soups & Stew
Black Bean Soup, 44
Chicken Stew, 49
Creamy Chicken Rice Soup, 43
Zippy White Chili, 46

CHOCOLATE
Caramel Chocolate Cheesecake Bites, 246
Chocolate Angel Food Cake, 220
Chocolate Banana Smoothies, 38
Chocolate Cappuccino Cookies, 206
Chocolate Macaroon Cupcakes, 232
Chocolate Marvel Cake, 225
Chocolate Swirl Cake, 244
Cocoa Chip Cookies, 212
Cream Cheese Swirl Brownies, 214
Double Chocolate Pie, 238
Fudgy Brownie Dessert, 228
Fudgy Fruit Dip, 36
Marshmallow Fudge, 244
No-Bake Chocolate Cheesecake, 240
Orange Chocolate Chip Bread, 59
Peanut Butter Chocolate Pudding, 222
Walnut Oat Brownies, 216

COOKIES & BARS
Apple Nut Bars, 215
Blondies with Chips, 218
Chocolate Cappuccino Cookies, 206
Cocoa Chip Cookies, 212
Cranberry Cheesecake Bars, 217
Cranberry Oat Cookies, 213
Cream Cheese Swirl Brownies, 214
Double Peanut Bars, 207
Frosted Pumpkin Bars, 206
Gingerbread Cookies, 210
Honey Spice Cookies, 208
Oatmeal Raisin Cookies, 212
Peanut Butter Cookies, 209
Pecan Cookies, 211
Pineapple Almond Bars, 215
Pineapple Coconut Squares, 208
Raspberry Nut Bars, 211
Soft Gingersnaps, 216
Walnut Oat Brownies, 216

COFFEE
Cappuccino Cupcakes, 239
Chocolate Cappuccino Cookies, 206
Light Tiramisu, 225

CORN & CORNMEAL
Green Bean Corn Casserole, 89
Jalapeno Corn Bread, 63
Sausage Corn Bread Dressing, 77

CORNISH HENS
Stuffed Cornish Hens, 128

CRANBERRIES
Apple Cranberry Bread, 57
Cran-Apple Crisp, 243
Cranberry Cheesecake Bars, 217
Cranberry Cheesecake Tart, 247
Cranberry-Mustard Pork Medallions, 162
Cranberry Oat Cookies, 213
Molded Cranberry Fruit Salad, 88

DESSERTS (also see Cookies & Bars)
Apple Cobbler, 231
Banana Cream Pie, 243
Banana Cupcakes, 241

Banana Split Cheesecake, 221
Banana Split Ice Cream, 238
Blueberry Crisp, 227
Blueberry Crumb Pie, 222
Cappuccino Cupcakes, 239
Caramel Chocolate Cheesecake Bites, 246
Caramel-Pecan Cheese Pie, 230
Cherry Meringue Dessert, 242
Chocolate Angel Food Cake, 220
Chocolate Macaroon Cupcakes, 232
Chocolate Marvel Cake, 225
Chocolate Mousse, 249
Chocolate Swirl Cake, 244
Cran-Apple Crisp, 243
Cranberry Cheesecake Tart, 247
Cream Cheese Bonbons, 235
Creamy Apple Crumb Pie, 226
Double Chocolate Pie, 238
Double-Decker Banana Cups, 233
Easy Cherry Cobbler, 245
Fluffy Pistachio Dessert, 249
Frosted Spice Cake, 226
Fudgy Brownie Dessert, 228
Gran's Apple Cake, 241
Lemon Chiffon Cake, 229
Light Tiramisu, 225
Maple Pumpkin Pie, 242
Marshmallow Fudge, 244
No-Bake Chocolate Cheesecake, 240
Orange Pineapple Torte, 227
Peach-Topped Cake, 237
Peanut Butter Chocolate Pudding, 222
Pineapple Upside-Down Cake, 234
Raisin Carrot Cake, 237
Raspberry Pear Crisp, 229
Refreshing Lime Pie, 232
Rhubarb-Topped Cheesecake, 224
Strawberry Banana Dessert, 248
Strawberry Cheesecake Ice Cream, 223
Strawberry Cream Cheese Pie, 234
Strawberry Lemon Trifle, 236
Sweet Potato Crisp, 246
Tart Cherry Pie, 230
Very Berry Pie, 220

EGGS & EGG SUBSTITUTE
Breakfast Bake, 23
Cream Cheese Ham Omelet, 19
Crustless Mushroom Spinach Tart, 204
Crustless Spinach Quiche, 17
Egg Foo Yong with Sauce, 192
Eggs Florentine, 19
Garden Frittata, 12
Ham and Apple Skillet, 11
Hash Brown Cheese Omelet, 20
No-Yolk Deviled Eggs, 34
Sausage Breakfast Wraps, 14
Seasoned Scrambled Eggs, 16
Skinny Crab Quiche, 177

FISH & SEAFOOD
Main Dishes
Breaded Orange Roughy, 184
Broccoli Tuna Roll-Ups, 180
Catfish Jambalaya, 164
Cilantro Lime Cod, 168
Confetti Salmon Steaks, 176
Crab Cakes, 165
Crab Rice Primavera, 183
Creole Catfish Fillets, 167
Crumb-Topped Scallops, 164
Grilled Halibut with
  Mustard Dill Sauce, 182
Homemade Fish Fingers, 170
Lemon Dill Walleye, 173
Lime Fish Tacos, 181

Maple-Glazed Grilled Salmon, 178
Mediterranean-Style Red Snapper, 183
Oven Fish 'n' Chips, 175
Perch with Cucumber Relish, 166
Salmon with Dill Sauce, 185
Salsa Tuna Salad, 178
Scallops and Asparagus Stir-Fry, 171
Sea Scallops and Mushrooms, 174
Shrimp 'n' Veggie Pizza, 172
Skinny Crab Quiche, 177
Snapper with Spicy Pineapple Glaze, 186
Spicy Haddock, 181
Stuffed Mountain Trout, 174
Taco Fish, 184
Tomato Baked Haddock, 177
Tomato-Topped Cod, 173
Tuna Noodle Casserole, 167
Tuna Patties with Dill Sauce, 168
Zippy Shrimp Linguine, 169
Sandwiches
Open-Face Tuna Melts, 171
Shrimp Salad Bagels, 170
Spicy Shrimp Wraps, 179
Snacks
Shrimp Tartlets, 37
Shrimp with Creole Sauce, 29
Smoked Salmon Spread, 33
Soups
Asian Shrimp Soup, 53
Mediterranean Seafood Chowder, 46

FRUIT (also see specific kinds)
Creamy Fruit Salad, 86
Fruit Kabobs, 21
Molded Cranberry Fruit Salad, 88

GROUND BEEF
Main Dishes
Beef Noodle Casserole, 105
Cabbage Rolls, 97
Flavorful Meat Loaf, 107
Hearty Taco Casserole, 113
Italian Shepherd's Pie, 110
Mediterranean Beef Toss, 100
Salisbury Steak with Gravy, 96
Skillet Ole, 98
Spaghetti with Italian Meatballs, 109
Tex-Mex Lasagna, 106
Tortilla Pie, 98
Turkey 'n' Beef Loaf, 138
Zucchini Beef Lasagna, 105
Sandwiches
Chuck Wagon Wraps, 110
Mushroom Pizza Burgers, 92
Open-Faced Meatball Sandwiches, 102
Zippy Burgers, 95
Soups & Stew
Beef Minestrone, 40
Harvest Soup, 42
Root Vegetable Beef Stew, 51
Taco Soup, 47

HAM
Breakfast & Brunch
Cream Cheese Ham Omelet, 19
Ham and Apple Skillet, 11
Main Dishes
Black Beans 'n' Rice, 152
Ham and Red Beans, 157
Ham Mushroom Fettuccine, 148
Ham Noodle Casserole, 161
Ham with Orange Sauce, 146
Light Chicken Cordon Bleu, 121
Moist Ham Loaf, 159
Sweet and Sour Ham, 150
Tomato Ham Pasta, 158

Sandwiches & Soup
  Asparagus Ham Rolls, 144
  Creamy Ham Turnovers, 158
  Ham and Lima Bean Soup, 50

LAMB
Irish Stew, 43

LEMONS & LIMES
Cilantro Lime Cod, 168
Lemon Chiffon Cake, 229
Lemon Dill Walleye, 173
Lemon Ginger Muffins, 11
Lime Fish Tacos, 181
Refreshing Lime Pie, 232
Strawberry Lemon Trifle, 236

LOW-FAT RECIPES
Breads & Rolls
  Apple Cranberry Bread, 57
  Bell Pepper Muffins, 58
  Buttermilk Biscuits, 69
  Buttermilk Dill Bread, 65
  Country Raisin Rye Bread, 64
  Garlic Cheese Breadsticks, 59
  Hot Cross Buns, 62
  Italian Bread Wedges, 60
  Jalapeno Corn Bread, 63
  Maple Oat Bread, 68
  Onion-Garlic Bubble Bread, 70
  Orange Chocolate Chip Bread, 59
  Peach Scones, 60
  Ribbon Pumpkin Bread, 66
  Spiced Pear Bread, 63
  Superb Herb Bread, 69
  Sweet Potato Yeast Rolls, 56
  Three Grain Pan Rolls, 65
  Walnut Wheat Bread, 62
Breakfast & Brunch
  Blueberry Waffles, 20
  Buttermilk Blueberry Muffins, 13
  Cinnamon Buns, 22
  Crispy French Toast, 10
  Crustless Spinach Quiche, 17
  Fruit Crepes, 10
  Fruit Kabobs, 21
  Hearty Brunch Potatoes, 23
  Home-Style Country Sausage, 17
  Lemon Ginger Muffins, 11
  Orange-Cinnamon French Toast, 13
  Raspberry Coffee Cake, 16
Cookies & Bars
  Apple Nut Bars, 215
  Chocolate Cappuccino Cookies, 206
  Cocoa Chip Cookies, 212
  Cranberry Cheesecake Bars, 217
  Cranberry Oat Cookies, 213
  Gingerbread Cookies, 210
  Honey Spice Cookies, 208
  Oatmeal Raisin Cookies, 212
  Peanut Butter Cookies, 209
  Pecan Cookies, 211
  Pineapple Almond Bars, 215
  Raspberry Nut Bars, 211
  Soft Gingersnaps, 216
Desserts
  Banana Split Ice Cream, 238
  Cappuccino Cupcakes, 239
  Cherry Meringue Dessert, 242
  Chocolate Angel Food Cake, 220
  Chocolate Macaroon Cupcakes, 232
  Chocolate Marvel Cake, 225
  Chocolate Swirl Cake, 244
  Double Chocolate Pie, 238
  Double-Decker Banana Cups, 233
  Easy Cherry Cobbler, 245

Lemon Chiffon Cake, 229
Marshmallow Fudge, 244
Peach-Topped Cake, 237
Peanut Butter Chocolate Pudding, 222
Pineapple Upside-Down Cake, 234
Raspberry Pear Crisp, 229
Strawberry Banana Dessert, 248
Strawberry Cheesecake Ice Cream, 223
Strawberry Lemon Trifle, 236
Sweet Potato Crisp, 246
Very Berry Pie, 220
Fish & Seafood Main Dishes
  Breaded Orange Roughy, 184
  Catfish Jambalaya, 164
  Cilantro Lime Cod, 168
  Crab Cakes, 165
  Crumb-Topped Scallops, 164
  Homemade Fish Fingers, 170
  Lemon Dill Walleye, 173
  Open-Face Tuna Melts, 171
  Oven Fish 'n' Chips, 175
  Salsa Tuna Salad, 178
  Scallops and Asparagus Stir-Fry, 171
  Sea Scallops and Mushrooms, 174
  Shrimp Salad Bagels, 170
  Spicy Haddock, 181
  Taco Fish, 184
  Tomato-Topped Cod, 173
  Tuna Patties with Dill Sauce, 168
Meatless Main Dishes
  Five-Veggie Stir-Fry, 201
  Great Grain Burgers, 196
  Three-Bean Cassoulet, 199
  Veggie Burgers, 204
  Veggie Pockets, 191
Pork Main Dishes
  Asparagus Ham Rolls, 144
  Black Beans 'n' Rice, 152
  Creole Sausage and Vegetables, 160
  Ham and Red Beans, 157
  Ham Noodle Casserole, 161
  Ham with Orange Sauce, 146
  Pepper-Crusted Pork Tenderloin, 147
  Sausage Bow Tie Salad, 151
  Tangy Pork Barbecue, 142
  Tomato Ham Pasta, 158
Poultry Main Dishes
  Chicken 'n' Bean Tacos, 130
  Chicken Jambalaya, 122
  Chicken Pasta Primavera, 130
  Chicken Pepper Fajitas, 136
  Grilled Breaded Chicken, 139
  Marinated Barbecued Chicken, 137
  Mushroom Cheese Chicken, 133
  Nostalgic Chicken and Dumplings, 120
  Oven-Fried Chicken, 125
  Seasoned Turkey Burgers, 120
  Spanish Chicken and Rice, 123
  Sweet-and-Sour Chicken, 129
  Tender Chicken Nuggets, 135
  Turkey Tetrazzini, 133
  Wild Rice Chicken Bake, 140
Side Dishes
  Au Gratin Red Potatoes, 87
  Baked Basil Fries, 72
  Broiled Parmesan Tomatoes, 90
  Cheese-Stuffed Potatoes, 89
  Confetti Barley Pilaf, 74
  Confetti Potato Pancakes, 85
  Creamy Broccoli Casserole, 88
  Creamy Fruit Salad, 86
  Crispy Baked Cauliflower, 81
  Dilly Potato Salad, 90
  Fried Rice, 85
  Garlic-Chive Mashed Potatoes, 75
  Home-Style Coleslaw, 78

Light Sweet Potato Casserole, 76
Maple-Glazed Parsnips and Carrots, 79
Mashed Potato Bake, 78
Molded Cranberry Fruit Salad, 88
Salsa Potato Salad, 81
Salsa Red Beans 'n' Rice, 76
Sausage Corn Bread Dressing, 77
Savory 'n' Saucy Baked Beans, 75
Southwestern Hominy, 79
Sweet 'n' Savory Apple Stuffing, 83
Tangy Onion Flowers, 82
Three-Bean Casserole, 84
Snacks & Beverages
  Cappuccino Shake, 31
  Caramel Apple Dip, 36
  Chocolate Banana Smoothies, 38
  Creamy Guacamole, 35
  Fudgy Fruit Dip, 36
  Iced Coffee, 28
  No-Yolk Deviled Eggs, 34
  Onion Cheese Ball, 34
  Pineapple Iced Tea, 26
  Ranch Tortilla Roll-Ups, 27
  Raspberry Cream Smoothies, 29
  Saucy Turkey Meatballs, 26
  Seasoned Snack Mix, 31
  Shrimp Tartlets, 37
  Shrimp with Creole Sauce, 29
  Smoked Salmon Spread, 33
  Spiced Tomato Drink, 35
  Strawberry Slush, 33
  Stuffed Mushrooms, 28
Soups & Stew
  Asian Shrimp Soup, 53
  Black Bean Soup, 44
  Cheesy Potato Soup, 53
  Chicken Stew, 49
  Ham and Lima Bean Soup, 50
  Italian Vegetable Soup, 52
  Mediterranean Seafood Chowder, 46
  Mexican Bean 'n' Barley Chili, 202
  Mushroom Barley Soup, 44
  Southwestern Broccoli Cheese Soup, 48
  Spiced Tomato Soup, 47
  Steak Chili, 50
  Three-Bean Chili, 54
  Turkey Noodle Soup, 40
  Zippy White Chili, 46

LOW-SALT RECIPES
Beef Main Dishes
  Autumn Pot Roast, 93
  Chicken-Fried Steak, 103
  Down-Home Pot Roast, 95
  Gingered Beef Stir-Fry, 101
  Oven Swiss Steak, 104
  Skillet Ole, 98
  Spiced Beef Roast, 114
  Tropical Tenderloin Steaks, 96
  Zucchini Beef Lasagna, 105
Breads & Rolls
  Apple Cranberry Bread, 57
  Bell Pepper Muffins, 58
  Buttermilk Dill Bread, 65
  Chive Garden Rolls, 61
  Country Raisin Rye Bread, 64
  Garlic Cheese Breadsticks, 59
  Hot Cross Buns, 62
  Jalapeno Corn Bread, 63
  Maple Oat Bread, 68
  Onion-Garlic Bubble Bread, 70
  Onion Herb Biscuits, 67
  Orange Chocolate Chip Bread, 59
  Peach Scones, 60
  Ribbon Pumpkin Bread, 66
  Spiced Pear Bread, 63

LOW-SALT RECIPES

Breads & Rolls (continued)
Superb Herb Bread, 69
Sweet Potato Yeast Rolls, 56
Three Grain Pan Rolls, 65
Walnut Wheat Bread, 62
Zucchini Bread, 66

Breakfast & Brunch
Buttermilk Blueberry Muffins, 13
Cinnamon Buns, 22
Cinnamon Pecan Ring, 24
Fruit Crepes, 10
Fruit Kabobs, 21
Hearty Brunch Potatoes, 23
Lemon Ginger Muffins, 11
Orange-Cinnamon French Toast, 13
Raspberry Coffee Cake, 16

Cookies & Bars
Apple Nut Bars, 215
Blondies with Chips, 218
Chocolate Cappuccino Cookies, 206
Cocoa Chip Cookies, 212
Cranberry Cheesecake Bars, 217
Cranberry Oat Cookies, 213
Cream Cheese Swirl Brownies, 214
Double Peanut Bars, 207
Frosted Pumpkin Bars, 206
Gingerbread Cookies, 210
Honey Spice Cookies, 208
Oatmeal Raisin Cookies, 212
Peanut Butter Cookies, 209
Pecan Cookies, 211
Pineapple Almond Bars, 215
Pineapple Coconut Squares, 208
Raspberry Nut Bars, 211
Soft Gingersnaps, 216
Walnut Oat Brownies, 216

Desserts
Apple Cobbler, 231
Banana Cream Pie, 243
Banana Cupcakes, 241
Banana Split Ice Cream, 238
Blueberry Crisp, 227
Blueberry Crumb Pie, 222
Cappuccino Cupcakes, 239
Caramel Chocolate Cheesecake Bites, 246
Caramel-Pecan Cheese Pie, 230
Cherry Meringue Dessert, 242
Chocolate Macaroon Cupcakes, 232
Chocolate Mousse, 249
Cran-Apple Crisp, 243
Cranberry Cheesecake Tart, 247
Cream Cheese Bonbons, 235
Creamy Apple Crumb Pie, 226
Frosted Spice Cake, 226
Fudgy Brownie Dessert, 228
Gran's Apple Cake, 241
Lemon Chiffon Cake, 229
Maple Pumpkin Pie, 242
Marshmallow Fudge, 244
Peach-Topped Cake, 237
Peanut Butter Chocolate Pudding, 222
Pineapple Upside-Down Cake, 234
Raspberry Pear Crisp, 229
Refreshing Lime Pie, 232
Rhubarb-Topped Cheesecake, 224
Strawberry Banana Dessert, 248
Strawberry Cheesecake Ice Cream, 223
Strawberry Cream Cheese Pie, 234
Sweet Potato Crisp, 246
Tart Cherry Pie, 230
Very Berry Pie, 220

Fish & Seafood Main Dishes
Cilantro Lime Cod, 168
Confetti Salmon Steaks, 176
Lemon Dill Walleye, 173
Maple-Glazed Grilled Salmon, 178
Perch with Cucumber Relish, 166
Salmon with Dill Sauce, 185
Salsa Tuna Salad, 178

Meatless Main Dishes
Great Grain Burgers, 196
Veggie Burgers, 204
Veggie Pockets, 191

Pork Main Dishes
Asparagus Ham Rolls, 144
Pork Chops with Red Cabbage, 147
Pork Picante, 142
Pork Soft-Shell Tacos, 155
Tangy Pork Barbecue, 142
Tomato Ham Pasta, 158

Poultry Main Dishes
Chicken 'n' Bean Tacos, 130
Chicken 'n' Biscuits, 139
Chicken Pepper Fajitas, 136
Savory Roasted Chicken, 116
Seasoned Turkey Burgers, 120
Spanish Chicken and Rice, 123
Tender Chicken Nuggets, 135

Side Dishes
Baked Basil Fries, 72
Broiled Parmesan Tomatoes, 90
Cheese-Stuffed Potatoes, 89
Cheesy Zucchini Medley, 86
Confetti Potato Pancakes, 85
Creamy Broccoli Casserole, 88
Creamy Fruit Salad, 86
Crispy Baked Cauliflower, 81
Dilly Potato Salad, 90
Fried Rice, 85
Home-Style Coleslaw, 78
Light Sweet Potato Casserole, 76
Maple-Glazed Parsnips and Carrots, 79
Molded Cranberry Fruit Salad, 88
Salsa Potato Salad, 81
Savory 'n' Saucy Baked Beans, 75
Southwestern Hominy, 79
Sweet Potato Apple Scallop, 72
Tangy Onion Flowers, 82
Veggie Macaroni Salad, 82

Snacks & Beverages
Cappuccino Shake, 31
Caramel Apple Dip, 36
Creamy Guacamole, 35
Fudgy Fruit Dip, 36
Iced Coffee, 28
No-Yolk Deviled Eggs, 34
Onion Cheese Ball, 34
Pineapple Iced Tea, 26
Raspberry Cream Smoothies, 29
Shrimp Tartlets, 37
Shrimp with Creole Sauce, 29
Strawberry Slush, 33
Stuffed Mushrooms, 28

Soups & Stew
Beef Minestrone, 40
Cheesy Potato Soup, 53
Chicken Stew, 49
Italian Vegetable Soup, 52
Steak Chili, 50

MUSHROOMS
Beef Fillets with Portobello Sauce, 101
Crustless Mushroom Spinach Tart, 204
Ham Mushroom Fettuccine, 148
Mushroom Barley Soup, 44
Mushroom Broccoli Pizza, 200
Mushroom Cheese Chicken, 133
Mushroom Chicken Pizza, 135
Mushroom Pizza Burgers, 92
Onion Beef Stroganoff, 107
Sea Scallops and Mushrooms, 174
Stuffed Mushrooms, 28
Turkey Tetrazzini, 133

NUTS & PEANUT BUTTER
Apple Nut Bars, 215
Caramel-Pecan Cheese Pie, 230
Cinnamon Pecan Ring, 24
Double Peanut Bars, 207
Peanut Butter Chocolate Pudding, 222
Peanut Butter Cookies, 209
Pecan Cookies, 211
Pecan Waffles, 14
Pineapple Almond Bars, 215
Raspberry Nut Bars, 211
Walnut Oat Brownies, 216
Walnut Wheat Bread, 62

OATS
Cranberry Oat Cookies, 213
Great Grain Burgers, 196
Hearty Oatmeal Pancakes, 18
Maple Oat Bread, 68
Oatmeal Raisin Cookies, 212
Three Grain Pan Rolls, 65
Walnut Oat Brownies, 216

ONIONS & CHIVES
Chive Garden Rolls, 61
Garlic-Chive Mashed Potatoes, 75
Onion Beef Stroganoff, 107
Onion Cheese Ball, 34
Onion-Garlic Bubble Bread, 70
Onion Herb Biscuits, 67
Tangy Onion Flowers, 82

ORANGES
Ham with Orange Sauce, 146
Orange Chocolate Chip Bread, 59
Orange-Cinnamon French Toast, 13
Orange Pineapple Torte, 227

PASTA
Baked Macaroni and Cheese, 194
Beef Noodle Casserole, 105
Chicken Lasagna, 125
Chicken Noodle Casserole, 123
Chicken Pasta Primavera, 130
Easy Beef Goulash, 108
Fettuccine Italiana, 124
Ham Mushroom Fettuccine, 148
Ham Noodle Casserole, 161
Italian Turkey and Noodles, 131
Mediterranean Pork and Orzo, 154
Onion Beef Stroganoff, 107
Pasta-Filled Peppers, 193
Penne Sausage Bake, 134
Pork Lo Mein, 143
Sausage Bow Tie Salad, 151
Smoked Sausage with Pasta, 117
Southwest Lasagna Rolls, 196
Spaghetti Casserole, 199
Spaghetti with Italian Meatballs, 109
Spinach Manicotti, 197
Tex-Mex Lasagna, 106
Tomato Ham Pasta, 158
Tortellini Primavera, 191
Tuna Noodle Casserole, 167
Turkey Noodle Soup, 40
Veggie Macaroni Salad, 82
Zippy Shrimp Linguine, 169
Zucchini Beef Lasagna, 105

PEACHES
Peach Scones, 60
Peach-Topped Cake, 237

PEARS
Raspberry Pear Crisp, 229
Spiced Pear Bread, 63

PEPPERS
Bell Pepper Muffins, 58
Black Bean Fajitas, 188
Chicken Pepper Fajitas, 136
Herbed Stuffed Green Peppers, 122
Italian-Sausage Pepper Sandwiches, 145
Jalapeno Corn Bread, 63
Pasta-Filled Peppers, 193
Roasted Garlic and Pepper Pizza, 194
Steak Fajitas, 92
Sweet Pepper Sandwiches, 195

PINEAPPLE
Orange Pineapple Torte, 227
Pineapple Almond Bars, 215
Pineapple Coconut Squares, 208
Pineapple Iced Tea, 26
Pineapple Upside-Down Cake, 234
Polynesian Kabobs, 152
Snapper with Spicy Pineapple Glaze, 186
Sweet-and-Sour Chicken, 129
Sweet and Sour Ham, 150

PORK (also see Bacon & Canadian Bacon; Ham; Sausage)
Baked Pork Chimichangas, 156
Breaded Pork Chops, 145
Caramelized Pork Slices, 149
Cranberry-Mustard Pork Medallions, 162
Herb-Stuffed Pork Loin, 161
Mediterranean Pork and Orzo, 154
Mexican Pork Stew, 41
Mustard-Glazed Pork Chops, 153
One-Pot Pork and Rice, 157
Pepper-Crusted Pork Tenderloin, 147
Pork 'n' Veggie Packets, 149
Pork Chops with Red Cabbage, 147
Pork Lo Mein, 143
Pork Picante, 142
Pork Soft-Shell Tacos, 155
Slow-Cooked Pork Roast, 154
Tangy Pork Barbecue, 142
Teriyaki Pork, 150

POTATOES (also see Sweet Potatoes)
Au Gratin Red Potatoes, 87
Baked Basil Fries, 72
Breakfast Bake, 23
Canadian Bacon Potato Skins, 30
Cheese-Stuffed Potatoes, 89
Cheesy Potato Soup, 53
Confetti Potato Pancakes, 85
Dilly Potato Salad, 90
Garlic-Chive Mashed Potatoes, 75
Hash Brown Cheese Omelet, 20
Hearty Brunch Potatoes, 23
Italian Shepherd's Pie, 110
Mashed Potato Bake, 78
Oven Fish 'n' Chips, 175
Salsa Potato Salad, 81

PUMPKIN
Frosted Pumpkin Bars, 206
Maple Pumpkin Pie, 242
Ribbon Pumpkin Bread, 66

QUICK-FIX RECIPES
Beef Main Dishes
Beef Fillets with Portobello Sauce, 101
Chicken-Fried Steak, 103
Chuck Wagon Wraps, 110
Easy Beef Goulash, 108
Gingered Beef Stir-Fry, 101
Mediterranean Beef Toss, 100
Mushroom Pizza Burgers, 92
Onion Beef Stroganoff, 107
Skillet Ole, 98
Steak Fajitas, 92
Tortilla Pie, 98
Zippy Burgers, 95
Breads & Rolls
Bell Pepper Muffins, 58
Ham 'n' Cheese Muffins, 56
Jalapeno Corn Bread, 63
Peach Scones, 60
Breakfast & Brunch
Blueberry Waffles, 20
Buttermilk Blueberry Muffins, 13
Cream Cheese Ham Omelet, 19
Crispy French Toast, 10
Eggs Florentine, 19
Fruit Kabobs, 21
Hash Brown Cheese Omelet, 20
Hearty Oatmeal Pancakes, 18
Home-Style Country Sausage, 17
Lemon Ginger Muffins, 11
Orange-Cinnamon French Toast, 13
Pecan Waffles, 14
Seasoned Scrambled Eggs, 16
Desserts
Chocolate Mousse, 249
Double-Decker Banana Cups, 233
Double Peanut Bars, 207
Peanut Butter Chocolate Pudding, 222
Fish & Seafood Main Dishes
Breaded Orange Roughy, 184
Catfish Jambalaya, 164
Confetti Salmon Steaks, 176
Crab Cakes, 165
Crab Rice Primavera, 183
Creole Catfish Fillets, 167
Crumb-Topped Scallops, 164
Grilled Halibut with
  Mustard Dill Sauce, 182
Lemon Dill Walleye, 173
Lime Fish Tacos, 181
Mediterranean-Style Red Snapper, 183
Open-Face Tuna Melts, 171
Perch with Cucumber Relish, 166
Salmon with Dill Sauce, 185
Salsa Tuna Salad, 178
Scallops and Asparagus Stir-Fry, 171
Sea Scallops and Mushrooms, 174
Shrimp 'n' Veggie Pizza, 172
Shrimp Salad Bagels, 170
Snapper with Spicy Pineapple Glaze, 186
Spicy Haddock, 181
Spicy Shrimp Wraps, 179
Taco Fish, 184
Zippy Shrimp Linguine, 169
Meatless Main Dishes
Black Bean Fajitas, 188
Egg Foo Yong with Sauce, 192
Five-Veggie Stir-Fry, 201
Sweet Pepper Sandwiches, 195
Toasted Veggie Sandwich, 202
Tortellini Primavera, 191
Veggie Burgers, 204
Veggie Pockets, 191
Pork Main Dishes
BLT Tortillas, 146
Caramelized Pork Slices, 149
Creamy Ham Turnovers, 158
Creole Sausage and Vegetables, 160
Ham Mushroom Fettuccine, 148
Italian-Sausage Pepper Sandwiches, 145
Mediterranean Pork and Orzo, 154
Mustard-Glazed Pork Chops, 153
Polynesian Kabobs, 152
Pork 'n' Veggie Packets, 149
Pork Chops with Red Cabbage, 147
Pork Picante, 142
Pork Soft-Shell Tacos, 155
Sausage Bow Tie Salad, 151
Sweet and Sour Ham, 150
Tomato Ham Pasta, 158
Poultry Main Dishes
Barbecued Turkey Sandwiches, 126
Chicken 'n' Bean Tacos, 130
Chicken in Creamy Gravy, 132
Chicken Pasta Primavera, 130
Fettuccine Italiana, 124
Hot Swiss Chicken Sandwiches, 136
Mushroom Chicken Pizza, 135
Salsa Chicken Skillet, 119
Smoked Sausage with Pasta, 117
Spanish Chicken and Rice, 123
Stir-Fried Chicken Marinara, 126
Sweet-and-Sour Chicken, 129
Tender Chicken Nuggets, 135
Side Dishes
Broiled Parmesan Tomatoes, 90
Cheesy Zucchini Medley, 86
Confetti Potato Pancakes, 85
Creamy Fruit Salad, 86
Fried Rice, 85
Garlic-Chive Mashed Potatoes, 75
Maple-Glazed Parsnips and Carrots, 79
Salsa Red Beans 'n' Rice, 76
Savory 'n' Saucy Baked Beans, 75
Snacks & Beverages
Cappuccino Shake, 31
Caramel Apple Dip, 36
Creamy Guacamole, 35
Iced Coffee, 28
No-Yolk Deviled Eggs, 34
Onion Cheese Ball, 34
Raspberry Cream Smoothies, 29
Shrimp Tartlets, 37
Spiced Tomato Drink, 35
Stuffed Mushrooms, 28
Soups
Asian Shrimp Soup, 53
Black Bean Soup, 44
Cheesy Potato Soup, 53
Creamy Chicken Rice Soup, 43
Italian Vegetable Soup, 52
Mediterranean Seafood Chowder, 46
Southwestern Broccoli Cheese Soup, 48
Spiced Tomato Soup, 47
Taco Soup, 47
Three-Bean Chili, 54

RAISINS
Country Raisin Rye Bread, 64
Oatmeal Raisin Cookies, 212
Raisin Carrot Cake, 237

RASPBERRIES
Fruit Crepes, 10
Raspberry Coffee Cake, 16
Raspberry Cream Smoothies, 29
Raspberry Nut Bars, 211
Raspberry Pear Crisp, 229
Very Berry Pie, 220

RHUBARB
Rhubarb-Topped Cheesecake, 224

RICE & BARLEY
Black Beans 'n' Rice, 152
Broccoli Rice Hot Dish, 80
Brown Rice 'n' Apple Stuffed Turkey, 119

RICE & BARLEY (continued)
Catfish Jambalaya, 164
Chicken Jambalaya, 122
Confetti Barley Pilaf, 74
Crab Rice Primavera, 183
Creamy Chicken Rice Soup, 43
Fried Rice, 85
Great Grain Burgers, 196
Mexican Bean 'n' Barley Chili, 202
Mushroom Barley Soup, 44
One-Pot Pork and Rice, 157
Salsa Red Beans 'n' Rice, 76
Spanish Chicken and Rice, 123
Spanish Rice with Bacon, 73
Wild Rice Chicken Bake, 140

SALADS
Creamy Fruit Salad, 86
Dilly Potato Salad, 90
Home-Style Coleslaw, 78
Molded Cranberry Fruit Salad, 88
Salsa Potato Salad, 81
Salsa Tuna Salad, 178
Sausage Bow Tie Salad, 151
Veggie Macaroni Salad, 82

SANDWICHES
Asparagus Ham Rolls, 144
Barbecued Turkey Sandwiches, 126
BLT Tortillas, 146
Chuck Wagon Wraps, 110
Creamy Ham Turnovers, 158
Great Grain Burgers, 196
Hot Swiss Chicken Sandwiches, 136
Italian-Sausage Pepper Sandwiches, 145
Mushroom Pizza Burgers, 92
Open-Face Tuna Melts, 171
Open-Faced Meatball Sandwiches, 102
Seasoned Turkey Burgers, 120
Shredded Beef Barbecue, 104
Shrimp Salad Bagels, 170
Spicy Shrimp Wraps, 179
Sweet Pepper Sandwiches, 195
Tangy Pork Barbecue, 142
Toasted Veggie Sandwich, 202
Turkey Sloppy Joes, 129
Veggie Burgers, 204
Veggie Pockets, 191
Zippy Burgers, 95

SAUSAGE
Creole Sausage and Vegetables, 160
Italian-Sausage Pepper Sandwiches, 145
Polynesian Kabobs, 152
Sausage Bow Tie Salad, 151

SIDE DISHES
Au Gratin Red Potatoes, 87
Baked Basil Fries, 72
Broccoli Rice Hot Dish, 80
Broiled Parmesan Tomatoes, 90
Cheese-Stuffed Potatoes, 89
Cheesy Zucchini Medley, 86
Confetti Barley Pilaf, 74
Confetti Potato Pancakes, 85
Creamy Broccoli Casserole, 88
Crispy Baked Cauliflower, 81
Fried Rice, 85
Garlic-Chive Mashed Potatoes, 75
Green Bean Corn Casserole, 89
Light Sweet Potato Casserole, 76
Maple-Glazed Parsnips and Carrots, 79
Mashed Potato Bake, 78
Salsa Red Beans 'n' Rice, 76
Sausage Corn Bread Dressing, 77
Savory 'n' Saucy Baked Beans, 75

Southwestern Hominy, 79
Spanish Rice with Bacon, 73
Sweet 'n' Savory Apple Stuffing, 83
Sweet Potato Apple Scallop, 72
Tangy Onion Flowers, 82
Three-Bean Casserole, 84

SNACKS & BEVERAGES
Bacon Ranch Dip, 32
Canadian Bacon Potato Skins, 30
Cappuccino Shake, 31
Caramel Apple Dip, 36
Chocolate Banana Smoothies, 38
Creamy Guacamole, 35
Fudgy Fruit Dip, 36
Iced Coffee, 28
No-Yolk Deviled Eggs, 34
Onion Cheese Ball, 34
Pineapple Iced Tea, 26
Ranch Tortilla Roll-Ups, 27
Raspberry Cream Smoothies, 29
Saucy Turkey Meatballs, 26
Seasoned Snack Mix, 31
Shrimp Tartlets, 37
Shrimp with Creole Sauce, 29
Smoked Salmon Spread, 33
Spiced Tomato Drink, 35
Strawberry Slush, 33
Stuffed Mushrooms, 28

SOUPS & STEWS
Asian Shrimp Soup, 53
Beef Minestrone, 40
Black Bean Soup, 44
Cheesy Potato Soup, 53
Chicken Stew, 49
Creamy Chicken Rice Soup, 43
Ham and Lima Bean Soup, 50
Harvest Soup, 42
Irish Stew, 43
Italian Vegetable Soup, 52
Lentil Sausage Soup, 49
Mediterranean Seafood Chowder, 46
Mexican Bean 'n' Barley Chili, 202
Mexican Pork Stew, 41
Mushroom Barley Soup, 44
Root Vegetable Beef Stew, 51
Southwestern Broccoli Cheese Soup, 48
Spiced Tomato Soup, 47
Steak Chili, 50
Taco Soup, 47
Three-Bean Chili, 54
Turkey Dumpling Stew, 45
Turkey Noodle Soup, 40
Zippy White Chili, 46

SPINACH
Crustless Mushroom Spinach Tart, 204
Crustless Spinach Quiche, 17
Eggs Florentine, 19
Spinach Burritos, 192
Spinach Cheese Enchiladas, 188
Spinach Manicotti, 197

STRAWBERRIES
Strawberry Banana Dessert, 248
Strawberry Cheesecake Ice Cream, 223
Strawberry Cream Cheese Pie, 234
Strawberry Lemon Trifle, 236
Strawberry Slush, 33

SWEET POTATOES
Light Sweet Potato Casserole, 76
Sweet Potato Apple Scallop, 72
Sweet Potato Crisp, 246
Sweet Potato Yeast Rolls, 56

TOMATOES
BLT Tortillas, 146
Brisket with Chunky Tomato Sauce, 100
Broiled Parmesan Tomatoes, 90
Chicken Cacciatore, 132
Spiced Tomato Drink, 35
Spiced Tomato Soup, 47
Stir-Fried Chicken Marinara, 126
Tomato Baked Haddock, 177
Tomato Ham Pasta, 158
Tomato-Topped Cod, 173

TURKEY
Breakfast & Brunch
Hearty Brunch Potatoes, 23
Home-Style Country Sausage, 17
Sausage Breakfast Wraps, 14
Main Dishes
Barbecued Turkey Pizza, 118
Brown Rice 'n' Apple Stuffed Turkey, 119
Fettuccine Italiana, 124
Herbed Stuffed Green Peppers, 122
Horseradish-Crusted Turkey Tenderloins, 116
Italian Turkey and Noodles, 131
Penne Sausage Bake, 134
Smoked Sausage with Pasta, 117
Turkey 'n' Beef Loaf, 138
Turkey Biscuit Potpie, 127
Turkey Tetrazzini, 133
Sandwiches
Barbecued Turkey Sandwiches, 126
Seasoned Turkey Burgers, 120
Turkey Sloppy Joes, 129
Side Dish
Sausage Corn Bread Dressing, 77
Snacks
Saucy Turkey Meatballs, 26
Soups & Stew
Lentil Sausage Soup, 49
Turkey Dumpling Stew, 45
Turkey Noodle Soup, 40

VEGETABLES (also see specific kinds)
Chicken Pasta Primavera, 130
Crab Rice Primavera, 183
Creole Sausage and Vegetables, 160
Five-Veggie Stir-Fry, 201
Garden Frittata, 12
Harvest Soup, 42
Italian Vegetable Soup, 52
Pork 'n' Veggie Packets, 149
Root Vegetable Beef Stew, 51
Shrimp 'n' Veggie Pizza, 172
Sirloin Veggie Kabobs, 94
Toasted Veggie Sandwich, 202
Tortellini Primavera, 191
Veggie Burgers, 204
Veggie Macaroni Salad, 82
Veggie Pockets, 191

ZUCCHINI
Cheesy Zucchini Medley, 86
Italian Zucchini Bake, 197
Zucchini Beef Lasagna, 105
Zucchini Bread, 66
Zucchini Crepes, 198